ANATOMY AND PHYSIOLOGY

CareerStep

ONLINE EDUCATION & TRAINING SOLUTIONS

Career Step, LLC
Phone: 801.489.9393
Toll-Free: 800.246.7837
Fax: 801.491.6645
careerstep.com

This text companion contains a snapshot of the online program content converted to a printed format. Please note that the online training program is constantly changing and improving and is always the source of the most up-to-date information.

Product Number: HG-PR-11-120
Generation Date: August 1, 2013

TABLE OF CONTENTS

UNIT 1

Introduction

INTRODUCTION TO ANATOMY AND PHYSIOLOGY

LEARNING OBJECTIVES

At the conclusion of this module, the learner will be able to:

1. Identify and describe the basic structure, organization, and functions of human body systems.
2. Identify anatomical structures of the body using anatomical orientation tools such as labels and assessment.
3. Discuss different online lookup tools such as Adam.
4. Utilize anatomical plate work to enhance learning experience.

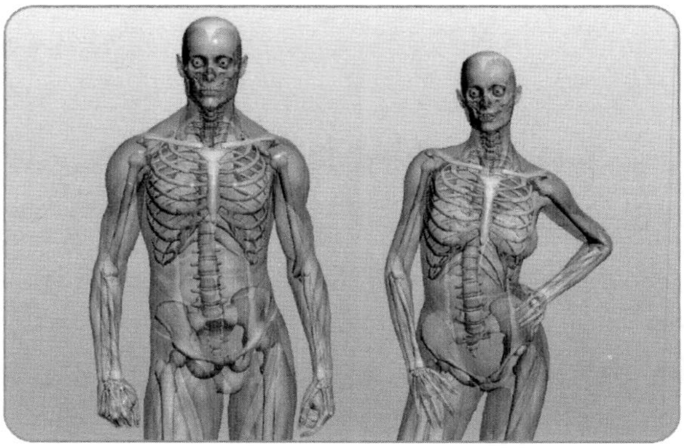

Medicine is about people—the minds and bodies of human beings. In the best-case scenario, everything works perfectly like a well-oiled machine. In reality, the human body and mind break down and suffer illness and injury. The ravages of the environment, aging, effects of childbirth, overuse, and emotional and physical trauma also affect the human body and mind.

Because medical records document the impact of disease and traumatic events on the body, human anatomy (structure), physiology (function), and disease processes are important parts of health information. A solid understanding of human anatomy and body systems is essential to interpreting medical documentation and the proper assignment of diagnosis and procedure codes.

Medical coding as a career deals largely with practical application of medical terms. As a medical coder, you will be deciphering the physical manifestation a patient has been experiencing, the treatment of any problems, their reaction to treatments, and any future suggetions for the patient— all from the medical documentation you are provided.

A basic understanding of the anatomy and physiology of the human body is essential to understanding key parts of medical reports for coding and billing.

In this setting, a basic understanding of bones, muscles, arteries and veins, ligaments, joints, and organs, as well as body functions (or physiology), such as the respiratory, digestive, and reproductive systems, becomes important. The more terms you are familiar with, the less time you will spend wandering aimlessly through your reference books.

The key word here is basic. Do not be overwhelmed by everything in this module. You are not expected to be a doctor or to know everything that a doctor knows. It is the case, however, that you may be able to easily locate a word in a report because you know the meaning of a word or the location in the body to which a specific term refers.

UNIT 2

Structural Organization of the Body

STRUCTURAL ORGANIZATION OF THE BODY – INTRODUCTION

It is important to review the structural organization of the body before studying the anatomical structures. The human body is divided several ways for medical professionals. This unit teaches some of the most common ways used to describe the structural organization of the body.

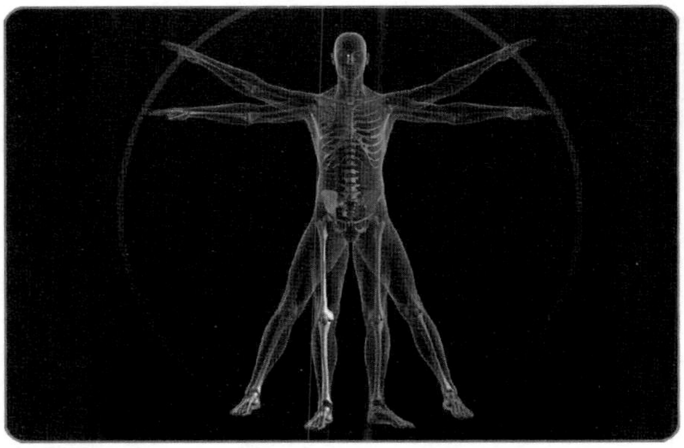

LEVELS OF STRUCTURAL ORGANIZATION

Anatomy refers to the study of the structure of the body. The human body is made up of six levels of structural organization. Each level of organization is composed of the previous levels.

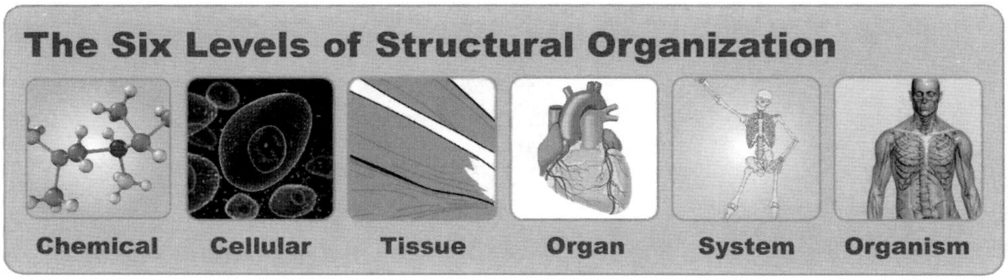

Level	Structure Definition
Chemical	The chemical level represents the smallest components of the body. Increasing in size from atoms such as carbon and oxygen, to molecules like water and carbon dioxide, to biological macromolecules like proteins, fats and carbohydrates, chemicals are the most basic building blocks of the body.
Cellular	Molecules combine together to form cells. The cells of the body are the basic structural and functional units of an organism. Examples of cells in the body include muscle cells, nerve cells, and blood cells.

Tissue	Tissues are made up of groups of cells and the materials surrounding them. They work together to perform specific functions. There are four types of tissues in your body. The four types of tissue are: **epithelial** – Protective tissue found in the linings of cavities and organs and as part of the integumentary system, or skin. This tissue helps to protect the structures it lines from injury and fluid loss. **muscle** – Responsible for all of the movement of the body. It is subdivided into divisions of skeletal muscle, smooth muscle, and cardiac muscle. Skeletal muscle is made of long fibers and is the tissue that allows for voluntary body movements. Smooth muscle lines the internal organs and carries out primarily involuntary body movements that assist in organ function. Cardiac muscle is found only in the heart and is specifically designed to maintain heartbeat and blood flow. **connective** – Tissue that binds the body together, supports structure and function, and is involved in the transport of metabolic products. Example of binding connective tissue are tendons and ligaments—thick strong tissue that binds muscle to bone and bones to each other. Supporting connective tissue consists of the bones and cartilage of the body, which give the body support and a foundational structural framework. Fibrous connective tissue is also a binding material, though instead of connecting other connective tissues, this tissue connects muscles together and binds the skin to the rest of the body. Adipose tissue (fat) and blood are examples of fibrous connective tissue. **nervous** – Composed of nerve cells. It is the communication system of the body. Nervous tissue conducts electrochemical signals to and from the brain. This allows for all motor functions, both voluntary and involuntary.
Organ	The different kinds of tissue discussed above combine to form the organ level. The organs are composed of two or more types of these tissues. Each organ has specific functions and recognizable shapes. Some examples of organs are the heart, lungs, brain, liver, and kidneys.
System	A system is made up of several organs that have a common function. For example, the organs that are a part of the digestive system break down and absorb food. These organs include the mouth, pharynx (throat), esophagus, stomach, small intestine, and large intestine. Some organs can be part of more than one system. For example, the pancreas is part of both the digestive system and the endocrine system.
Organism	The largest structural level is the organism level. All the parts which make up the body and function with each other form the total organism (one living individual).

I. MATCHING.
Match the correct term to the definition.

1. ____ system
2. ____ muscle
3. ____ tissue
4. ____ cellular
5. ____ connective
6. ____ epithelial

A. molecules combine together to form this level
B. responsible for all of the movement of the body
C. protects cavities and organ structures from injury and fluid loss
D. made up of several organs which have a common function
E. supports structure and function
F. made up of groups of cells and the materials surrounding them

ANATOMICAL POSITION

The human body can be looked at from many angles or viewpoints. Therefore, it is necessary for medical personnel to refer to the human body in a fixed or standard position when referring to specific body areas. Descriptive terms for parts of the body are referenced according to this fixed or "anatomical position." The anatomical position refers to the human body as erect (standing), facing forward with eyes straight ahead, arms at the sides with palms open and facing forward, and feet parallel and flat on the floor.

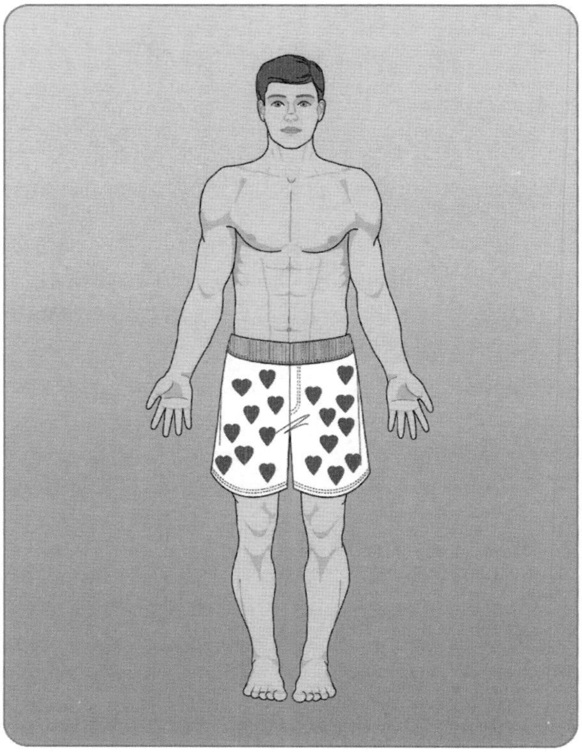

The Anatomical Position

Note that these relative positions are actually used frequently in medical reports. Not only are they used as descriptive words throughout human anatomy, doctors must use them when describing any findings on a physical exam, within an operative note, or when describing an x-ray (where great detail must be provided). In order to achieve clarity of reference, it is necessary for dictators to use standard directional indicators.

In anatomical terms, any veins, muscles, ligaments, bones, tendons, or other structures that utilize one of these descriptive terms will be specifically related to this anatomical position. If you know and can determine for yourself whether something is above, below, in front of, behind, beside, or near another structure, you can be relatively certain that you are using the correct descriptive term.

PLANES OF THE BODY

Frontal or **coronal plane** divides the body into front and back sections.

Sagittal or **lateral plane** divides the body in right and left sections.

Median or **midsagittal plane** divides the body into right and left equal sections.

Transverse or **cross-sectional plane** divides the body into top and bottom sections.

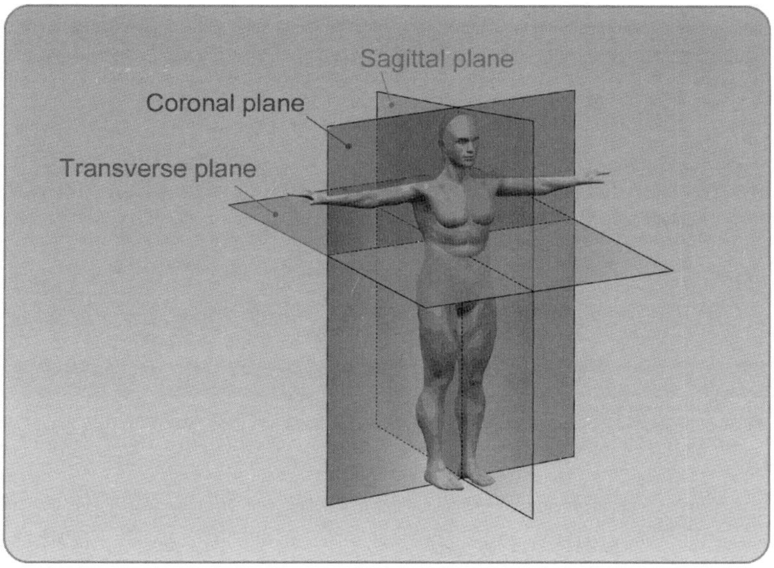

DIRECTIONAL TERMS

anterior – Situated in front of or toward the front of a body part or organ. This term is also used in reference to a ventral or belly surface of the body. Frontal is a common synonym for anterior.

coronal – Division of the body into anterior and posterior sections. Also called frontal plane. Can mean pertaining to the head or the crown.

distal – Remote; farther from the center of the body or point of attachment to the body; opposite of proximal. (The elbow is distal to the shoulder, but proximal to the wrist.)

dorsal – Pertaining to the back of the body; also used to denote a position that is more toward the back than another object of reference. Sometimes called posterior.

inferior – Situated below a structure or directed downward; also used to denote the lower portion of an organ or the lower of two structures.

lateral – Pertaining to the side; denoting a position farther from the midline (median plane) of a structure.

medial – Pertaining to the middle; closer to the midline of a body; pertaining to the middle layer.

posterior – Situated in the back; also used in reference to the back or dorsal surface of the body.

proximal – Nearest; closer to the center of the body or point of attachment to the body; opposite of distal. (The elbow is distal to the shoulder but proximal to the wrist.)

sagittal – Division of body into left and right sides in a vertical lengthwise fashion.

superior – Situated above, or directed upward; in official anatomic nomenclature, used in reference to the upper surface of an organ or other structure, or to a structure occupying a higher position.

transverse – A horizontal plane situated at right angles to the long axis, or sagittal and coronal planes; placed crosswise.

ventral – Pertaining to the abdomen; used to denote a position that is more toward the belly/ abdominal surface than some other object of reference.

bilateral – Occuring on both sides of the body.

superficial (external) – Near the outer surface.

deep (internal) – Situated further inward, away from the surface.

I. MULTIPLE CHOICE.
Choose the best answer.

1. Pertaining to the belly-side or the abdomen.
   - ○ posterior
   - ○ ventral
   - ○ inferior
   - ○ superior

2. Means to the side.
   - ○ medial
   - ○ lateral
   - ○ inferior
   - ○ anterior

3. Situated in front of.
   - ○ inferior
   - ○ transverse
   - ○ coronal
   - ○ anterior

4. Denoting the lower of two structures.
   - ○ inferior
   - ○ superior
   - ○ sagittal
   - ○ coronal

5. Nearest to midline.
   - ○ distal
   - ○ inferior
   - ○ lateral
   - ○ proximal

6. Pertaining to the back.
   - ◯ dorsal
   - ◯ superior
   - ◯ inferior
   - ◯ ventral

7. Pertaining to the middle layer.
   - ◯ medial
   - ◯ lateral
   - ◯ inferior
   - ◯ posterior

8. Also pertaining to the back.
   - ◯ posterior
   - ◯ coronal
   - ◯ sagittal
   - ◯ ventral

COMBINING DIRECTIONAL TERMS

Term	Combining Form	Examples
anterior	antero	anteroinferior anterolateral anteromedial anteroposterior
distal	disto	distobuccal distocervical distolabial
dorsal	dorso*	dorsoanterior dorsolateral dorsomedial dorsoposterior
inferior	infero	inferolateral inferomedial inferoposterior
lateral	latero	lateroposition lateroversion
medial	medio	mediocarpal mediolateral
posterior	postero	posteroinferior posterolateral posteromedial
superior	supero	superolateral superomedial
ventral	ventro*	ventrodorsal ventrolateral ventroposterior

**dorso- and ventro- can be designed dorsi- and ventri- in certain instances. However, these forms are generally not used in combination with other positional or anatomical planes. Examples would be dorsiflexion and ventriflexion (which mean bending towards the extensor surface of a limb and bending toward the belly, respectively).*

Notice that several of the terms can be combined in both directions, such as *inferoposterior* and *posteroinferior.*

To precisely describe the position of a structure it is often necessary to combine directional terms. For example, a big scrape on your leg is much better described as an abrasion on the anterolateral aspect of the right leg, two inches distal to the knee.

To join directional and positional adjectives, use the combining vowel.

I. **FILL IN THE BLANK.**

Combine the following directional and positional adjectives.

1. ventral + lateral = ________________
2. inferior + posterior = ________________
3. posterior + inferior = ________________
4. superior + lateral = ________________
5. lateral + posterior = ________________
6. medial + lateral = ________________
7. inferior + medial = ________________
8. superior + inferior = ________________
9. anterior + medial = ________________
10. dorsal + flexion = ________________
11. distal + cervical = ________________
12. anterior + lateral = ________________

REGIONS, QUADRANTS, AND LANDMARKS

Often there are abdominal-pelvic regions referred to by some physicians in their documentation. The nine regions are shown in the image. Note that the nine regions do not include any thoracic organs.

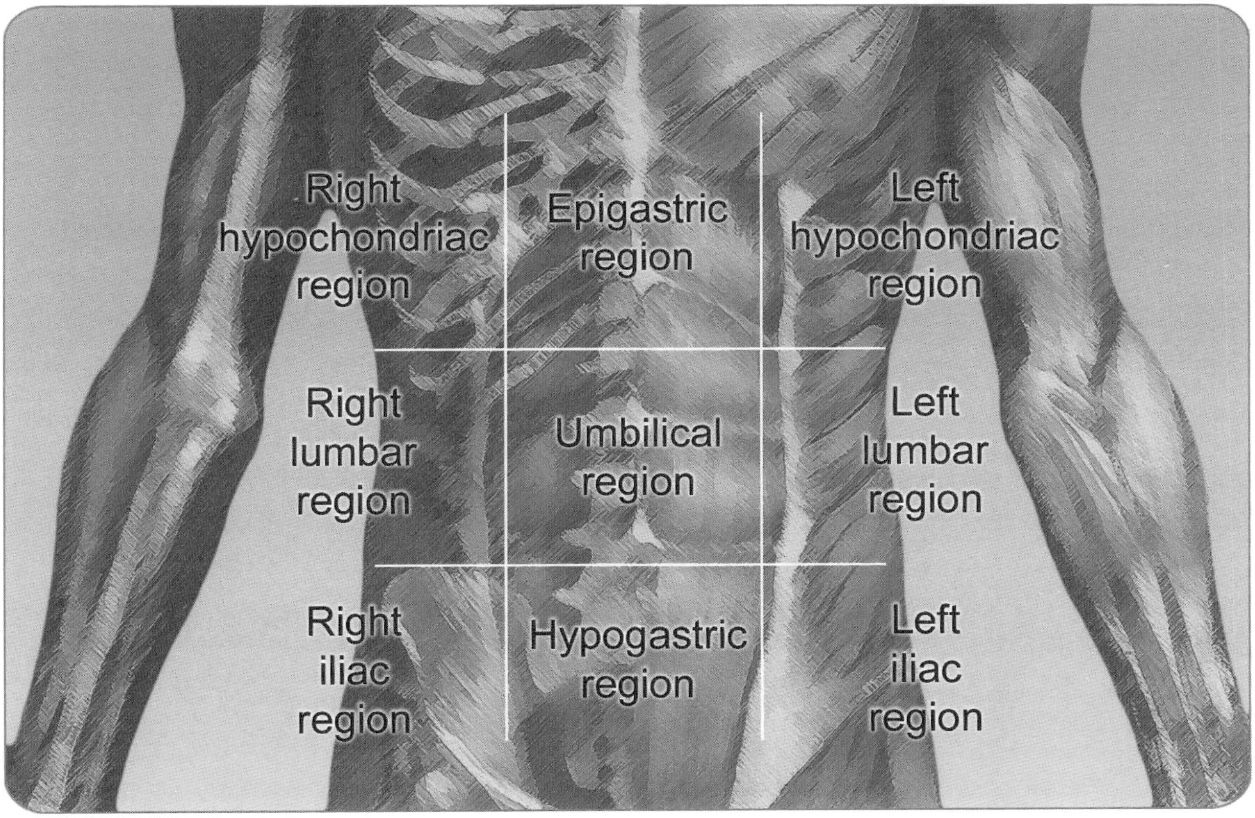

There are four quadrants that are also used as reference points for the location of specific organs.

Body Quadrants:

- RUQ (liver, gallbladder, pancreas, small intestine, and large intestine)
- LUQ (left lobe liver, stomach, spleen, pancreas (majority), and parts of small and large intestine)
- RLQ (small and large intestines, right ovary, right fallopian tube, appendix, and right ureter)
- LLQ (small and large intestines, left ovary, left fallopian tube, and left ureter)

Anatomical landmarks are used to identify regions of the body where technical or descriptive names are used. The landmarks are illustrated here.

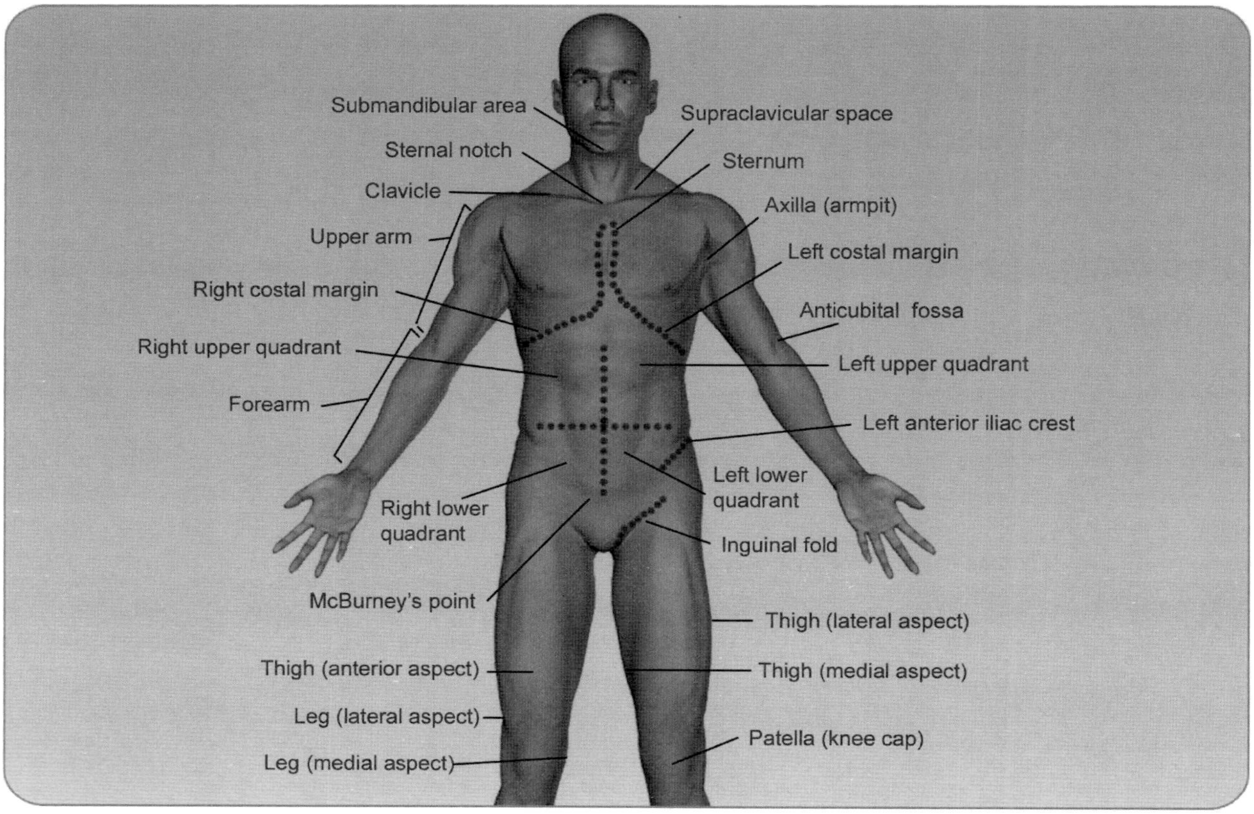

REFERENCES AND ADDITIONAL ACTIVITIES FOR CODERS

http://shs2.westport.k12.ct.us/mjvl/anatomy/intro/nine_abdominal_regions.htm

www.mgccc.edu

www.anatomy.tv/StudyGuides/StudyGuide.aspx?guideid=9&nextID=0&maxID=0&customer=primal

www.wiley.com/college

EXAMPLES OF ANATOMICAL LANDMARKS ARE AVAILABLE AT MEDLINE PLUS:

Back View: www.nlm.nih.gov/medlineplus/ency/imagepages/1069.htm

Side View: www.nlm.nih.gov/medlineplus/ency/imagepages/1071.htm

Front View: www.nlm.nih.gov/medlineplus/ency/imagepages/1070.htm

Eponyms

An **eponym** is a word derived from the name of a real, fictional, mythical or spurious character or person. Anatomists and medical professionals are moving away from the use of eponyms toward terms that are more descriptive and universal. Some eponyms are still in common use; therefore, it is beneficial for you to be familiar with them as well as their proper anatomical names. The occurrence of common eponyms, in this curriculum, will be noted by the anatomical name followed by its eponym in parentheses. A short list of these appears below for a few examples:

- calcaneal tendon (Achilles tendon)
- glomerular capsule (Bowman's capsule)
- vestibular gland (Bartholin gland)
- uterine tube (Fallopian tube)
- renal column (columns of Bertin)
- nephron loop (loop of Henle)
- cerebral arterial circle (circle of Willis)

I. MULTIPLE CHOICE.
Choose the best answer.

1. The spleen is located in the _____.
   - ◯ left upper quadrant
   - ◯ left lower quadrant
   - ◯ right lower quadrant
   - ◯ right upper quadrant

2. The submandibular anatomic landmark refers to the area _____.
   - ◯ below the jaw
   - ◯ under the arms
   - ◯ above the clavicle
   - ◯ below the clavicle

3. The epigastric anatomical region refers to the _____.
   - ◯ lower middle third of the abdominal-pelvic region
   - ◯ middle third of the abdominal-pelvic region
   - ◯ upper middle abdominal-pelvic region
   - ◯ lateral middle third of the abdominal-pelvic region

UNIT 3

The Skeletal System

THE SKELETAL SYSTEM - INTRODUCTION

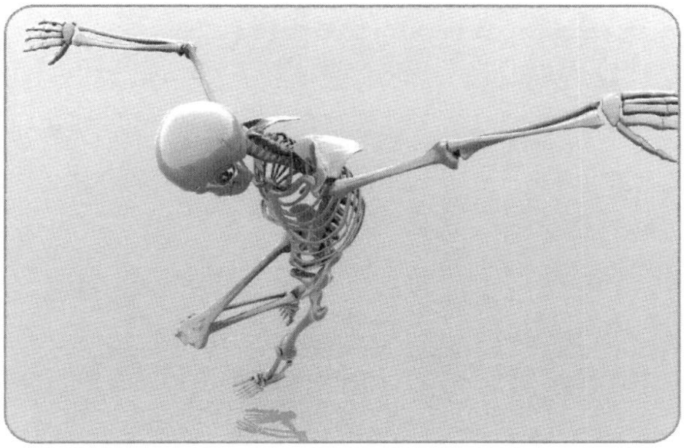

Your study of anatomy began with a high-level description of the structural levels of human anatomy—chemical, cellular, tissue, organ, system, and organism. You are also able to use directional terms to describe an anatomical structures' location in the body. Building on your understanding of those concepts, you are going to learn more about each of the organ systems that make up the human body. You'll be starting with the skeletal system. In the following unit we will discuss:

- the purpose, composition, formation, and development of bones
- the types of bones found in the body
- the names, locations, and any special markings or purposes for specific bone types

BONE FORMATION AND DEVELOPMENT

During the eighth week (or so) of development, the human embryo begins the process of ossification (bone formation). This early bone formation produces immature bone, which is rather different from mature bone found in the adult skeleton. Immature bone is similar to bone tissue that forms during repair of bone fractures—it contains many fibers and cells, and less of the cement and mineral substances found in mature bone. Over time, the bulk of immature bone is replaced by mature bone.

Highlights

The process of bone formation is called ossification. Bone is made up of three different cell types:

1. osteoblasts
2. osteocytes
3. osteoclasts

Bone is made up of three different cell types: osteoblasts, osteocytes, and osteoclasts.

Bone formation (ossification) begins when osteoblasts, originating from stem cells, appear in the body. Osteoblasts secrete an extracellular (outside the cells) matrix composed of collagen fibers onto which bone salts (hydroxyapatite) are deposited to initiate the process of calcification (hardening). The matrix in which young bone is formed, as well as the young bone itself that is created, is called osteoid. The term *osteoid* means "resembling bone."

When the osteoblasts become surrounded by the extracellular matrix, they become osteocytes (former osteoblasts). The purpose of osteocytes is to regulate the increased bone metabolism that occurs with growth and development. The tiny pits within bone matrix that contain osteocytes are called lacunae. Osteocytes receive blood supply and communicate with other bone cells by extending cellular processes through microscopic channels called canaliculi.

Osteoblasts continue to form immature bone while bone growth and development ensure that immature bone is replaced by mature bone. Replacement occurs when osteoclasts attach themselves to mature bone, dissolve it, and then reabsorb it. Throughout the process, there is a constant turnover of bone matrix, which results in the continuous remodeling of bone tissue.

Two similar forms of ossification, intramembranous and intracartilaginous (endochondral), have the same purpose: to replace membrane and cartilage with bone. Ossification in the human body is completed by about age 25. This progressive ossification is the reason why fractures, breaks, or ruptures in bone tissue heal much more easily and with fewer complications in a young person's skeleton than they do in an older person's skeleton.

Term	Definition
bone cells	Cells the body has programmed to create bones
canaliculi	channels in calcified bone matrix through which osteocytes extend cellular processes
immature bone	the first formation of bone
lacunae	tiny pits within calcified bone matrix that contain osteocytes
mature bone	bone that has ossified and calcified
ossification	bone formation
osteoblasts	bone-forming cells that secrete a matrix which becomes calcified
osteoclasts	large multinucleated cells that reabsorb bone matrix
osteocytes	former osteoblasts that are surrounded by bone matrix and have calcified

I. MATCHING.
Match the correct term to the definition.

1. ____ bone cells
2. ____ osteoblasts
3. ____ osteocytes
4. ____ immature bone
5. ____ osteoclasts
6. ____ mature bone
7. ____ ossification

A. bone-forming cells that secrete a matrix which becomes calcified
B. former osteoblasts that are surrounded by bone matrix and have calcified
C. large multinucleated cells that reabsorb bone matrix
D. the first formation of bone
E. bone that has ossified and calcified
F. bone formation
G. cells that the body has programmed to create bones

BONE TISSUE TYPES AND STRUCTURE

There are two types of bone tissue found in mature bones: cortical (compact) bone and cancellous (spongy) bone.

Cortical Bone

Cortical (compact) bone represents almost 80% of the skeletal mass of the human body. It is called "compact" because it forms a protective outer layer around every bone in the body.

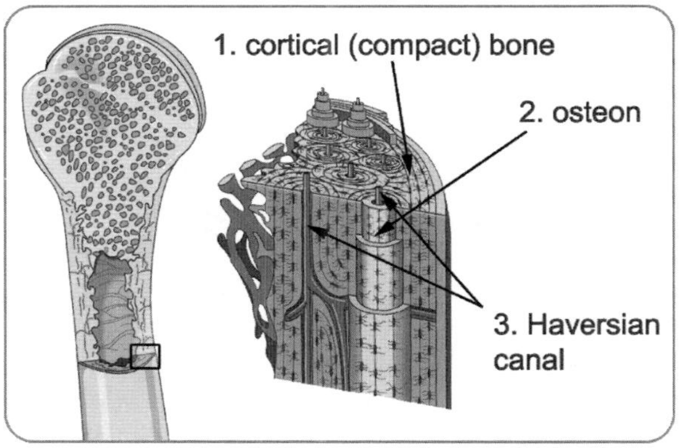

The structural unit of compact bone is the **osteon**. If you were to examine a cross section of cortical bone with a microscope, you would see what appear to be groupings of bullseyes. Each bullseye is an osteon. The circular rings of the bullseye are called **concentric lamellae** (meaning layer or plate). Within the lamellae are thousands of lacunae that house osteocytes. In the center of the bullseye, the **central canal of the osteon** or **Haversian canal** (eponym) transmits nerves and vascular tissue.

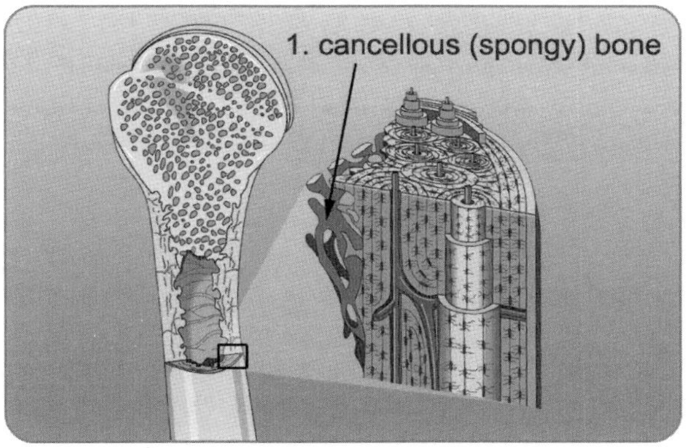

Between the osteons are **interstitial lamellae** (3–15 layers of mineralized bone) and around the outside layer of the bone are **circumferential lamellae**. The overall structural pattern of cortical (compact) bone gives it a plywood-like strength that is highly resistant to bending, torsion, and breakage. Cortical bone has a very slow turnover rate but is in a constant state of remodeling by osteoclast and osteoblast activity. This activity level is high in children and early adolescents and decreases with the progression of age.

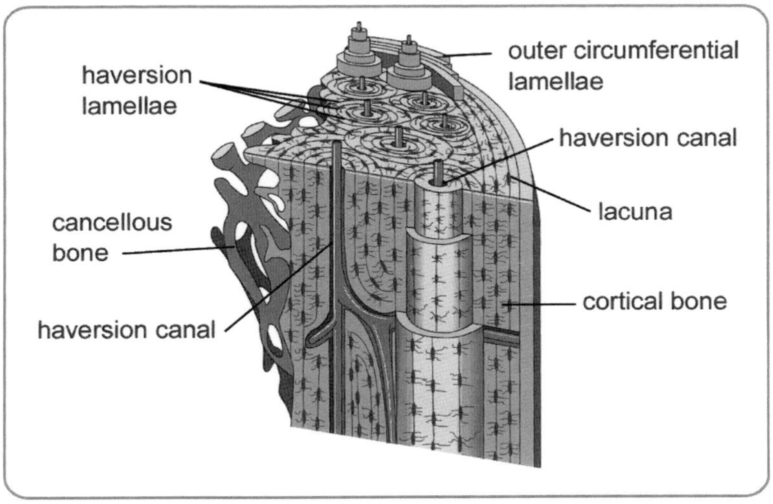

Cancellous Bone

Cancellous (spongy) bone represents only about 20% of the skeletal mass.

Cancellous bone contains a trabecular (mesh-like) network of bone tissue that allows it to maintain its shape despite compressive forces. The structural unit of cancellous bone has several characteristics:

1. it does not contain osteons
2. it is less dense than cortical bone
3. it is very elastic
4. it has a higher turnover rate than cortical bone

The area containing cancellous bone maintains an intricate balance of bone cells, extracellular matrix (collagenous fibers), marrow, and other tissues vital for bone formation. Cancellous bone is as hard as cortical bone, but it is formed in such a way as to appear spongy or mesh-like. Most of the bones in the axial skeleton, including the bones of the skull, ribs, ears, and spine are composed mainly of cancellous bone.

Bone is an intricate and dynamic part of the human body. Not only does bone tissue regulate hematopoesis (the production of blood cells), it performs other important functions as well. Bone is not "dead" tissue. An example of its dynamic nature is its ability to heal itself quickly when fractures occur. This healing is a demonstration of the constant tissue remodeling mentioned above.

SKELETAL FUNCTION

The skeleton has multiple functions, three of which are:

- To form the framework of the human body.
- To serve as a means of attachment for muscles.
- To protect vital organs such as the heart, lungs, and brain.

These functions are likely self-explanatory given your personal experience having your own human body. Unlike jellyfish, humans have a solid framework that encases important organs and gives people substance and shape. The skeletal system also has functions that are not so apparent in everyday life (unless they stop working!) but that are equally important:

- Bone marrow and cell formation
- Mineral storage

The internal soft tissues of the bones contain marrow, which is responsible for erythropoiesis (the formation of red blood cells) and the formation of white blood cells.

Erythropoietic marrow is found in:

- hip bones
- proximal ends of the thigh and arm bones
- bones of the skull
- vertebrae
- sternum

This erythropoietic marrow is the medium for the development and storage of about 95% of the body's blood cells. Erythropoietic bone marrow contains hematopoietic stem cells that are precursor cells and are capable of producing all other types of blood cells. From the hematopoietic stem cells, red blood cells, white blood cells and megakaryocytes, from which platelets are derived, are formed. These cells are very important and serve the following specific functions:

Red blood cells, also called erythrocytes, carry oxygen from the lungs to the rest of the body and return carbon dioxide and other waste products.

White blood cells, also called leukocytes, help fight infections and generally support the immune system.

> **Highlights**
>
> Red blood cells carry oxygen and return waste products. White blood cells help fight infections and support the immune system.

There are many different types of white blood cells, including:

- lymphocytes
- monocytes
- eosinophils
- basophils
- neutrophils (granulocytes)

All blood cells form from stem cells found in the bone marrow.

Platelets or thrombocytes circulate in the bloodstream and are involved in hemostasis, leading to the formation of blood clots and the control of bleeding.

Measurement of the body's red blood cells and white blood cells is extremely important in the identification, diagnosis, and treatment of diseases.

Bones also store minerals, such as calcium and phosphorus, which are released into the blood stream as needed. These minerals provide bones with their rigidity and strength. The lack of these minerals or improper absorption by the blood stream can cause a variety of maladies of the skeleton, such as osteoporosis, in which the bones break easily even when there has been minimal trauma.

TYPES OF BONES

The human skeleton consists of bones of many different shapes and sizes. Here are a few of them.

Long bones

Long bones are bones whose length is greater than their width, such as the bones of the extremities (tibia, fibula, femur, radius, ulna, humerus).

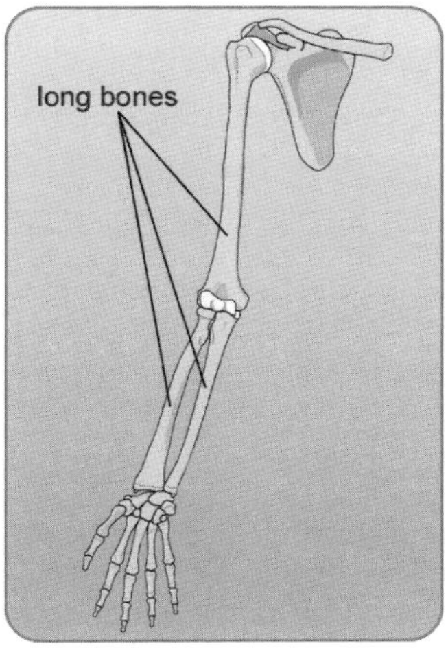

Short bones

Short bones are shaped more like cubes and are generally found in the ankle and wrist (carpus and tarsus).

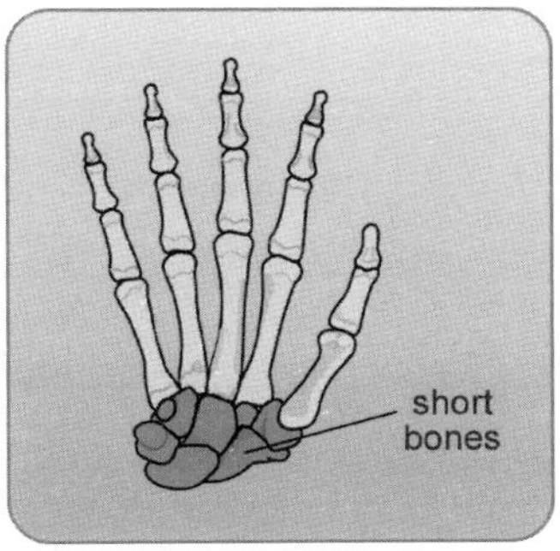

Flat bones

Flat bones are found in the cranial vault, sternum (breastbone), shoulder blades, and ribs. Flat bones are made up of a layer of marrow (diploe) sandwiched between two layers of compact bone.

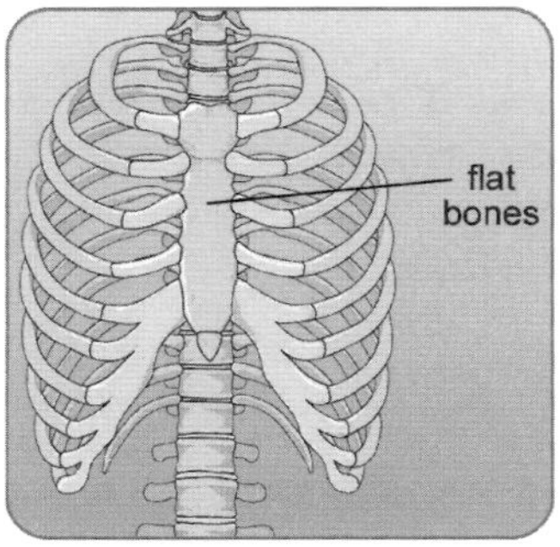

Irregular bones

Irregular bones are a mix of irregularly shaped bones that do not fall into any of the other bone-type categories. They are found in the face, spinal column, and hips.

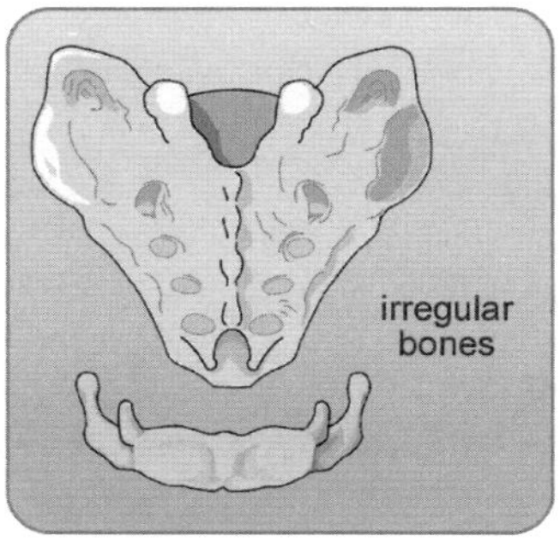

Sesamoid bones

Sesamoid bones are mostly rounded masses embedded in certain tendons and are usually related to the surfaces of joints. Included in this group are the patella (kneecap), metacarpophalangeal joints of the hands, and metatarsophalangeal joints of the toes.

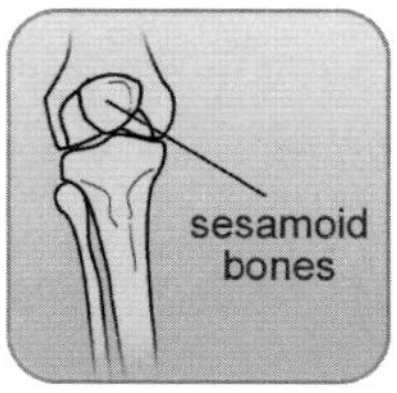

Wormian bones

Wormian bones are small bones found between suture lines of the skull where the edges of the skull bones are joined together.

BONE LANDMARKS AND FEATURES

Besides knowing the types, functions, and shapes of bones, there are also markings that differentiate bones. For example, some bones have parts with a "scooped out" look. Depending on the size of the scooped out area, this feature is known as a **fossa**, groove, or pit. Other bones have an opening or hole in them referred to as a **foramen**. Many bone markings, or landmarks, are locations of muscle attachment such as the radial **tuberosity**. Others, such as the foramen magnum, depicted in the figure on the right, transmit nerves and vascular tissue. The foramen magnum, specifically, allows the passage of the spinal cord to the base of the brain.

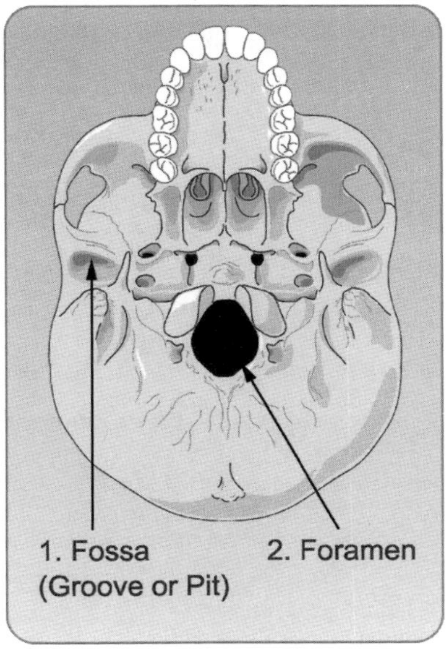

You will also become familiar with terms such as: **articulate**, connected at a joint or junction; **epiphysis**, the terminal end of a long bone (each long bone has 2 epiphyses); **diaphysis**, the elongated middle portion or shaft of a long bone, often referred to as the **body**; **condyles** or **epicondyles**, rounded projections that are often part of the articular surface of a bone. The **metaphysis**, commonly known as the growth plate, is "sandwiched" between the epiphysis and diaphysis. You will encounter these terms as well as others in the list below.

sinuses: Cavities inside a bone.

head: Rounded end of a long bone (the rounded tip).

foramen: Opening or hole in a bone.

tubercle: Small rounded projections.

fossa/groove/pit: Indentation of a bone, also called a depression.

condyles/epicondyles: Rounded bone projections.

neck: Constricted end of a long bone before the head or rounded end.

canal/meatus: Long or deep hole in a bone.

facets: Small, smooth, and flat areas.

tuberosity: Large rounded projections.

process: Prominence or projection, as of bone.

articulate: Connected at a joint or junction.

epiphysis: The terminal end of a long bone (each long bone has 2 epiphyses).

diaphysis: The elongated middle portion or shaft of a long bone, often referred to as the body.

metaphysis: The growing portion of a bone located in between the epiphysis and diaphysis.

condyles or epicondyles: Rounded projections that are often part of the articular surface of a bone.

I. MULTIPLE CHOICE.

Determine if the following terms are a bone marking or a type of bone.

1. condyles
   - ◯ Bone marking
   - ◯ Bone type
2. long
   - ◯ Bone marking
   - ◯ Bone type
3. neck
   - ◯ Bone marking
   - ◯ Bone type
4. sinuses
   - ◯ Bone marking
   - ◯ Bone type
5. short
   - ◯ Bone marking
   - ◯ Bone type
6. cavity
   - ◯ Bone marking
   - ◯ Bone type
7. sesamoid
   - ◯ Bone marking
   - ◯ Bone type
8. wormian
   - ◯ Bone marking
   - ◯ Bone type
9. facets
   - ◯ Bone marking
   - ◯ Bone type
10. tubercle
    - ◯ Bone marking
    - ◯ Bone type

11. irregular
    - ◯ Bone marking
    - ◯ Bone type

12. tuberosity
    - ◯ Bone marking
    - ◯ Bone type

13. flat
    - ◯ Bone marking
    - ◯ Bone type

14. foramen
    - ◯ Bone marking
    - ◯ Bone type

15. meatus
    - ◯ Bone marking
    - ◯ Bone type

16. fossa
    - ◯ Bone marking
    - ◯ Bone type

17. process
    - ◯ Bone marking
    - ◯ Bone type

REVIEW: BONES

I. MATCHING.
Match the correct term to the definition.

1. ____ condyles
2. ____ foramen
3. ____ epiphysis
4. ____ diaphysis
5. ____ articulate
6. ____ cortical bone
7. ____ cancellous bone

A. also called spongy bone, it contains a mesh-like network of bone tissue that is not composed of osteons
B. the terminal end of a long bone
C. also called compact bone, it forms the protective outer layer around every bone in the body and is composed of osteons
D. connected at a joint or junction
E. an opening or hole in a bone that allows the passage of nervous and/or vascular tissue
F. rounded projections that are often part of the articular surface of a bone
G. the elongated middle portion or shaft of a long bone

II. MULTIPLE CHOICE.
Choose the best answer.

1. Erythrocytes
   - ◯ red blood cells
   - ◯ white blood cells

2. Lymphocytes
   - ◯ red blood cells
   - ◯ white blood cells

3. Red blood cells
   - ◯ carry oxygen from the lungs to the rest of the body
   - ◯ help fight infections and aid the immune system
   - ◯ are capable of producing all other types of blood cells

4. White blood cells
   - ◯ carry oxygen from lungs to rest of body
   - ◯ help fight infections and aid the immune system
   - ◯ are capable of producing all other types of blood cells

5. Stem cells
   - ◯ carry oxygen from lungs to rest of body
   - ◯ help fight infections and aid the immune system
   - ◯ are capable of producing all other types of blood cells

6. Monocytes
   - ◯ red blood cells
   - ◯ white blood cells

7. Neutrophils
   - ◯ red blood cells
   - ◯ white blood cells

8. Phosphorus is a _____.
   - ◯ red blood cell
   - ◯ white blood cell
   - ◯ mineral

9. Helps control bleeding
   - ◯ thrombocytes
   - ◯ lymphocytes
   - ◯ minerals

10. Minerals provide bones with _____.
    - ◯ marrow
    - ◯ rigidity and strength
    - ◯ immunization against infection

AXIAL AND APPENDICULAR SKELETON

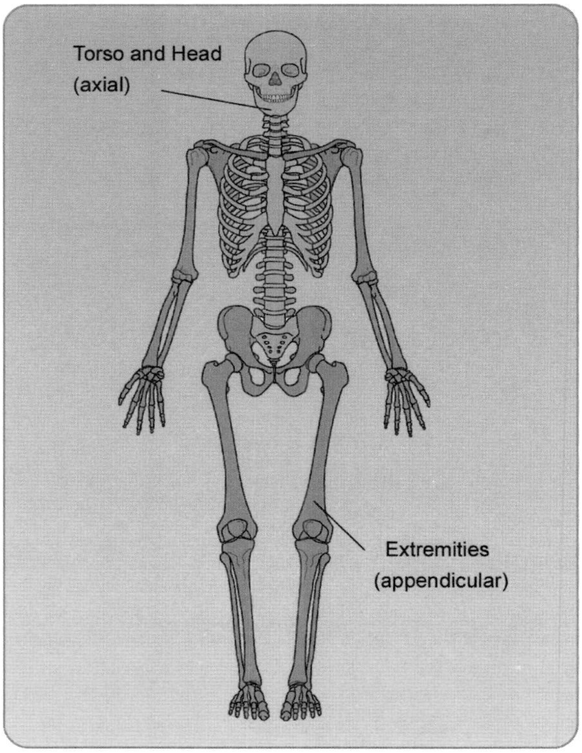

The human skeleton is made of densely packaged and calcified connective tissue. At birth, the human body has anywhere from 275–350 bones. As the body matures, some bones in the wrists, ankles, sacrum, coccyx, etc. fuse together, reducing that number to 206 bones. All of these bones working together are classified as the skeletal system.

The bones of the human skeleton are placed into two divisions: the axial skeleton and the appendicular skeleton.

Axial skeleton: The axial skeleton has 80 bones and includes the bones of the skull, vertebral column, thoracic cage, sternum, hyoid, and ears.

- skull 28 (8 paired and 6 unpaired cranial and facial bones and 6 ossicles of the ears)
- hyoid bone (only floating bone)
- vertebrae 26 bones
- chest 25 bones
- total 80

Appendicular skeleton: The appendicular skeleton has 126 bones and includes the bones of the upper and lower extremities.

- upper extremities 64 bones
- lower extremities 62 bones
- total 126

REVIEW: AXIAL AND APPENDICULAR SKELETON

I. MULTIPLE CHOICE.
Choose whether the portions of the body belong to the axial or appendicular skeleton.

1. forearm
   ◯ axial
   ◯ appendicular

2. thighbone
   ◯ axial
   ◯ appendicular

3. skull
   ◯ axial
   ◯ appendicular

4. ossicles (ear bones)
   - ◯ axial
   - ◯ appendicular

5. calf
   - ◯ axial
   - ◯ appendicular

6. upper arm
   - ◯ axial
   - ◯ appendicular

7. vertebrae
   - ◯ axial
   - ◯ appendicular

8. feet
   - ◯ axial
   - ◯ appendicular

9. lower jaw
   - ◯ axial
   - ◯ appendicular

10. neck
   - ◯ axial
   - ◯ appendicular

11. elbow
   - ◯ axial
   - ◯ appendicular

12. chest
   - ◯ axial
   - ◯ appendicular

13. knees
   - ◯ axial
   - ◯ appendicular

14. ankles
   - ◯ axial
   - ◯ appendicular

AXIAL SKELETON - CRANIAL AND FACIAL BONES

The axial skeletal system consists of, as previously noted, the bones of the skull, vertebral column, thoracic cage, sternum, hyoid, and ears. This creates the structure for most of the vital areas of the body, providing support and protection for the inner organs, as well as movement through the neck and the spine.

Bones of the Skull

There are 8 sets of paired bones and 6 unpaired bones that make up the bones of the skull.The cranium contains 6 main bones, the face has 16 bones, and the ossicles of the ears have 6 bones (3 per ear).

Paired bones (8 sets for a total of 16):

- nasal concha
- lacrimal bone
- maxilla
- nasal bone
- palatine bone*
- parietal bone
- temporal bone
- zygomatic bone

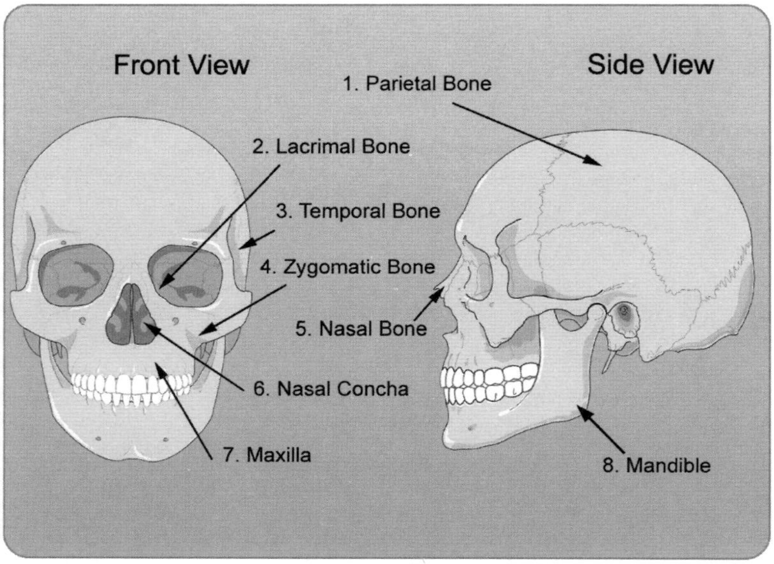

**Palatine bone is the bone of the "roof of the mouth" and is not depicted.*

Unpaired Bones (6 for a total of 6):

- ethmoid*
- frontal bone
- occipital bone
- sphenoid bone
- vomer
- mandible

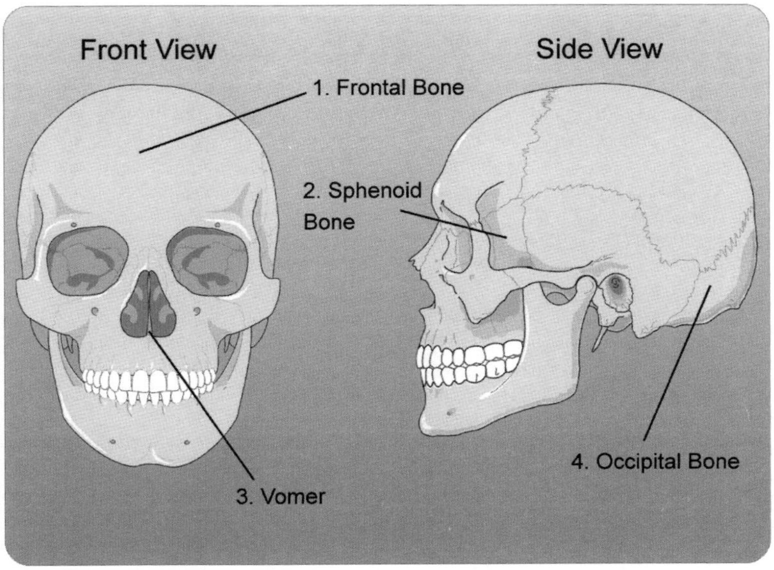

The ethmoid bone separates the nasal cavity from the brain and is not depicted.

MAIN CRANIAL BONES AND SUTURES

After birth, the bones of the cranium continue to grow until the fontanels are no longer present. The posterior and anterolateral fontanels usually fill in 2–3 months after birth. The posterolateral fontanels usually fill in at the end of the first year. The anterior fontanel (the largest fontanel) usually fills in by the middle of the second year after birth.

The cranial bones are 6 (2 paired sets and 2 unpaired) flat bones bound together by fibrous joints called sutures. Although sutures are technically joints, which will be discussed later in the module, we will identify them here due to their intricate placement between the cranial bones.

Term	Definition
coronal suture	Joins the frontal bone to the two parietal bones
frontal bone	Bone that closes the anterior part of the cranial cavity and forms the skeleton of the forehead
lambdoid suture	Joins the two parietal bones to the occipital bone
occipital bone	Bone situated at the posterior and inferior part of the cranium; articulating with the two parietal and two temporal bones
parietal bones	Bones forming part of the superior and lateral surfaces of the skull, and joining each other in the midline at the sagittal suture
sagittal suture	Joins one parietal bone to the other parietal bone

squamous suture	Joins the parietal bones to the temporal bones
temporal bones	Bones forming part of the lateral surfaces and the base of the skull, and containing the organs of hearing

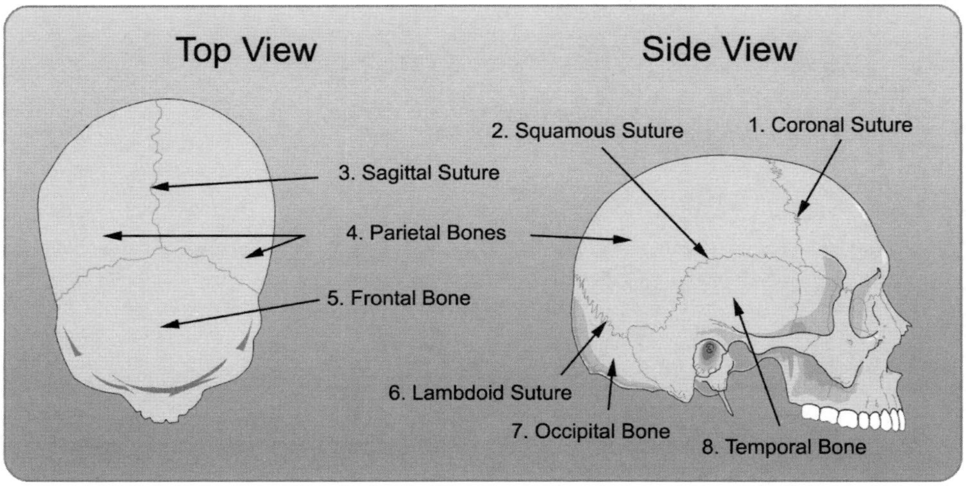

The cranial bones consist of:

- frontal bone
- parietal bones
- occipital bone
- temporal bones

The sutures that join these bones together are:

- coronal suture
- squamous suture
- lambdoid suture
- sagittal suture

I. FILL IN THE BLANK.

Looking at the figure further up on this page, please list the names of the cranial bones that are joined by the specified suture. Remember that parietal and temporal bones are bilateral. Bilateral means that there is one on each side (bi = two, lateral = side).

1. The sagittal suture joins one parietal bone to the other ________________ bone.
2. The squamous sutures join the parietal bones to the ________________ bones.
3. The coronal suture joins the ________________ bone to the two parietal bones.
4. The lambdoid suture joins the two parietal bones to the ________________ bone.

II. FILL IN THE BLANK.

Using the words in the box, label the diagram.

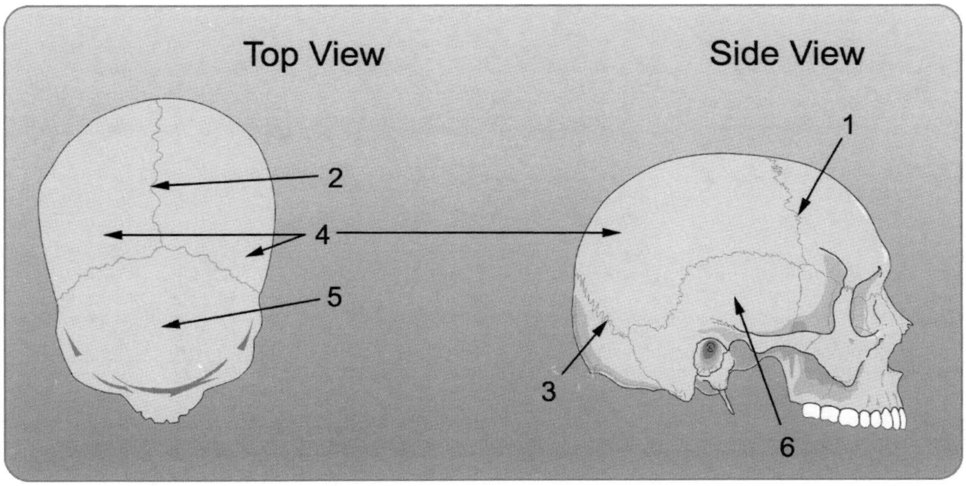

1. ______________
2. ______________
3. ______________
4. ______________
5. ______________
6. ______________

frontal bone
sagittal suture
temporal bone
lambdoid suture
coronal suture
parietal bone

CRANIAL FONTANELS

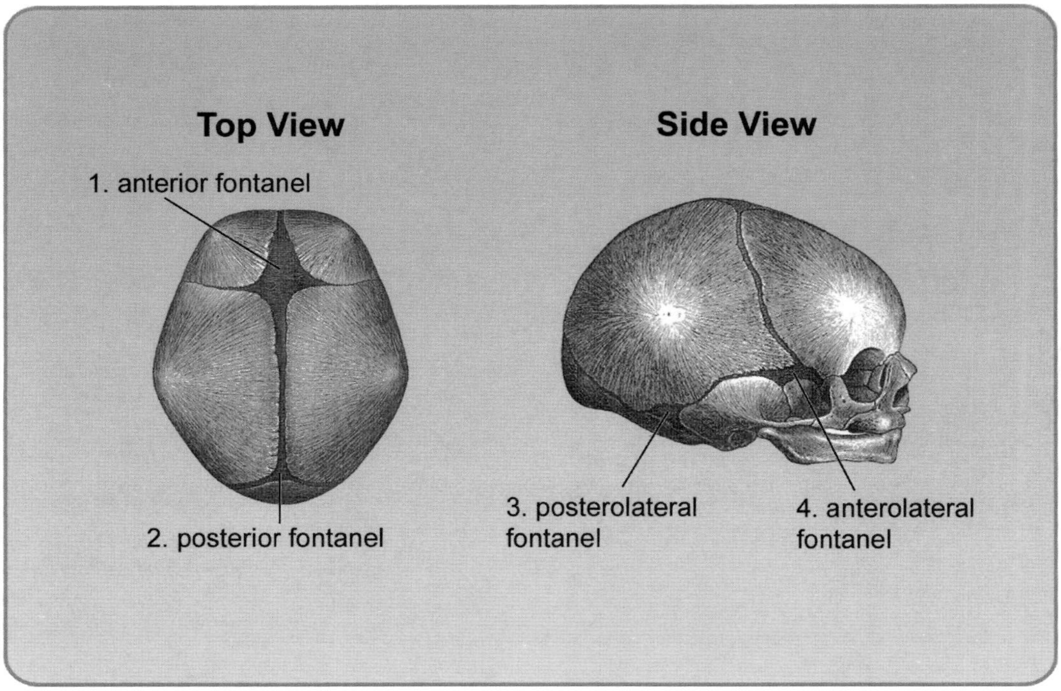

Fontanels

At birth, the bones of the head are not completely formed. As a result, there is adequate space between them to allow the baby's head to be molded enough to fit through the birth canal. These 6 spaces are known as fontanels or “soft spots.”

anterior fontanel: The space where the frontal angles of the parietal bones meet the two ununited halves of the frontal bone.

posterior fontanel: The space where the occipital angles of the parietal bones meet the occipital.

posteriolateral fontanels: The interval on either side of the head between the mastoid angle of the parietal bone, the temporal bone, and the occipital bone.

anterolateral fontanels: An interval on either side of the head where the frontal angle of the temporal bone and greater wing of the sphenoid meet.

LANDMARKS OF THE SKULL

Finally, let's cover a few easy-to-identify markings of the bones of the skull. Remember the definitions of *foramen* and *process*? (Sneak a peek at the sticky note if you forgot.)

Use your fingers to trace your eye sockets, jaw, and behind your ears. See if you can feel the openings, projections, and prominences listed below:

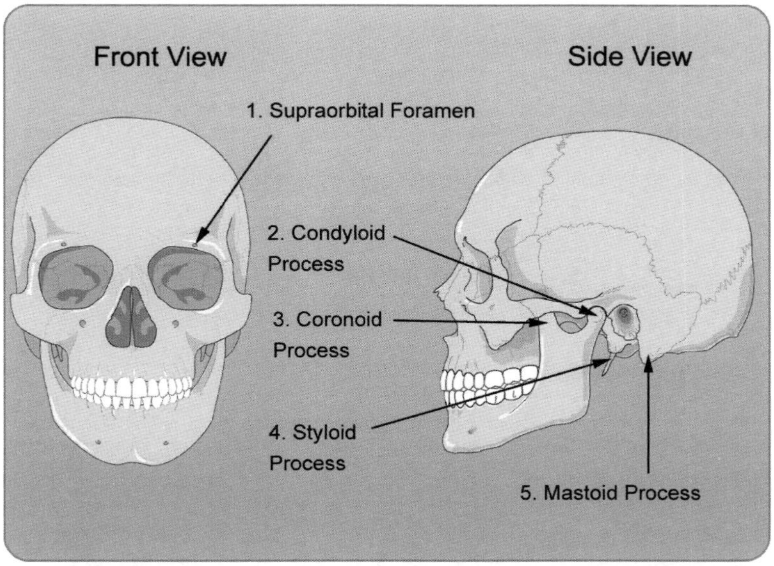

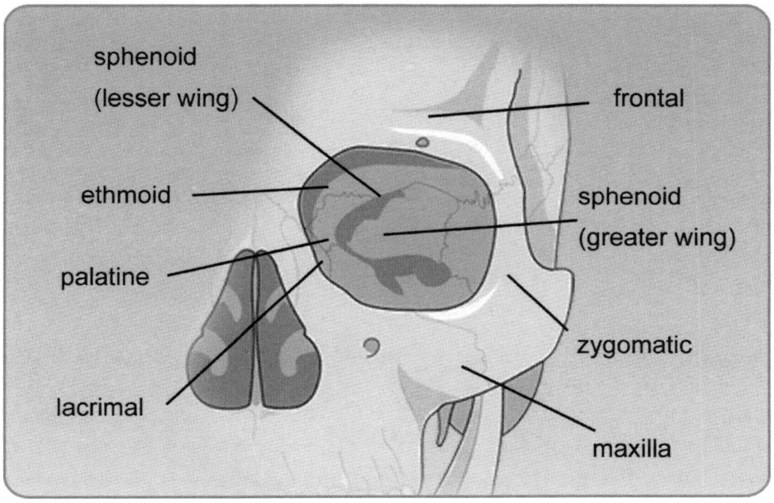

orbit — the paired bony depressions in the skull that house the eyes.

supraorbital foramen — as the name suggests "supra" - above, "orbital" - referring to the orbit or the bones that make up the eye socket (shown below). Opening directly superficial to the eyebrow, the supraorbital foramen allows passage of the supraorbital nerve and the supraorbital artery and vein.

supraorbital process of the frontal bone — the bony ridge along the inferior aspect of the forehead.

external acoustic meatus — this is the exterior skeletal opening of the ear canal. The external acoustic meatus is located inferiorly on the temporal bone and is situated between the mastoid process and the codyloid process of the mandible.

mastoid process — located postero-inferior to the external acoustic meatus, the mastoid process serves as the attachment point for several muscles including the sternocleidomastoid muscle.

styloid process (of the temporal bone) — lies inferior to the external acoustic meatus at the base of the temporal bone. The styloid process is a thin, pointed projection pointing antero-inferiorly that is the attachment site for small ligaments and muscles of the face and neck.

nasal turbinates — (nasal conchae) curved bone projections into the nasal cavity. There are three turbinates on each side creating four air passages per side.

zygomatic Arch — composed of the zygomatic bone anteriorly, and the zygomatic process of the temporal bone posteriorly, the zygomatic arch is a flat bridge of bone that extends from the "cheekbone" to the superior aspect of the external acoustic meatus. It serve as an attachment site for the masseter muscle.

occipital condyle — articular processes at the base of the skull. These articulate with the atlas vertebra to allow the head to nod.

foramen magnum — the large foramen at the base of the skull that transmits the spinal cord.

Process: prominence or projection, as of bone.

Foramen: opening or hole in a bone.

MANDIBLE, AUDITORY OSSICLES, AND HYOID

The Mandible

The mandible is the largest of the facial bones. It is largely composed of hard compact bone and holds the lower teeth within landmarks called alveolar processes. It articulates with the temporal bone at the temporomandibular joint being moved by the strong muscles of mastication

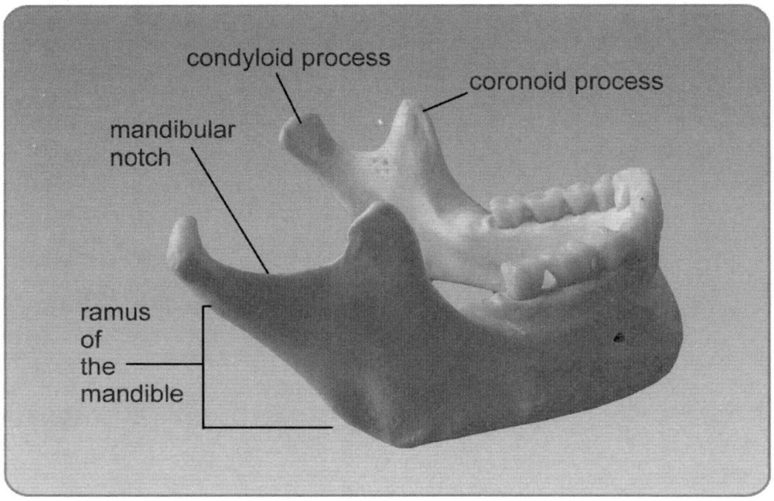

Source: Wikipedia

ramus of the mandible—These are the bilateral upward projections posterior to the teeth. Each ramus terminates in two processes, the coronoid process anteriorly and the condyloid process posteriorly, with the u-shaped mandibular notch between them.

condyloid process of the mandible—the condyliod (resembling a condyle) process of the mandible lies anterior to the external acoustic meatus. It forms the articular surface joining the temporal bone to form the temporomandibular joint.

coronoid process of the mandible—located anterior to the condyloid process on the superior portion of the mandible, the coronoid process provides an attachment site for the temporalis muscle of the lateral skull.

mandibular notch —the "U"-shaped depression at the superior boarder of the ramus located between the condyloid and coronoid processes.

The Inner Ear

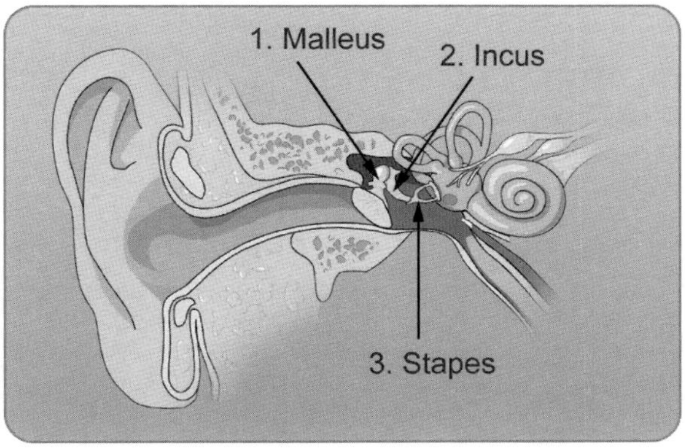

Each ear contains three auditory ossicles. An ossicle is simply a small bone. We refer to them as "auditory" because they are essential for hearing. There are 3 ossicles per side, for a total of 6. Each is given a name that is derived from the Latin word for its shape, the English translations being hammer, anvil, and stirrup:

malleus (hammer)—this ossicle remains in direct contact with the tympanic membrane (ear drum), transmitting the vibrations of sound waves on to the incus with which it articulates.

incus (anvil)—the incus lies between the malleus and the stapes, articulating with both bones to transmit sound vibrations from the malleus to the stapes.

stapes (stirrup)—the stapes transmits sound vibrations from the incus to the membranous oval window, leading to the inner ear.

The neck contains the only "floating" bone of the entire body. This floating bone, or **hyoid** bone, is shaped like a U and is supported by the muscles of the neck.

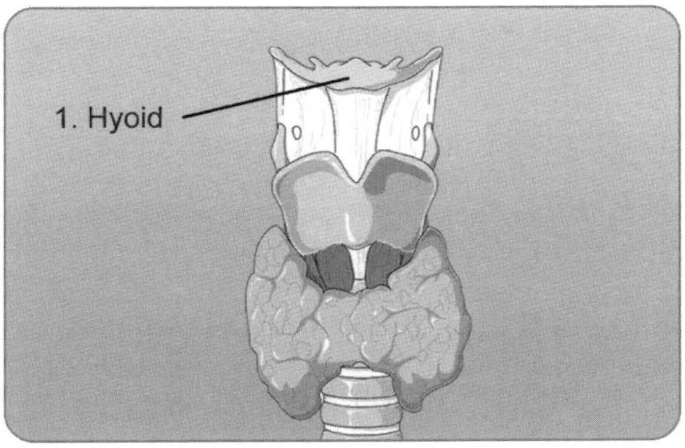

Notice the hyoid bone is at the top of the tracheal tube.

REVIEW: THE SKULL

I. FILL IN THE BLANK.

Use the word(s) in the box to fill in the blanks.

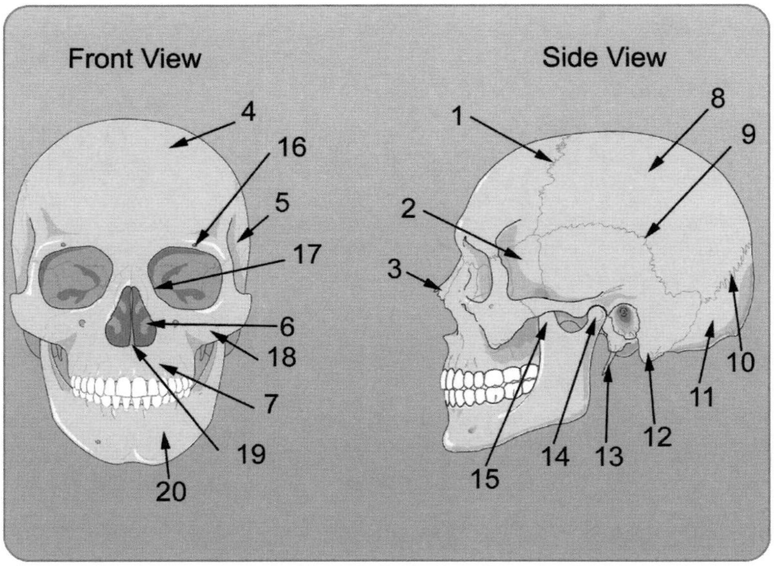

squamous suture
sphenoid bone
mandible
maxilla
supraorbital foramen
temporal bone
coronoid process
nasal concha
coronal suture
mastoid process
frontal bone
parietal bone
condyloid process
lambdoid suture
nasal bone
zygomatic bone
occipital bone
vomer
styloid process
lacrimal bone

1. ________________
2. ________________
3. ________________
4. ________________
5. ________________
6. ________________
7. ________________
8. ________________
9. ________________
10. ________________
11. ________________
12. ________________
13. ________________
14. ________________
15. ________________

16. ______________

17. ______________

18. ______________

19. ______________

20. ______________

VERTEBRAL COLUMN

The vertebral column consists of 26 total bones, differentiated below. The last lumbar vertebra connects to the sacrum, which connects to the coccyx (or tailbone).

- cervical vertebrae (7)
  - atlas vertebra (the first cervical vertebra)
  - axis vertebra (the second cervical vertebra)
- thoracic vertebrae (12)
- lumbar vertebrae (5)
- sacrum
- coccyx

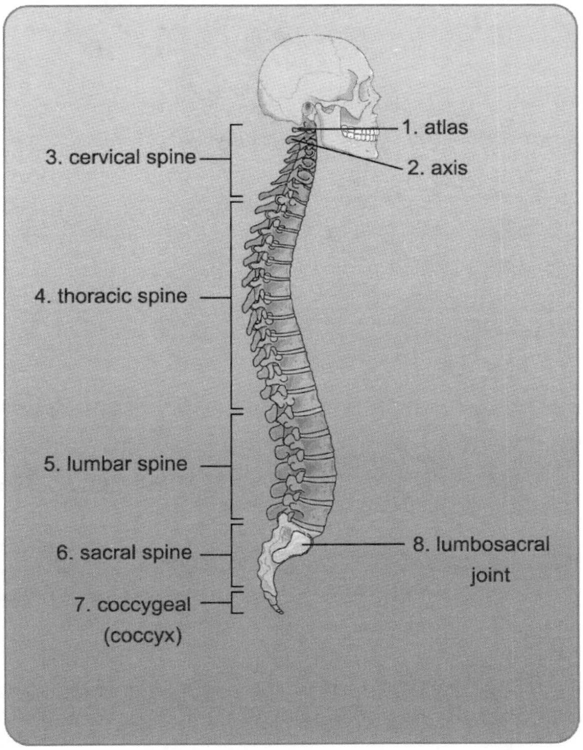

The vertebral column is a major support structure for the human body. It consists of 26 bones that are stacked upon one another, but separated by **intervertebral discs**. A designated space for passage of the spinal cord is made by the **intervertebral foramina** (plural of foramen). In other words, the spinal cord runs right through the center of the bony vertebral column, protecting it from injury.

The vertebral column is not straight like a stack of checkers. The spine has 4 important curvatures - cervical, thoracic, lumbar, and pelvic - that contribute to the overall posture of the human body and the ability to walk upright. To allow these curvatures each vertebra is unique in shape and highly specialized for its respective function. For example, each of the 5 lumbar vertebrae has a thick, bulky **body** designed to support a heavy weight. The body of a lumbar vertebra is also taller than the dorsal portion of the bone, contributing to the lumbar curvature. Each of the 26 vertebrae is likewise individually shaped to build a highly specialized system to support the human upper body.

The vertebral column has many processes and landmarks that protect and assist in the function of the spine. Some of these are depicted in the figure below.

As mentioned previously, the bones of the vertebral column are separated by intervertebral discs (except between the atlas and the axis). These discs act as a shock absorber keeping the vertebrae separate during the impact of body activity. Their structure consists of 2 important sections. The outer section, the annulus fibrosus, is annular (like a ring), as its name suggests, and is composed of several layers of dense fibrocartilage. These annular layers hold in the inner section, the nucleus pulposus, which is composed of loose cartilaginous fibers surrounded by a jelly-like protein gel. Although the intervertebral discs are not bone tissue and not technically part of the skeletal system, they play an integral role in the proper construction and function of the spine.

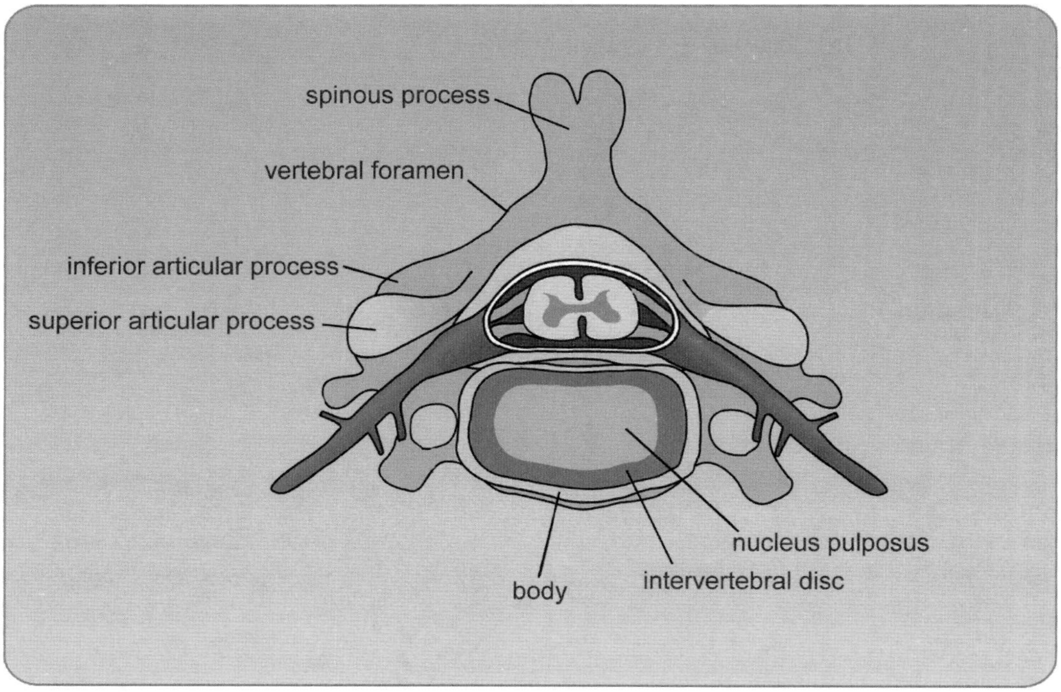

cervical spine: The cervical spine contains 7 vertebrae located in the neck area. In medical reports this spine is abbreviated C1-C7. The cervical spine curve is concave. With the ability to raise the head and stand with erect posture comes the development of this curve, which is why infants are not born with the cervical spine curve.

thoracic spine: The thoracic spine contains 12 vertebrae located in the chest area, which connect to the ribs. In medical reports this spine is abbreviated T1-T12. The thoracic spine curve is convex and is already formed at the time of birth.

articulate: The uniting or association of skeletal components (bone, cartilage) to form a union or joint.

lumbar spine: The lumbar spine contains 5 vertebrae located in the lower back. The lumbar spine curve is concave. Like the thoracic spine, it is already formed at the time of birth.

sacral spine: The sacral spine consists of 5 fused sacral vertebrae. It is easily distinguishable as an upside-down triangular shape. The two lateral surfaces (sides) are smooth for articulation (loose connection) with the iliac bones of the pelvis.

coccyx (coccygeal spine): The coccyx or "tailbone" is a single bone formed by fusion of 4-5 coccygeal vertebrae. When pressure is placed on the coccyx, it moves forward and acts like a shock absorber. Sitting down or falling on it too hard can cause it to become fractured. The adjectival form of coccyx is coccygeal.

intervertebral discs: Intervertebral discs (also correctly spelled disks) are composed of fibrous tissue and cartilage located between the vertebrae. Their function is to form strong joints and absorb spinal compression and shock.

body: The rounded mass of bone that composes the anterior portion of the vertebrae. The vertebral bodies are separated from one another by the intervertebral discs.

spinous process: The pointed projection that extends dorsally from the vertebrae.

transverse process: Bilateral bony processes that project laterally from the vertebrae to articulate with the ribs.

vertebral foramen: The opening in the center of the vertebrae that houses and transmits the spinal cord.

nucleus pulposus: The jelly like substance on the inside of the intervertebral discs that acts as a shock absorber to prevent compression of the spine.

annulus fibrosus: The annular ring of fibrocartilage that composes the outside margin of the intervertebral discs. This ring houses the nucleus pulposus.

I. MATCHING.
Match the correct term to the definition.

1. ____ lumbar spine
2. ____ intervertebral discs
3. ____ cervical spine
4. ____ thoracic spine
5. ____ articulate
6. ____ sacral spine
7. ____ coccyx

A. triangular shaped
B. the neck
C. tailbone
D. join
E. connects to the ribs
F. between the bones of the spine
G. lower back

STERNUM AND RIBS

The last sections of the axial skeleton to be covered are the sternum and ribs. This portion of the axial skeleton contains:

12 ribs

- true ribs (1–7)
- false ribs (8–10)
- floating (false) ribs (11–12)

sternum

- manubrium
- body
- xiphoid process

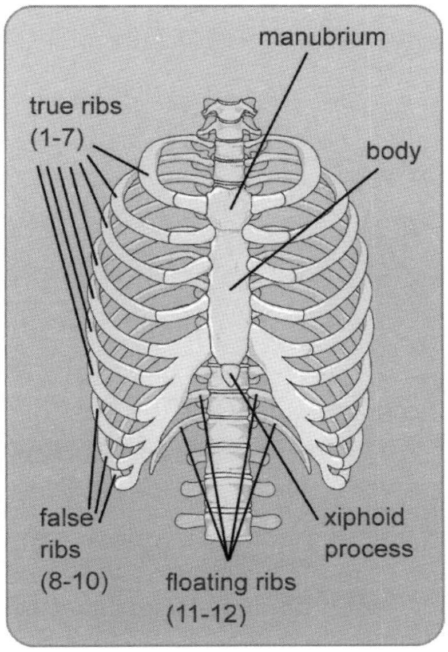

There are 12 pairs of ribs in the human body. These are long, curved bones that attach posteriorly to the thoracic vertebrae. Anteriorly rib pairs 1–7 connect to the sternum with costal (meaning rib) cartilage and are called true ribs. Ribs 8–10 connect to costal cartilage anteriorly and are called false ribs. The remaining two ribs, 11–12, are also connected to the thoracic spine posteriorly, but are free from connection anteriorly. Although ribs 11–12 are technically considered false ribs, they are also called floating ribs.

The sternum (breastbone) is a dagger-shaped bone located anteriorly in the middle of the chest. It has three divisions: the upper portion is the manubrium (handle); the middle section (which is the longest part) is the body; and the smallest, most distal portion (i.e., farthest from the handle) is the xiphoid process. The xiphoid process does not ossify until adulthood.

The area on the sternum where the manubrium and the body join is a significant landmark of the chest. It is called the sternal angle.

manubrium: Upper portion (handle) of the sternum.

body: Middle section of the sternum.

xiphoid process: Distal portion of the sternum.

sternal angle: Area of sternum where the manubrium and body join.

REVIEW: AXIAL SKELETON

I. FILL IN THE BLANK

It is important to have the ability to combine terms (like you did in the Medical Word Building unit). Some answers may require more than one word to be complete. Use the word(s) in the box to fill in the blanks.

1. The uppermost (neck) portion of the vertebral column is the ________________ spine.
2. The spine that corresponds to the chest is the ________________ spine.
3. The shock absorbers of the spinal column are the ________________.
4. Another name for the tailbone is ________________.
5. The curve of the ________________ spine does not form until the head can be raised and the body stands erect.
6. The sternum is easily identifiable because it is shaped like a ________________.
7. Because false ribs 11-12 are connected only to the thoracic spine, they are also called ________________ ribs.

floating
xiphoid process
cervical
cervical
spinal cord
thoracic
manubrium
intervertebral discs
dagger
coccyx

8. The sternal angle is a very significant landmark of the chest and is located on the sternum at the junction of the ________________ and the body.
9. The ________________, a part of the sternum, does not ossify until adulthood.
10. The vertebral foramen is the area of the spine where the ________________ passes through.

II. MATCHING.
Match the correct term to the definition.

1. ___	Skull	A.	26 bones
2. ___	ossicles of ears	B.	27 bones
3. ___	vertebrae	C.	7 bones
4. ___	cervical vertebrae	D.	6 bones

APPENDICULAR SKELETON

The human skeleton displays bilateral symmetry. The means that left side of the skeleton is the mirror image of the right side, and vice versa. This is important when describing anatomical structures. You have probably heard stories of surgeons operating on the correct body part, only on the wrong side of the body. Many surgeons will now write their initials on the correct side and structure they are to perform a procedure on to eliminate any possibility of these errors. We will not be performing surgery on patients; however, it is important for us to correctly describe right and left in anatomical terms.

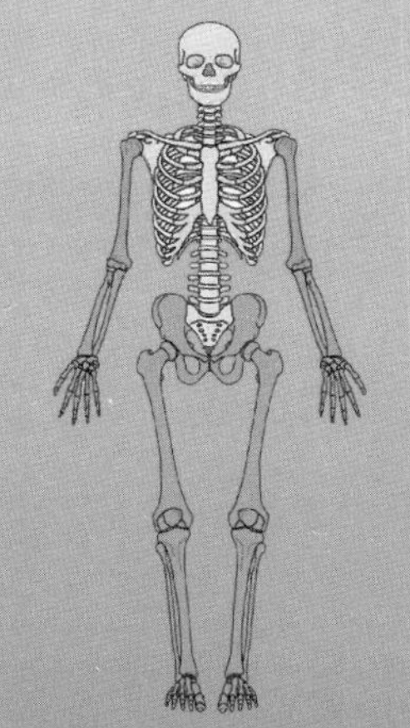

Appendicular Skeleton

Here is the rule: when using left and right to target one side of the body, you must always think of them in terms of the patient's left and right side and not your own.

Keep this in mind as you study the appendicular skeleton and notice that every structure we study has both a left and a right.

The appendicular skeleton, as shown to the right, gets its name from the fact that it consists of all the parts that append (hang on) to the axial skeleton. In fact, the arms and legs are known as the appendages.

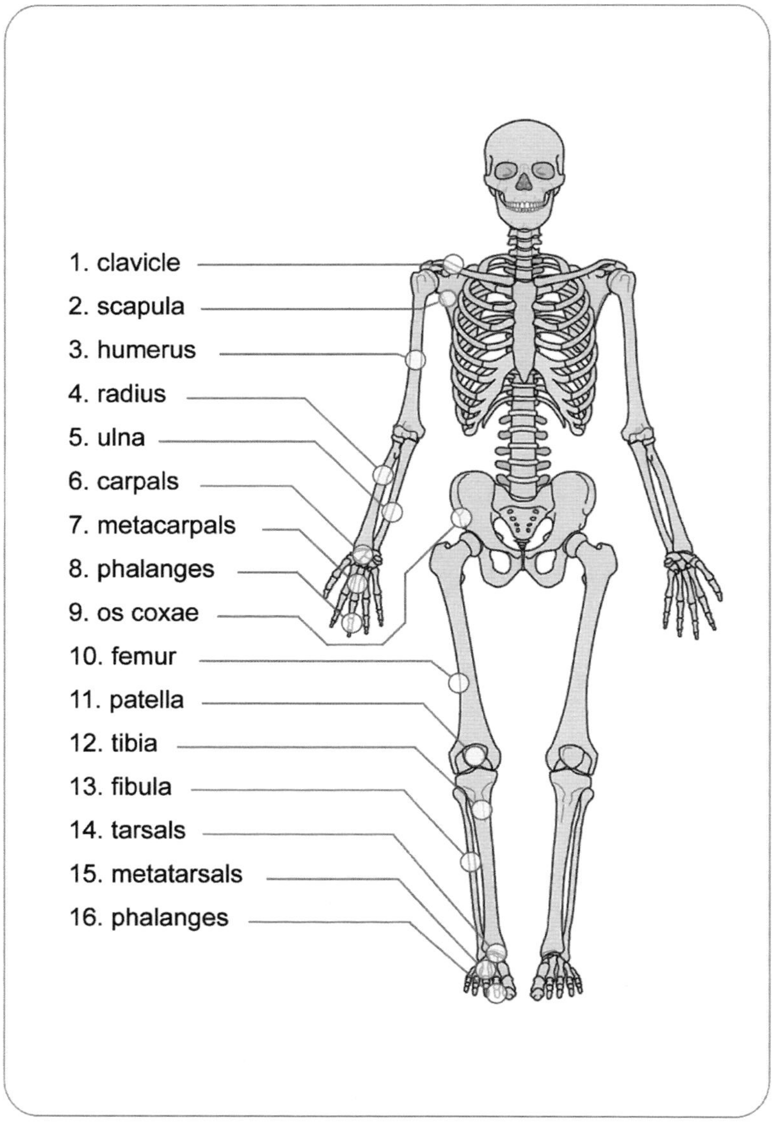

You may find it helpful to review terminology like anterior, distal, lateral, inferior, posterior, superior, and medial, as these terms are often used in anatomy for orientation.

In addition to the now-familiar bones of the axial skeleton, the human skeleton has appendicular bones of many shapes and sizes. Take a few minutes to study the bones of the appendicular skeleton.

clavicle: collarbone (1 per side for a total of 2)

scapula: shoulder bone (1 per side for a total of 2)

humerus: upper arm (1 per side for a total of 2)

radius: forearm (1 per side for a total of 2)

ulna: forearm (1 per side for a total of 2)

carpal: wrist (8 per side for a total of 16)

metacarpal: hand (5 per side for a total of 10)

phalanges: fingers (14 per side for a total of 28)

os coxae: hip/pelvic bone (1 per side for a total of 2)

femur: thigh (1 per side for a total of 2)

patella: kneecap (1 per side for a total of 2)

tibia: leg (1 per side for a total of 2)

fibula: leg (1 per side for a total of 2)

tarsal: ankle (7 per side for a total of 14)

metatarsal: foot (5 per side for a total of 10)

phalanges: toes (14 per side for a total of 28)

BONES OF THE SHOULDER

Clavicle

The **clavicle**, or collarbone, is the most frequently fractured bone in the body. Shaped like an elongated S, it allows the arm to move freely by holding the other bones of the shoulder away from the chest. To perform this function, the clavicle articulates with the acromion of the scapula at its lateral or **acromial extremity** and the manubrium of the sternum at its medial or **sternal extremity**. It is important to note that although the clavicle performs an important function in holding the upper appendages in place, it does not actually articulate with the upper arm bone (humerus). The clavicle is composed of cancellous bone covered by cortical bone with no bone marrow. It is the first bone of the human body to ossify.

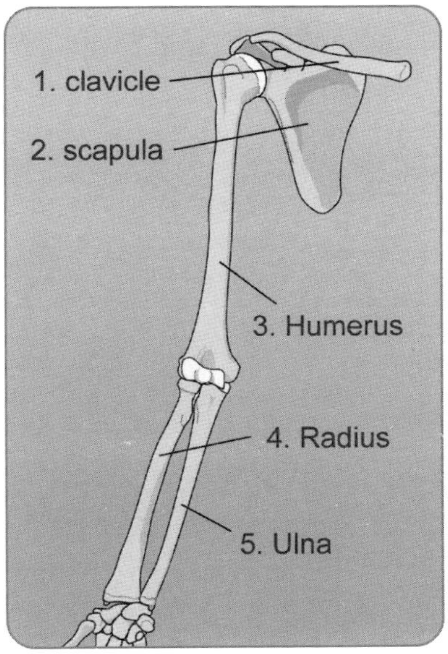

Scapula

The **scapula**, or shoulder blade, is positioned over ribs 2-7 and lies against the posterior aspect of the ribcage. There are several prominent landmarks on the scapula. The **spine of the scapula** is a long ridge that divides the scapula's posterior surface and ends in an extended process called the acromion. The **acromion** articulates with the lateral aspect of the clavicle to form the point of the shoulder. The **coracoid**

process arises from the superior aspect of the scapula and projects anterolaterally to serve as an attachment for 1 pectoral muscle and 2 upper arm muscles. The **glenoid cavity**, is a depressed area at the lateral angle where the head of the humerus articulates to form the basis of the shoulder joint.

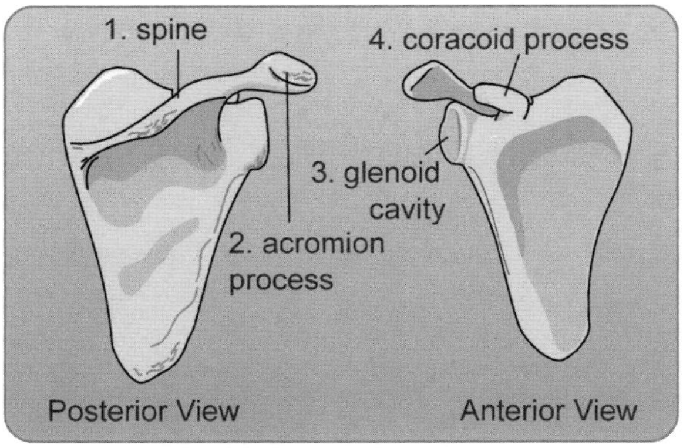

Humerus

The **humerus** is the only bone of the **brachium**, or upper arm. It is a long bone with two ends. The superior end, or the **head** of the humerus, is the rounded end that occupies the glenoid cavity of the scapula to form the shoulder joint. Below the head is the **anatomical neck** of the humerus, which has a small groove/ indentation located just beneath the head. On the extreme lateral aspect of the humerus, just below the anatomical neck, is a rounded process for muscle attachment called the **greater tuberosity**. The smaller, **lesser tuberosity** of the humerus lies medial to the greater tubercle and projects anteriorly. Inferior to the greater and lesser tubercles is the **surgical neck**, then the long diaphysis, or **body** of the humerus, and finally the inferior end of the bone. The distal epiphysis has **lateral** and **medial epicondyles** that are insertion points for muscles of the forearm, and the **trochlea** anteromedially which serves as the point of articulation with the ulna.

clavicle: The collarbone; the first bone in the human body to ossify.

sternal extremity: The end of the clavicle that is attached to the sternum.

acromial extremity: The end of the clavicle that is attached to the acromion.

scapula: Another name for the shoulder blade.

acromion: Process that helps form point of the shoulder.

coracoid process: Process that helps form point of the shoulder.

glenoid cavity: Cavity where the humerus rests.

humerus: Upper arm bone.

brachium: Term for the portion of the upper extremity that lies between the elbow joint and the shoulder joint; upper arm.

spine of the scapula: The bony ridge that projects posteriorly from the superior aspect of the dorsal surface of the scapula and gives rise to the acromion process.

head of the humerus: The rounded, proximal epiphysis of the humerus that articulates with the glenoid cavity of the scapula.

medial epicondyle: The medial, rounded projection on the distal epiphysis of the humerus.

lateral epicondyle: The lateral, rounded projection on the distal epiphysis of the humerus.

anatomical neck: A small groove/indentation located just beneath the head of the humerus.

surgical neck: The narrowing portion of the humerus just inferior to the greater and lesser tuberosity.

body of the humerus: The elongated diaphysis of the humerus.

trochlea of the humerus: The anteromedial projection from the distal epiphysis that articulates with the ulna in the elbow joint.

I. MATCHING.
Match the correct term to the definition.

1. ___ clavice
2. ___ glenoid cavity
3. ___ humerus
4. ___ scapula
5. ___ sternal end

A. upper arm bone
B. collar bone
C. medial end
D. where the head of the humerus rests
E. shoulder blade

II. MULTIPLE CHOICE.
Choose the best answer.

1. The humerus is a_____.
   - ◯ long bone
   - ◯ short bone
   - ◯ wormian bone
   - ◯ irregular bone

2. The clavicle is shaped like the letter _____.
   - ◯ A
   - ◯ N
   - ◯ S
   - ◯ X

3. The upper arm bone is called the _____.
   - ◯ humerus
   - ◯ femur
   - ◯ scapula
   - ◯ clavicle

4. Which of the following is NOT related to the scapula?
   - ◯ glenoid cavity
   - ◯ acromion
   - ◯ epicondyle
   - ◯ coracoid

5. Which bone lies against the rib cage, between ribs 2 and 7?
   - ◯ clavicle
   - ◯ scapula
   - ◯ humerus
   - ◯ acromion

BONES OF THE ANTEBRACHIUM

The forearm is made up of two separate bones known as the **radius** and the **ulna**.

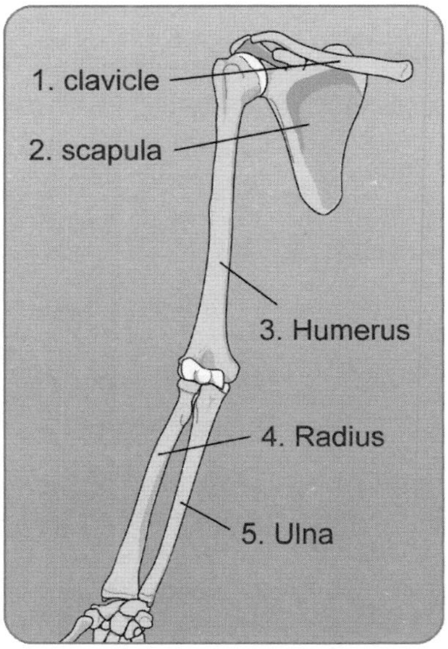

The **radius** is the bone positioned laterally of the two bones of the **antebrachium** in anatomical position. It is located on the thumb side of the forearm. It has a flattened head at the superior portion where it articulates with the humerus and the ulna. Further down, just below the **neck** on the anteromedial aspect of the **body** of the radius, is the **radial tuberosity**, a roughened bony prominence that is the insertion site for the biceps brachii muscle. At the inferior end lies the **styloid process** of the radius for articulation to the carpals. It forms a margin for the tendons of two muscles to the thumb.

The **ulna** is the longer bone of the antebrachium and is located on the medial or little finger side in anatomical position. The proximal end of the ulna articulates with the head of the radius and with the distal, or condylar, epiphysis of the radius to form the elbow joint. Although the radius also articulates with the humerus, the ulna has a much more extensive connection due to its highly specialized processes. The **olecranon** projects from the superior aspect of the ulna to form the top of the "C" shaped ulnar epiphysis. The bottom curve of the "C" is formed by the **coronoid process** of the ulna. This "C" shape forms a half-circle around the trochlea of the humerus to form the elbow joint. On the superficial aspect of the elbow joint, the olecranon forms the bony point of the elbow. Other notable landmarks of the ulna include the **trochlear notch**, the inside of the "C" shaped process that receives the trochlea of the radius; the **radial notch**, where the ulna and radius articulate at the elbow; the **head** of the ulna, which articulates with the wrist and hand; and the **styloid process** of the ulna, a bony prominence that can be palpated on the ulnar aspect of the wrist when the hand is palm down.

Take a few minutes to feel the olecranon by bending your elbow and using your fingers to find the "point." Then, putting your palm down, run your fingers along the ulnar (outer) aspect of your wrist. Do you feel the styloid process? Study the graphic of the radius and ulna. Do you see where the ulna and radius articulate (join) at the radial notch? Can you identify the head, where the radius articulates with the wrist and hand? Finally, think about the definition of **trochlea** (see the highlight box) as you flex and extend your elbow. In addition to the elbow (trochlear notch), where else might your body have pulley-shaped parts or structures? There is a fibrocartilaginous pulley in the frontal bone through which passes the tendon that controls the movement of the superior oblique eye muscle, known as the trochlea musculi obliqui, superioris oculi. You used an ocular pulley system to read this.

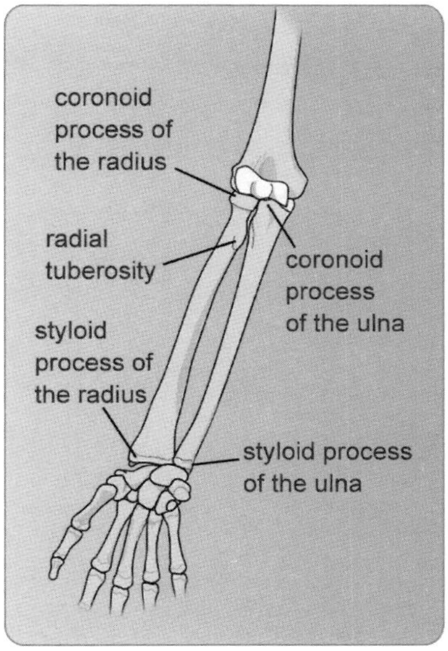

styloid process: Forms a margin for the tendons of two muscles to the thumb.

ulna: Forearm bone located on the medial side.

olecranon: The large process at the proximal end of the ulna which projects behind the articulation with the humerus and forms the bony prominence of the elbow.

trochlear notch: Pulley-shaped structure of the elbow.

radial notch: Point at which the radius and ulna articulate.

antebrachium: Term for the portion of the upper extremity between the elbow and the wrist; forearm.

coronoid process of the ulna: Anterior projection of the proximal ulnar epiphysis, along with the olecranon, the coronoid process forms a half-circle to articulate with the trochlea of the humerus.

styloid process of the radius: Projection on the lateral, distal epiphysis of the radius that articulates with the carpal bones in the wrist.

styloid process of the ulna: A bony prominence that can be palpated on the ulnar aspect of the wrist when the hand is palm down.

radial tuberosity: A roughened bony prominence just below the neck of the radius on the anteromedial aspect of the body of the radius that is the insertion site for the biceps brachii muscle.

Highlights

In anatomy and physiology, articulation is the place of junction between two different parts or objects. *Trochlea* is a general term for a pulley-shaped part or structure.

I. MATCHING.
Match the correct term to the definition.

1. ____ ulna
2. ____ tuberosity
3. ____ olecranon
4. ____ radial notch
5. ____ radius

A. thumb-side bone
B. pinky-side bone
C. point of the elbow
D. joint of ulna and radius
E. prominence

II. MULTIPLE CHOICE.
Choose the best answer.

1. The forearm bone closest to the pinky.
   - ◯ ulna
   - ◯ radius

2. The forearm bone closest to the thumb.
   - ◯ ulna
   - ◯ radius

3. Which of the following is not part of the ulna?
   - ◯ coronoid process
   - ◯ olecranon
   - ◯ malleolus
   - ◯ styloid process

4. The boney prominence of the elbow.
   - ◯ ulna
   - ◯ tuberosity
   - ◯ radial notch

5. Allows articulation with the carpals.
   - ◯ olecranon
   - ◯ styloid process

HAND AND WRIST BONES

Human wrists, hands, and fingers have incredible dexterity and range of motion. The fine motor ability of the human hand is due, in large part, to the framework of bones with their many muscle and tendon attachments.

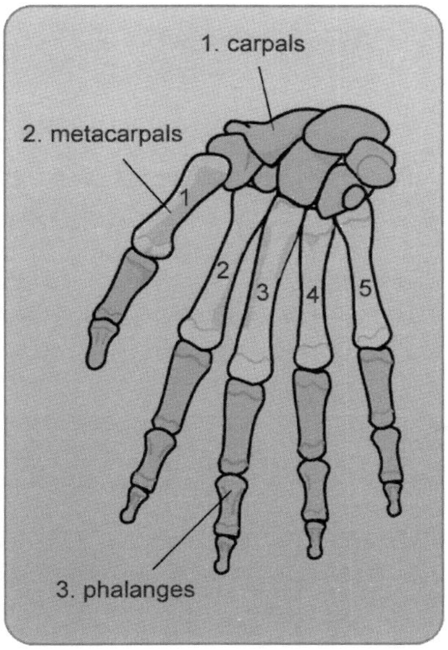

- carpals
- metacarpals
- phalanges

The **carpals** are the wrist bones. Carpals are generally made up of 2 rows of 4 bones each and are held in place by ligaments. The 8 carpal bones are the **hamate**, **scaphoid**, **trapezium**, **pisiform**, **trapezoid**, **lunate**, **triquetrum**, and **capitate** bones.

The **metacarpal bones** are the bones of the hands. They consist of 5 bones that form the structure of the hand and articulate with the carpals. These metacarpals are numbered from 1–5, with the thumb being first and the little finger fifth.

The **phalanges** articulate with the metacarpals to form the fingers. There are 5 fingers, and each has 3 phalanges (the distal, medial, and proximal phalanges), with the exception of the thumb, which has only 2.

The metacarpals and the phalanges (**phalanx** is the singular form) are not individually named apart from a descriptive numerical system. The metacarpal proximal to the ring finger, for example, is simply referred to as the 4th metacarpal. The phalanges are named by position (proximal, middle, distal) and by number. The phalanges of the ring finger are named 4th proximal phalanx, 4th middle phalanx and 4th distal phalanx respectively. This descriptive numerical system is repeated in the corresponding bones of the feet.

I. FILL IN THE BLANK.

Enter the word in the blank provided.

1. hamate ________________
2. scaphoid ________________
3. trapezium ________________
4. pisiform ________________
5. trapezoid ________________
6. lunate ________________
7. triquetrum ________________
8. capitate ________________

II. **MATCHING.**
Match the correct term to the definition.

1. ____	carpals	A.	hands
2. ____	metacarpals	B.	fingers
3. ____	phalanges	C.	wrists

HIP BONES AND FEMUR

Os Coxae

The hip bone, also called the **os coxae**, is formed by the fusion of three other bones:

- ilium
- ischium
- pubis

> **Highlights**
>
> Remember sound alike terms from medical terminology? Note the bone of the hip (spelled I-L-I-U-M). There is an organ of the gastrointestinal system called the ileum (spelled I-L-E-U-M). If you know that I-um is in the hip and E (eat)-um is next to the stomach, it can save you precious time spent looking in a medical dictionary.

The ilium articulates with the sacrum bilaterally at the posterior of the os coxae to form the pelvic girdle. If you view the pelvic girdle anteriorly, it resembles the mask of a superhero. It looks like a hat with wings sitting on top of a mask to cover the eyes. The wings are the ilium, the top of which is the **iliac crest** which is palpable as the anterior bony structure of the hips at the bottom of the waistline. The part of the mask that goes over the eyebrows is formed by the pubic bones. The lower part of the eye mask is formed by the ischium bones, and the portion between the eyes is the **symphysis pubis**, which is a fibrocartilaginous joint that joins the bones of the os coxae anteriorly. The symphysis pubis lies medially on the superior aspect of the **pubic arch**. Other notable os coxae landmarks include; the **acetabulum**, two depressions that lie on the lateral aspects of the ischium just below the inferior margin of the iliac crest. The acetabulum receives the head of the femur in the hip joint; the **obturator foramina** (singular form is foramen) are the eye holes in the mask, they are mostly occluded by a strong membrane but remain open in a specific location to transmit the obturator nerve and vascular tissue out of the pelvis.

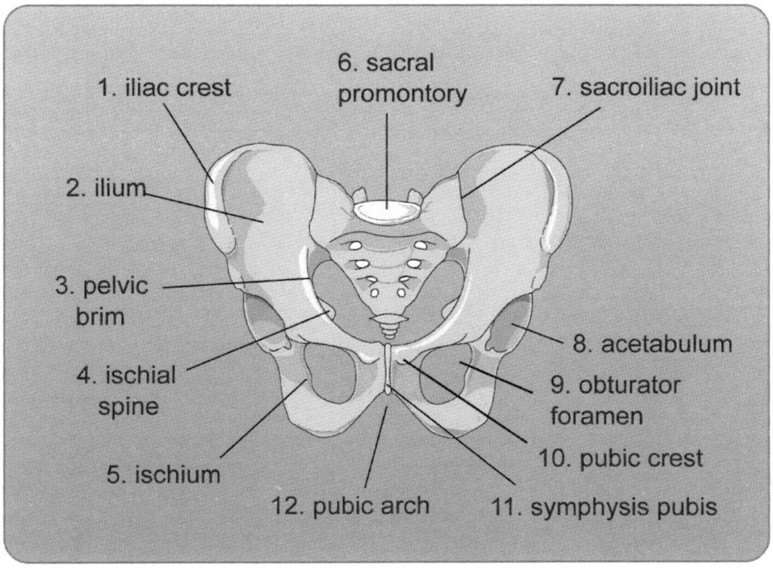

To support childbearing, the female pelvis is larger than the male pelvis. Unlike the male pelvic structure, the female pelvis has a wide subpubic arch and a forward tilt; the ischial bones are turned outwards and the symphysis pubis is shallow. In addition, the bones of the female pelvis are thin.

Femur

The **femur** (thigh bone) is the longest and strongest bone in the body. It articulates with the pelvis and two smaller leg bones to form the thigh. At its most superior point the femur consists of a **head**, **neck**, **greater trochanter**, and **lesser trochanter**. The head of the femur is knob-like and fits perfectly into the acetabulum of the os coxae (to form a ball and socket joint). The greater and lesser trochanters are bony prominences where muscles attach.

The **body** of the femur is the long diaphysis that is shaped like a rounded shaft. Situated at the most inferior end of the shaft are two lateral protrusions (to which ligaments and tendons attach) called the **medial epicondyle** and the **lateral epicondyle**. Situated between these two epicondyles is the patellar surface, where the **patella** or kneecap connects. The distal epiphysis of the femur terminates in the **medial condyle** and the **lateral condyle** which compose the femur's articular component of the knee joint.

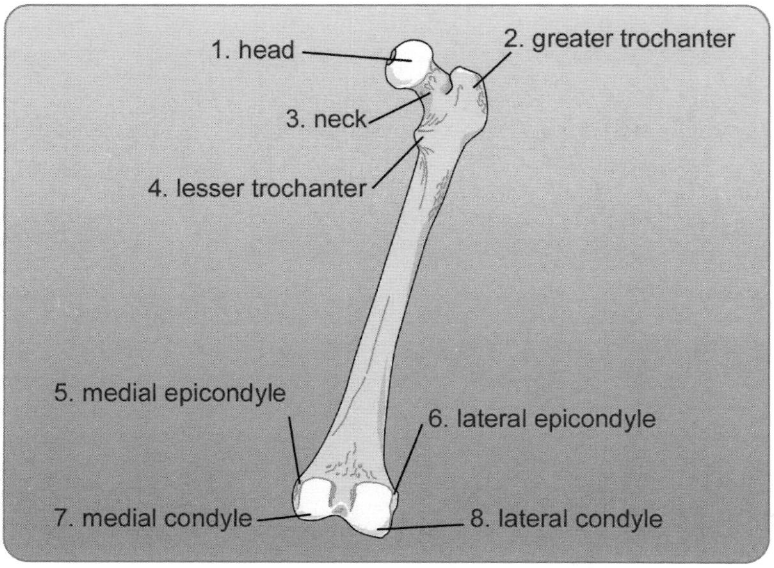

os coxae: The hip bone.

femur: The thigh bone.

ilium: Wings of the hip bone.

ischium: Lower part of the "eye mask" of the hip bone.

symphysis pubis: The portion of the hip bone between the "eyes".

greater trochanter: Bony prominence where muscles attach to the femur.

lesser trochanter: Bony prominence where muscles attach to the femur.

acetabulum: A groove in the hip bone.

medial epicondyle: A protrusion to which ligaments and tendons attach on the inferior end of the rounded shaft of the femur.

lateral epicondyle: A protrusion to which ligaments and tendons attach on the inferior end of the rounded shaft of the femur.

patella: The kneecap.

obturator foramen: The large, bilateral openings occurring on the inferior portion of the os coxae. The obtuator foramina are mostly occluded by a strong membrane but remain open in specific locations to transmit nerves and vascular tissue.

head of the femur: The knob-like proximal epiphysis of the femur that fits perfectly into the acetabulum of the os coxae to form the hip joint.

neck of the femur: The constricted portion of bone located just inferior to the head of the femur.

medial condyle of the femur: The medial, rounded prominence on the distal epiphysis of the femur that articulates with the tibia in the knee joint.

lateral condyle of the femur: The lateral, rounded prominence on the distal epiphysis of the femur that articulates with the tibia in the knee joint.

body of the femur: The elongated diaphysis of the femur.

pubic arch: The structure formed where the bilateral bones of the pubis meet at the mid-sagittal plane and are connected by the symphysis pubis.

I. MATCHING.
Match the correct term to the definition.

1. ____ femur		A. kneecap
2. ____ ischium		B. thigh bone
3. ____ acetabulum		C. the head of the femur fits into this
4. ____ os coxae		D. lower part of the "eye mask"
5. ____ patella		E. hip bone

II. MULTIPLE CHOICE.
Choose the best answer.

1. The superior portion of the femur consists of all but which ONE of the following?
   - ◯ neck
   - ◯ greater trochanter
   - ◯ lesser trochanter
   - ◯ ischium

2. Which of the following is NOT part of the hip bones?
   - ◯ os coxae
   - ◯ trochanter
   - ◯ ilium
   - ◯ symphysis pubis

3. The socket portion of the femur ball-and-socket joint.
   - ◯ acetabulum
   - ◯ patella
   - ◯ ischium
   - ◯ os coxae

4. Protrusions at the inferior end of the femur.
   - ◯ medial and lateral trochanters
   - ◯ medial and lateral epicondyles
   - ◯ greater and lesser trochanters
   - ◯ greater and lesser epicondyles

5. Thigh bone.
   - ◯ os coxae
   - ◯ patella
   - ◯ femur

LOWER LEG AND FOOT BONES

The lower legs, ankle, feet, and toes are the last part of the lower extremities. Like the hands and fingers, there are many small bones that allow mobility and flexibility. Running, jumping, climbing, and walking are made possible by the amazing lower extremity bone structure.

Tibia

The **tibia** is the largest of the two lower leg bones and the second longest bone in the human body. It articulates with the femur to form the knee joint and is located on the medial (or big toe) side of the leg. At the knee joint the epiphysis of the tibia widens to form a platform like articular surface. The top of the platform is divided into the **lateral condyle** and **medial condyle** of the tibia. These condyles are covered with pads of articular cartilage called meniscus that will be further reviewed later with joints. The tibia has a sharp, bony ridge that runs lengthwise down the anterior portion of its triangular shaft to form the edge of the shinbone (which can be felt through the skin on the front of the leg). Superiorly the sharp edge of the shinbone terminates at a bony prominence called the **tibial tuberosity** that is easily palpable below the patella and serves as an attachment for the patellar ligament. The most distal point on the medial side of the tibia has a bony extension that is called the **medial malleolus** (or ankle bone). This protrudes sharply and can be felt on the inner side of the ankle. The tibia is the weight-bearing bone of the lower leg.

Fibula

The **fibula** is a long, skinny lower leg bone that looks rather fragile. It is situated on the lateral (or little toe) side of the leg. It is not a weight-bearing bone. The **head** of the fibula occurs at its superior end and forms the lateral part of the knee joint. It is palpable below the knee and directly lateral to the tibial tuberosity. At the distal epiphysis the **lateral malleolus** forms and protects the lateral portion of the ankle.

Tarsals, Metatarsals, and Phalanges

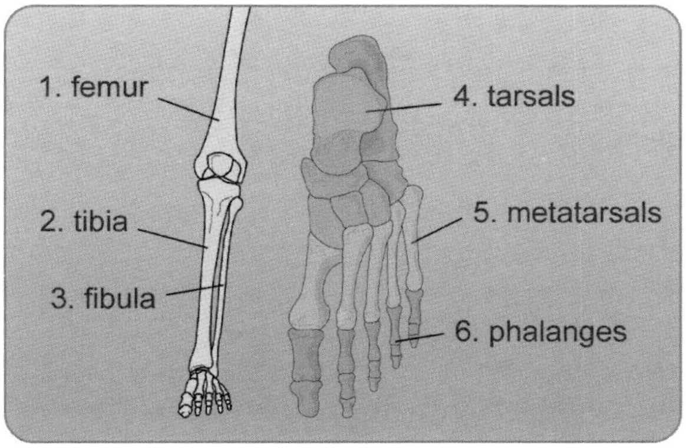

The **tarsals** are ankle bones and, along with the other bones in the foot (the metatarsals and phalanges), support weight and act as shock absorbers for the body. There are 7 tarsal bones in each foot: the **talus**, **calcaneus**, **cuboid**, **navicular**, and **medial**, **intermediate**, and **lateral cuneiform**. The talus articulates with the tibia and fibula to bear weight from the legs. The medial malleolus (on the tibia) and the lateral malleolus (on the fibula) protect the talus on both sides of the ankle.

The **metatarsals** are the bones of the feet that form the arches. The arches are designed to flatten and spread out during weight bearing activity. There are 5 metatarsals in each foot. These correspond to the metacarpals in the hand and are similarly numbered.

The **phalanges** or toes lie distal to the metatarsals. There are 14 phalanges per foot-2 in the great toe, or **hallux**, and 3 each in the remaining toes. The separations between the phalanges are identified as follows: the distal phalanx (tip of the toe), the middle phalanx, (in the middle) and the proximal phalanx (nearest the point of connection to the metatarsals). Notice that the medical term for toes is the same as for fingers.

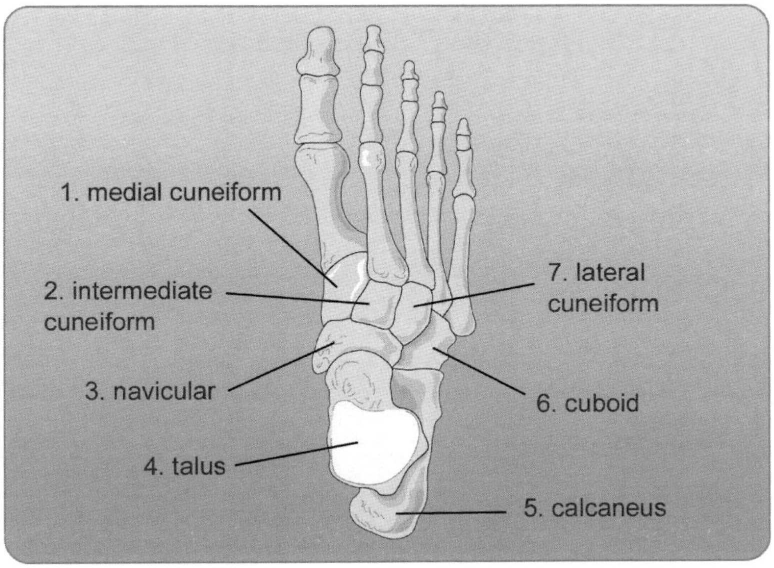

I. MATCHING.
Match the correct term to the definition.

1. ____ metatarsals
2. ____ tarsals
3. ____ phalanges
4. ____ medial and lateral malleolus
5. ____ tibia

A. ankle bone(s)
B. feet bones
C. larger lower leg bone
D. toes
E. protects the ankle

II. MULTIPLE CHOICE.
Choose the best answer.

1. How many phalanges are in the foot?
   - ◯ 2
   - ◯ 6
   - ◯ 14
   - ◯ 9

2. The more fragile of the lower leg bones.
   - ◯ tibia
   - ◯ fibula

3. The stronger and bigger of the lower leg bones.
   - ◯ tibia
   - ◯ fibula

4. Which is not a tarsal bone?
   - ◯ 2nd cuneiform
   - ◯ talus
   - ◯ navicular
   - ◯ epicondyle

5. The primary weight-bearing bone of the leg.
   - ◯ tibia
   - ◯ fibula

UNIT 4

The Muscular System

THE MUSCULAR SYSTEM - INTRODUCTION

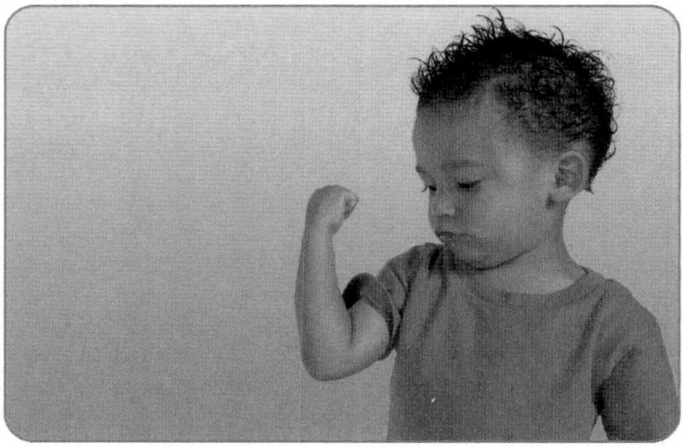

The joints and skeletal system give the body the framework for movement and mobility, but skeletal muscle provides the power. The muscles of the heart contract without voluntary control to deliver nutrient-rich blood to the tissues and cells of the body. The muscles of the digestive tract keep food products and waste moving. A muscle is an organ that contracts to produce movement. Muscle contraction in conjunction with skeletal flexibility makes movement possible in human beings. Without muscles there would be no voluntary movement of the body whatsoever and many internal systems and organs would be unable to function.

In our examination of the muscular system we will first discuss muscle tissue function and types. We will then take a closer look at each muscle type, and finally, we will identify many of the skeletal muscles that power the locomotion of the human body.

FUNCTION AND TYPES

Muscle tissue has the following functions:

Movement: Muscles that attach to the human skeleton allow us to walk, run, jump, and otherwise voluntarily move about. Muscles imbedded in the walls of many visceral organs produce movement by involuntarily contracting and relaxing, thereby squeezing body fluids and other substances through various organs (e.g., the esophagus, stomach, intestines, blood vessels, etc.).

Posture: In order for the body to maintain an erect posture or a sitting position, certain muscles must contract or remain contracted.

Stabilization of joints: As discussed briefly in the skeletal system, muscles and ligaments are vital to joint stabilization and allow for smooth movement when bending or twisting.

Body temperature maintenance: When muscles contract, they produce heat. Even when the body is at rest, muscles are constantly contracting and producing heat which plays a role in maintaining a normal body temperature of 98.6 degrees Fahrenheit.

There are three different types of muscle tissue found throughout the human body:

Skeletal muscle: The primary muscle used to allow voluntary movement of the body; they are usually attached to the skeleton by tendons.

Smooth muscle: The muscle that lines the walls of internal organs. This muscle is usually short in its strands and allows for the movement of body fluids and waste through the internal systems.

Cardiac muscle: This type of muscle is found only in the heart.

Muscles receive their instructions (stimuli) for movement from the nerves. The nerves contain motor fibers that transmit the impulses from the brain, spinal cord, and sensory fibers for proprioception (perception of the stimuli) to the muscles and connecting tissues. This is the case for both voluntary and involuntary muscle contraction.

I. MATCHING.
Match the correct muscle functions and types to the definition.

1. ____ movement
2. ____ posture
3. ____ stabilization of joints
4. ____ body temperature maintenance
5. ____ skeletal muscle
6. ____ smooth muscle
7. ____ cardiac muscle

A. Muscle found only in the heart
B. When muscles contract and produce heat
C. Primary muscles allowing voluntary movement of the body
D. Allow human skeleton movement
E. Allow for smooth movement when bending or twisting joints
F. Maintain a sitting position
G. Muscles lining the walls of internal organs

SKELETAL MUSCLE

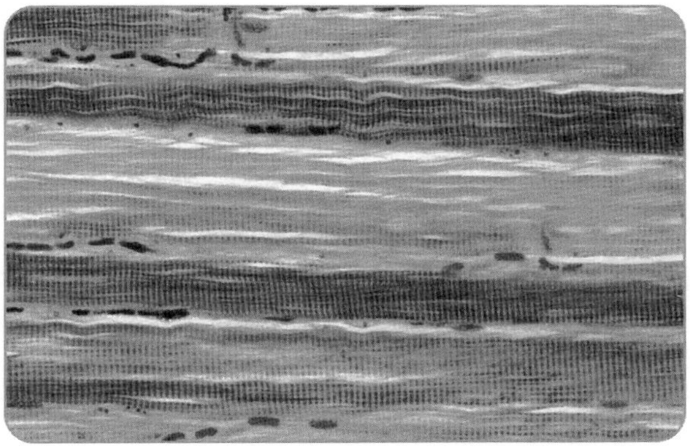

Skeletal muscles are voluntary muscles that connect to the bones of the skeleton. They are termed voluntary because in a normal functioning body, skeletal muscles move when we direct them to move. The cells of skeletal muscle tissue are usually large and have more than one nucleus. Because of their length and thin appearance, these muscle cells are often referred to as **muscle fibers** (and not cells). Skeletal muscles come in varying shapes and sizes and are called "striated" because of their striped (or band-like) appearance. Although cardiac muscle also appears striped, striated is normally a synonym for voluntary skeletal muscle.

Each muscle is made up of muscle fibers, blood vessels, connective tissue, and nerves. Skeletal muscle fibers are long and thin, often resembling a bunch of sticks that have been grouped together. Each muscle is supplied by at least one nerve, one artery, and (one or more) vein near the center or middle of the muscle.

Most skeletal muscles extend from one bone to another, crossing over at least one joint. When a skeletal muscle crosses a joint and contracts, one bone moves and the other bone remains stationary. The less moveable attachment of a muscle is called the **origin**. The more moveable attachment of a muscle is called the **insertion**. The insertion is always pulled towards the origin.

The less moveable attachment of a muscle is called the origin. The more moveable attachment of a muscle is called the insertion.

Muscles attach to their origins or insertions via connective tissue that is strong and fibrous. There are two basic types of attachments: direct (fleshy) attachments and indirect attachments. Direct attachments have such short strands of connective tissue that muscles appear to be directly connected to the bone. Indirect attachments are the opposite, with long strands of connective tissue extending far beyond the muscle. These long strands form either a rope-like structure called a **tendon**, or a flat tissue sheet called an **aponeurosis**, which connects to the bone. Bones generally have raised markings (tubercles, trochanters, crests) to which tendons attach. Most muscles attach by tendons rather than aponeuroses.

Highlights

Bone markings such as tubercles, trochanters, and crests are the places on bone where muscles attach with rope-like tendons. Less commonly, muscles attach with a flat tissue sheet called an aponeurosis.

Skeletal muscles are under our direct control. We decide if we want to move an arm or leg, tap our fingers on the table, run, bend, lift, or walk somewhere. Skeletal muscles contract and relax very quickly and are subject to fatigue, depending upon how often or how long they are in use.

origin: The less movable attachment of a muscle.

insertion: The more movable attachment of a muscle.

direct (fleshy) attachments: Short strands of connective tissue that make muscles appear as if they are directly connected to the bone.

indirect attachments: Long strands of connective tissue extending beyond the muscle.

tendon: A rope-like structure that binds muscles to bone.

aponeurosis: A flat tissue sheet that connects muscle to bone.

SMOOTH MUSCLE

Smooth muscles are found in the internal organs and inside blood vessels. Smooth muscles are involuntary: they contract with stimuli from the nervous system, but without conscious thought. Spindle-like (i.e., length greater than width) and fragile in appearance, smooth muscle cells have a single nucleus. Smooth muscle tissue has no striations. Functions such as blood flow, digestion, and pupillary response are due to smooth muscle contractions.

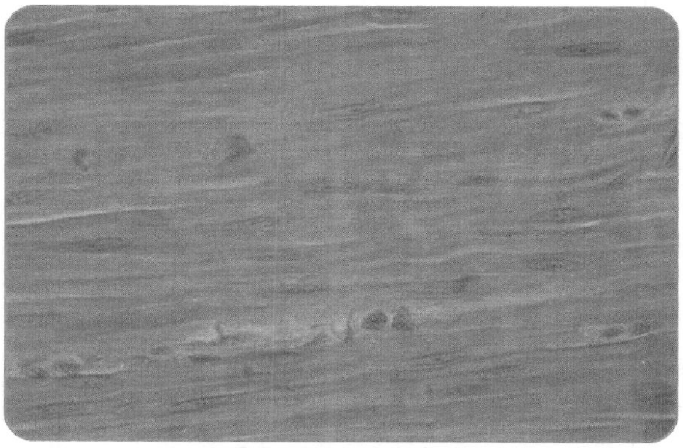

Smooth muscle occupies six major location sites:

- walls of the circulatory vessels
- digestive tubes
- urinary organs
- reproductive organs
- respiratory tubes
- inside the eye

Smooth muscle contraction is slow, sustained, and very resistant to fatigue.

In the hollow visceral organs (such as the digestive tubes), muscle fibers are often grouped into two sheets of smooth muscle. The muscle fibers of the longitudinal layer run parallel to the length of the organ. The muscles of the circular layer wrap around the circumference of the organ. During contraction, the longitudinal layer contracts or shortens the length of the organ, and the circular layer contracts or constricts the hollow organ. These waves of contraction and relaxation cause substances (in the case of the digestive tubes, food, and liquids) to be propelled through these tubes. This process of propelling substances through hollow visceral organs is called **peristalsis**.

Smooth muscle contraction is slow, sustained, and very resistant to fatigue. Smooth muscle has a slower contraction rate (about 30 times longer than skeletal muscle) but is required to hold such contractions much longer than skeletal muscle. This is important because in many of the internal organs mentioned above, smooth muscle needs to maintain a constant level of contraction.

I. MULTIPLE CHOICE.
Choose the best answer.

1. Smooth muscles are very _____.
   - ◯ easily tired
   - ◯ weak
   - ◯ resistant to fatigue
   - ◯ wide

2. Smooth muscle tissue has no _____.
   - ◯ strength
   - ◯ fibers
   - ◯ tubes
   - ◯ striations

3. Other than in circulatory vessels, smooth muscles can be found in _____.
   - ◯ the legs
   - ◯ the eye
   - ◯ the brain
   - ◯ the back

4. The process of propelling substances through hollow visceral organs is called _____.
   - ◯ peristalsis
   - ◯ hyperstalsis
   - ◯ contraction
   - ◯ expansion

5. Smooth muscles are spindle-like, which means they have _____.
   - ◯ spindled fibers
   - ◯ faster contractions
   - ◯ greater width than length
   - ◯ greater length than width

CARDIAC MUSCLE

Cardiac muscle is the third type of muscle found in the human body and forms the majority of the walls of the heart. It is similar in appearance to skeletal muscle with respect to its striated appearance, but it has a single-cell nucleus. This is an involuntary muscle and direct stimuli from the central nervous system (CNS) is not required for contraction. However, the CNS does modify (not initiate) contraction of cardiac muscle.

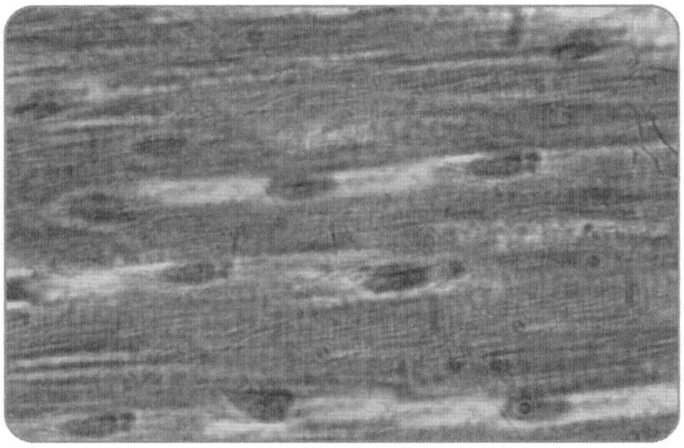

NAMING MUSCLES

The names of muscles are descriptive, as are the names of tendons. Therefore, it will help you to learn and remember them if you have an understanding of how they are named. There are seven (7) primary ways the names assigned to muscles are derived.

Term	Definition	Examples
Shape	Muscle names are often derived from the actual physical shape of the muscle itself or a defining physical characteristic, such as the number of heads that it has.	**Rhomboideus:** A muscle of the back that is shaped like a rhomboid. **Triangularis:** A muscle of the face that is triangular in shape. **Triceps:** A muscle with three (tri-) heads. **Biceps:** A muscle with two (bi-) heads.
Location	A muscle may be named for its actual location within the body relative to other body structures.	**Pectoralis:** Chest muscle located within the pectoral girdle. **Intercostal:** Muscle located between ribs (intercostal literally means between ribs). **Abdominis:** Located in the abdominal area.
Attachment	Many muscles are named for the bones to which they are attached. The muscle name may combine more than one name when more than one bone is involved.	**Zygomaticus:** Attached to the zygoma (bone of the face). **Sternocleidomastoid:** Attached to the sternum, clavicle, and mastoid process of the skull.

Size	The actual size of the muscle or its relative size to a similar muscle may be used in naming a muscle.	**Maximus or Major:** Both of these terms mean larger or largest. **Minimus or Minor:** Meaning smaller or smallest. **Longus:** Meaning long. **Brevis:** Meaning short.
Orientation of fibers	This is the direction that the individual fibers of a muscle extend.	**Oblique:** In a slanting or inclined direction. **Rectus:** Meaning straight. **Transverse:** Meaning across or placed crosswise.
Relative position	These delineations contain basic directional planes and are used on similar muscles to designate a slightly different orientation. Often a "medial" will have a corresponding "lateral"; likewise, an "internal" will have a corresponding "external."	**Lateral:** Something that is further from the midpoint or to the side. **Medial:** Something closer to the middle or the midline. **Internal:** Situated or occurring within or on the inside. **External:** Situated or occurring on the outside.
Function	Muscles are responsible for movement. However, there are several different types of movements, and muscles are often classified according to the actual movement that they produce.	**Adductor:** Movement to draw toward a medial plane. **Extensor:** General term for a muscle that extends a joint. **Flexor:** General term for a muscle that flexes a joint. **Levator:** A muscle that elevates or lifts an organ or structure.

Skeletal muscles and bones are so integral to each other in function that they are often referred to as the musculoskeletal system. We have already introduced the bones of the skeleton. The muscles and bones of the body are so interrelated; in fact, they depend upon each other to carry out their individual functions. There are over 600 skeletal muscles in the human body.

I. MATCHING.
Match the muscle to the descriptive term that gives it its name.

1. ____ biceps
2. ____ abdominis
3. ____ zygomaticus
4. ____ longus
5. ____ rectus
6. ____ internal
7. ____ levator

A. orientation of fibers
B. shape
C. location
D. attachment
E. size
F. function
G. relative position

MUSCLES OF THE FACE AND HEAD

The following figures are provided as a visual guide. Concentrate on body placement of the various muscle groups. We will start at the head and work our way down.

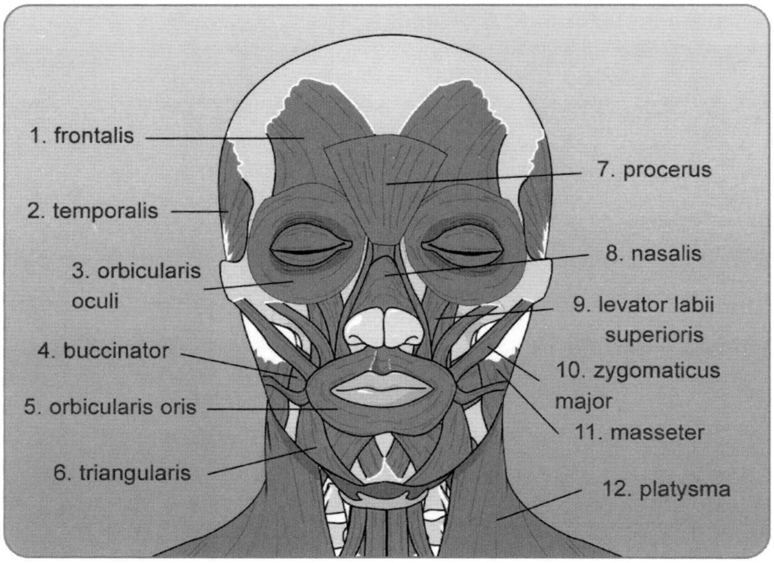

I. FILL IN THE BLANK.

In the blanks provided below, refer to the above diagram and enter the term corresponding to the following numbers. Use the word(s) in the box to fill in the blanks.

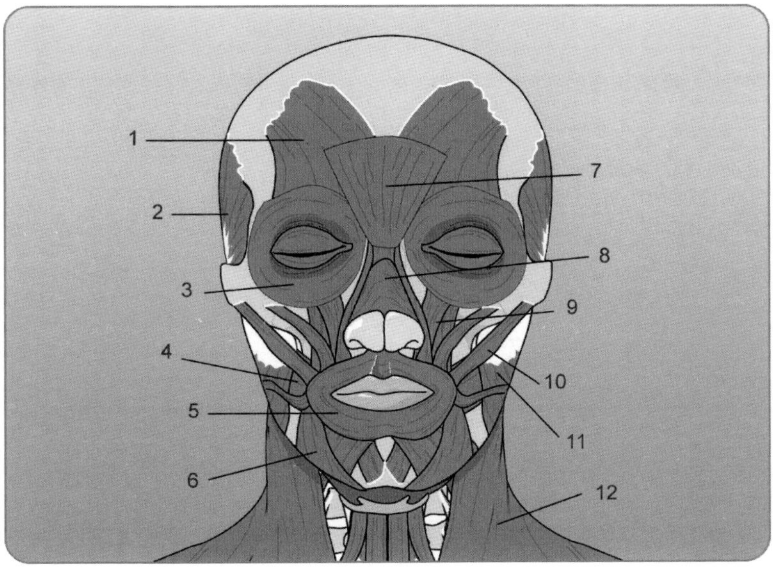

1. ____________
2. ____________
3. ____________
4. ____________
5. ____________
6. ____________
7. ____________
8. ____________
9. ____________
10. ____________
11. ____________
12. ____________

zygomaticus major
buccinator
orbicularis oculi
levator labii superioris
orbicularis oris
masseter
frontalis
platysma
procerus
temporalis
nasalis
triangularis

II. MULTIPLE CHOICE.
Choose the best answer.

1. The muscle surrounding the eye.
   - ◯ frontalis
   - ◯ orbicularis oris
   - ◯ orbicularis oculi
   - ◯ masseter

2. Lower jaw muscle in the shape of a triangle.
   - ◯ triangularis
   - ◯ temporalis
   - ◯ platysma
   - ◯ frontalis

3. Muscle located above the eye.
   - ◯ buccinator
   - ◯ procerus
   - ◯ frontalis
   - ◯ temporalis

4. Muscle that runs from the lower jaw down the neck.
   - ◯ platysma
   - ◯ levator labii superioris
   - ◯ zygomaticus major
   - ◯ triangularis

5. Cheek muscle.
   - ◯ platysma
   - ◯ temporalis
   - ◯ masseter
   - ◯ buccinator

6. Muscle found in the nose.
   - ◯ procerus
   - ◯ nasalis
   - ◯ platysma
   - ◯ zygomaticus major

7. A muscle that lifts and is above the lips.
   - ◯ nasalis
   - ◯ buccinator
   - ◯ orbicularis oris
   - ◯ levator labii superioris

8. Muscle surrounding the mouth.
   - ◯ orbicularis oris
   - ◯ orbicularis oral
   - ◯ orbicularis oculi
   - ◯ triangularis

9. Muscle found in the lower jaw.
   - ◯ maseter
   - ◯ masseter
   - ◯ massetter
   - ◯ massiter

10. The larger of the zygomaticus muscles.
    - ◯ lesser zygomatic
    - ◯ greater zygoma
    - ◯ zygomaticus major
    - ◯ platysma

11. Muscle located on the side of the head, just above both ears.
    - ◯ frontalis
    - ◯ temporalis
    - ◯ procerus
    - ◯ nasalis

12. Muscle located on the forehead; it creates the "worry lines" or wrinkling of the brow associated with frowning.
    - ◯ procerus
    - ◯ corugator
    - ◯ corrugater
    - ◯ currogator

MUSCLES OF FACIAL EXPRESSION AND MASTICATION

You will notice that some of the muscles included in these activities do not appear in the image. This is because these muscles are quite deep in relation to the facial bones.

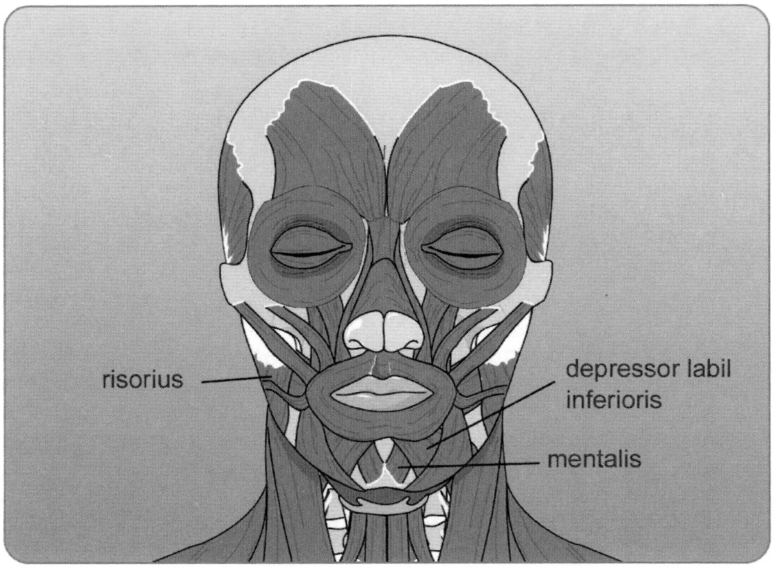

lateral pterygold: This is a muscle of mastication. It originates on the pterygoid process of the sphenoid bone. It moves the mandible and limits sideways jaw movement.

medial pterygold: Also a muscle of mastication. Both pterygoid muscles are on the inside of the mandible. The medial pterygoid elevates the jaw and provides sideways jaw movement.

risorius: The risorius originates on the side of the face and inserts on the orbicularis oris muscle. It draws the angle of the mouth laterally (to the side) and enables the human being to smile.

mentalis: The mentalis muscle originates on the chin and goes into the orbicularis oris muscle. It elevates and protrudes the lower lip. Basically it allows for pouting.

depressor labil inferioris: This muscle also originates on the mandible and inserts on to the orbicularis muscle. It depresses the bottom lip. (Names: depressor=depress, labii=lips, inferioris=below or bottom)

depressor anguli oris: This muscle originates on the lower part of the mandible. It pulls down the angle of the mouth. (Names: depressor=depress, anguli=angle, oris=mouth)

I. **SPELLING.**
Determine if the following words are spelled correctly. If the spelling is correct, leave the word as it has already been entered. If the spelling is incorrect, provide the correct spelling.

1. mentalis ____________________
2. depressor ____________________
3. terygoid ____________________
4. labi ____________________
5. risorius ____________________
6. angguli ____________________
7. inferioris ____________________

MUSCLES OF THE NECK

Muscles of the neck are used to support and move the head. Many of them are named based on the skeletal components they are associated with. Examples include: sternoceidomastoid, attaches at the sternum and the mastoid process of the temporal bone; sternohyoid, attaches at the sternum and the hyoid bone.

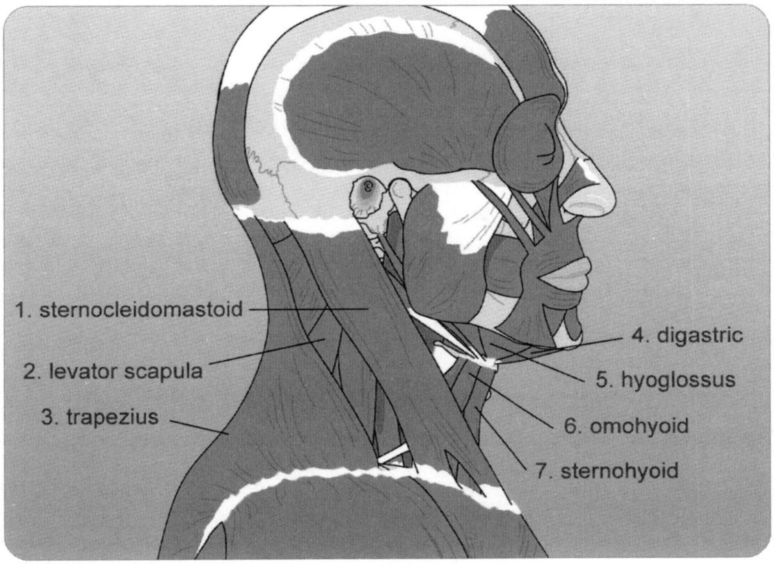

I. FILL IN THE BLANK.

In the blanks provided below, refer to the above image, and enter the term corresponding to the following numbers. Use the word(s) in the box to fill in the blanks.

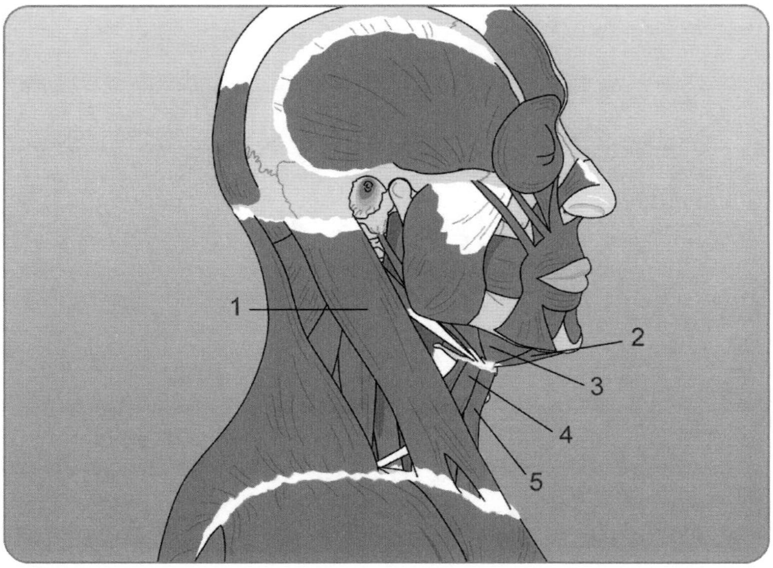

1. ________________
2. ________________
3. ________________
4. ________________
5. ________________
6. ________________
7. ________________

hyoglossus
sternohyoid
levator scapula
digastric
sternocleidomastoid
trapezius
omohyoid

MUSCLES OF THE ANTERIOR TORSO

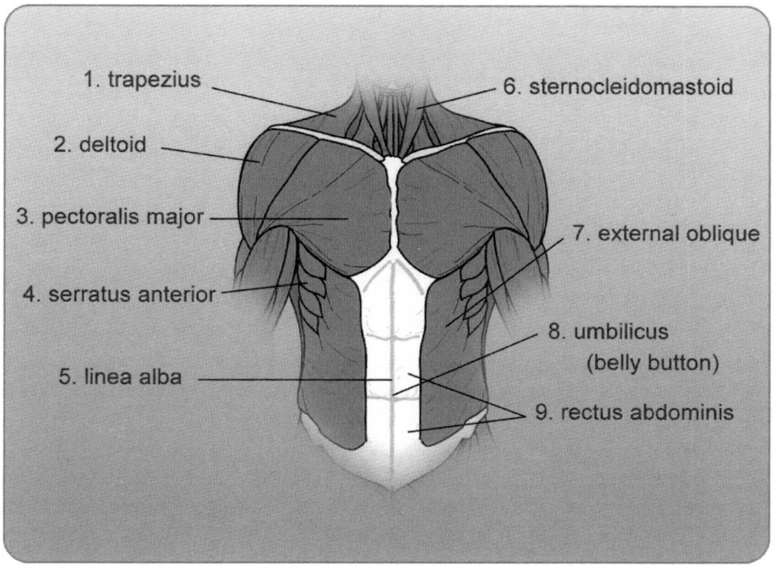

The pectoralis major are the bilateral pair of muscles that lie on the superior aspect of the torso, or chest. These muscles have three sub-portions named for their attachment locations: clavicular, sternocostal, and abdominal. The pectoralis major is the most powerful flexor of the shouder joint. The comparatively diminutive pectoralis minor (not depicted in the figure) lie deep and are completely covered by the pectoralis major.

The muscles of the abdomen that lie inferior to the pectoralis major (with the exception of the serratus anterior) are functionally responsible for the abdominal press, drawing the ribcage toward the pelvis. Beginning on the midsagittal plane, the linea alba and umbilicus are labeled in the figure on this page. These structures are not muscles but they represent significant landmarks for the muscles that surround them. Linea alba literally means "white line" and is the term for the tendinous line down the middle of the anterior abdominal wall directly between the two rectus abdominis muscles. The rectus abdominis are transversely crossed by tendinous intersections which create the "six pack" look in some physically fit individuals. Lateral to the rectus abdominis on both sides are the abdominal obliques. There are three layers of obliques, all of which have muscle fibers oriented in different directions to provide stability in support of the trunk and to power movement in multiple directions. The three layers of obliques, (superficial to deep: external, internal, and tranverse) as well as the rectus abdominis, are each individually covered by a sheath of tendinous connective tissue. Each of the individual sheaths converge and become continuous at the linea alba. The umbilicus, in the middle of the linea alba, as annotated, is the belly button.

The muscles and terms found on the figure are for the superficial muscles of the torso only. There are many additional muscles located in this region of the body, like the internal obliques and the transversus abdiminus mentioned before, that lie deep to the external obliques. If you come across a term that is not delineated above, look in your medical dictionary to find it. The trapezius and sternocleidomastoid muscles are muscles of the neck as shown on the previous page. They are depicted here for reference only.

I. FILL IN THE BLANK.

Refer to the figure below and use the word(s) in the box to fill in the blanks.

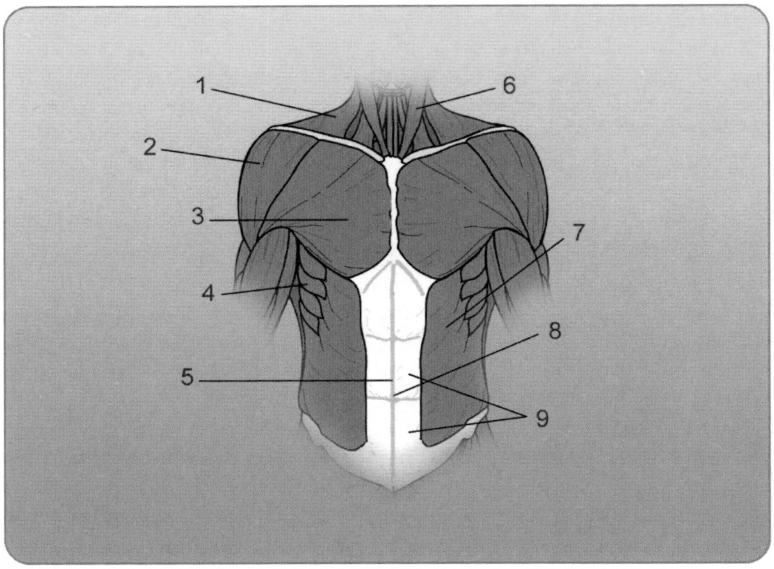

1. ____________
2. ____________
3. ____________
4. ____________
5. ____________
6. ____________
7. ____________
8. ____________
9. ____________

sternocleidomastoid
rectus abdominis
serratus anterior
pectoralis major
external oblique
deltoid
umbilicus (belly button)
linea alba
trapezius

MUSCLES OF THE POSTERIOR TORSO

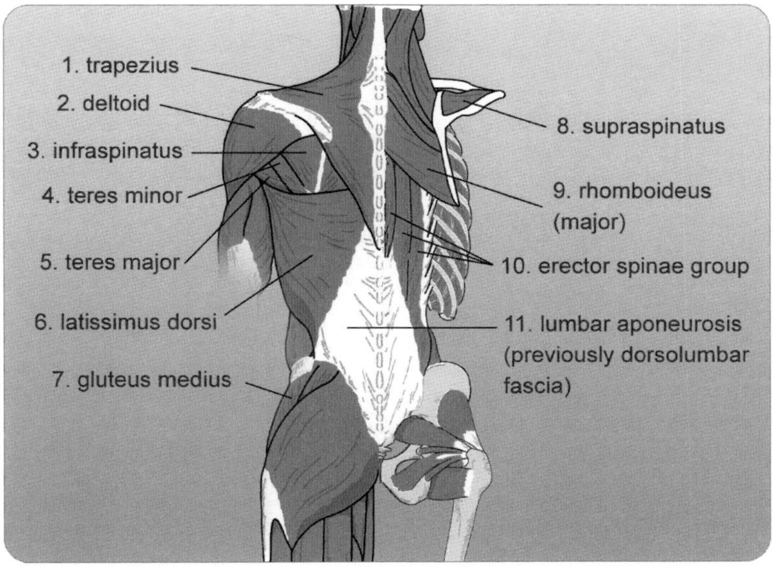

As with the earlier figures, these are not all the muscles of the back. These are the superficial ones, and they are the most commonly dictated terms. Notice the term *lumbar aponeurosis*. This is not a muscle. An aponeurosis, as previously stated, is a white, flattened tendinous expansion, serving mainly to connect a muscle with the parts that it moves.

The **trapezius** is so named for its trapezoidal shape when viewing both sides of the pair. Its origins begin at the external protuberance of the occipital bone and continue down to the spinous processes of each of the thoracic vertebrae. The belly of the muscle extends laterally to attach to the spine and acromion of the scapula and the clavicle. It functions in elevating the shoulder joint toward the head, like a shrugging gesture, and bringing the scapulae dorsally and toward the midline, or adduction.

The trapezius acts powerfully on the scapula, as does the **rhomboideus major** and minor and the levator scapulae (not depicted in the figure). The **rhomboid** muscles retract, rotate, fix, and elevate the scapula. The **teres major** and the large **latissimus dorsi** attach to the humerus to act on the shoulder joint in the adduction (movement toward the midline) of the arm.

Two groups of muscles that require further mention here are the erector spinae muscles and the muscles that comprise the rotator cuff.

Three distinct muscles make up the **erector spinae** group. From medial to lateral they are named **spinalis**, **longissimus**, and **iliocostalis**. This muscle group has an extensive tendinous origin at the posterior aspect of the sacrum and spans the vertical length of the spine to attach at the external protuberance of the occipital bone and the mastoid process of the temporal bone. Having numerous tendinous attachments to the spinous processes of the vertebrae all along vertebral column, these muscles extend the spine and are essential for maintaining upright posture for bipedal motion.

I. FILL IN THE BLANK.

In the blanks provided below, refer to the figure and enter the term that corresponds to the following numbers. Use the word(s) in the box to fill in the blanks.

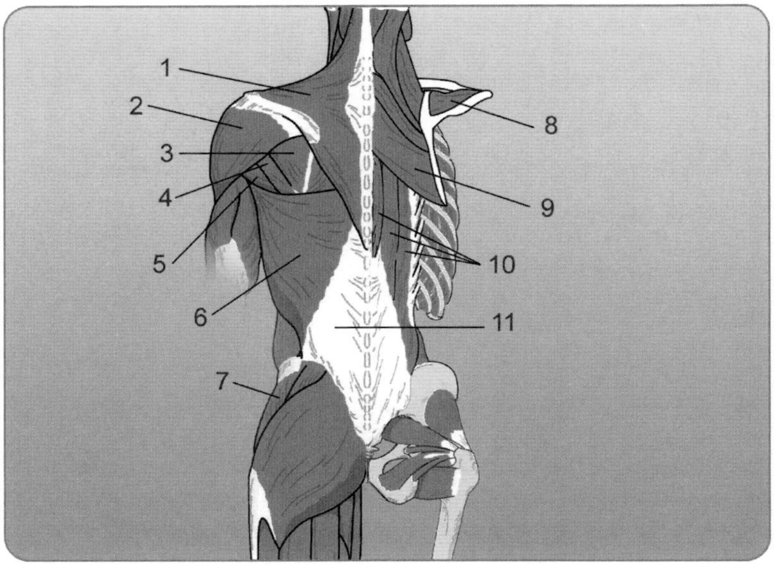

1. ________________
2. ________________
3. ________________
4. ________________
5. ________________
6. ________________
7. ________________
8. ________________
9. ________________
10. ________________
11. ________________

erector spinae group
teres major
lumbar aponeurosis
infraspinatus
gluteus medius
trapezius
supraspinatus
teres minor
latissimus dorsi
deltoid
rhomboideus (major)

MUSCLES OF THE SHOULDER GIRDLE

Most of the muscles around the shoulder originate in the spine or the head. We discussed the trapezius muscle with the muscles of the back, which raises or lowers the shoulders and is what allows us to "shrug" our shoulders. We also discussed a number of muscles that act on the scapula, an essential component of the shoulder girdle. Finally, the serratus anterior and pectoralis minor muscles pull the shoulder girdle down and forward. They were reviewed with the muscles of the anterior chest.

Highlights

A rotator cuff tear happens when the ligaments around the humerus are torn away from the bone.

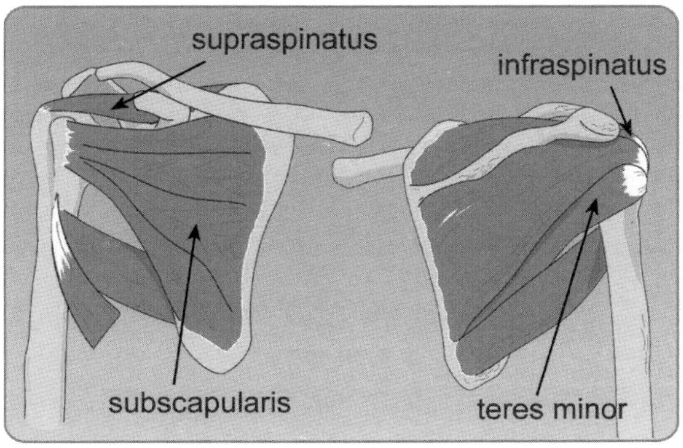

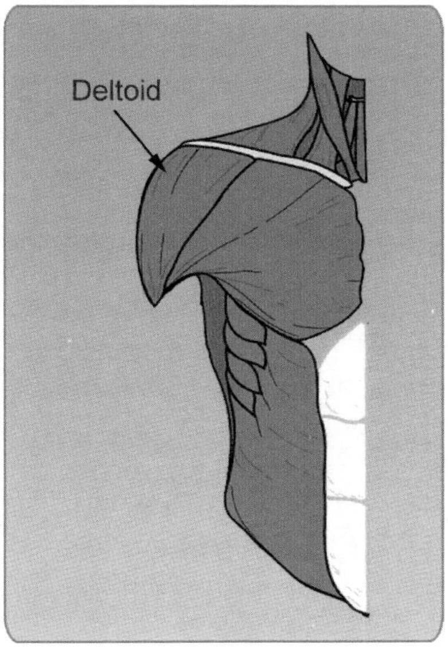

The deep muscles of the shoulder girdle are four muscles that comprise what is commonly called the **rotator cuff**: **supraspinatus**, **infraspinatus**, **subscapularis**, and **teres minor**. Each of these muscles originate on the scapula. They insert thier thick, flat tendons on the greater and lesser tuberosities of the humerus, strengthening the glenohumeral joint capsule and forming a "cuff" around the shoulder joint. Functionally, they are not the primary movers of the joint though they do contribute to some rotational motion. Their primary function is to stabilize and strengthen the joint against dislocation. The image above shows the four muscles and how their tendons surround the head of the humerus.

The superficial muscle of the shoulder is the **deltoid** muscle. It abducts and assists with flexion and extension of the upper arm and is responsible for powering the majority of the movements of the shoulder joint.

MUSCLES OF THE ARM

The deep muscles of the brachium are depicted in the first figure. The **coracobrachialis** is so named for its origin on the coracoid process of the scapula and its insertion and action on the brachium (upper arm). The **brachialis** flexes the elbow joint and lies deep to the inferior portion of the biceps brachii, just superior to the elbow joint.

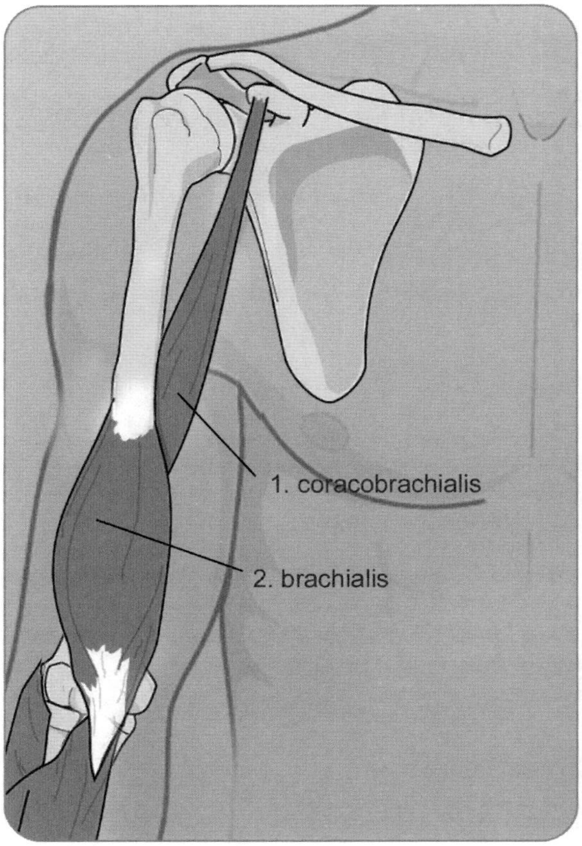

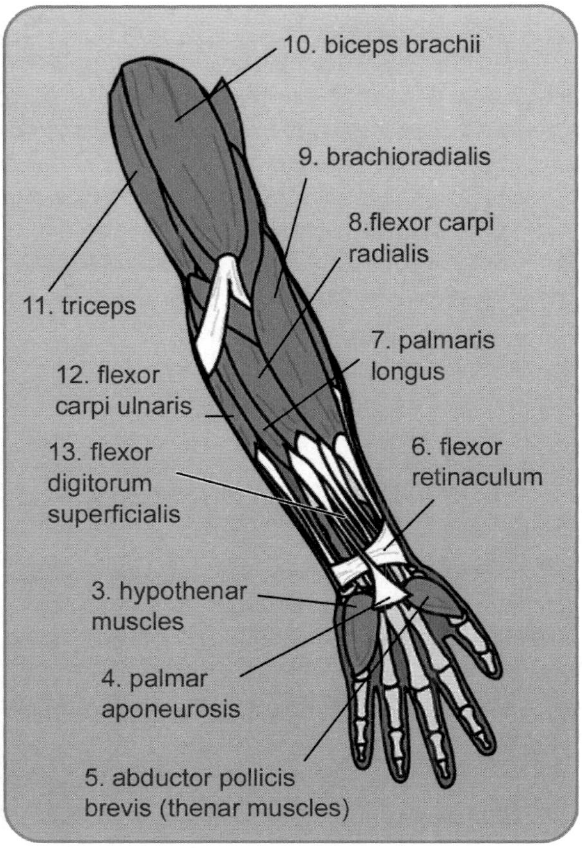

"Biceps", meaning two heads, is the origin for the name of the largest anterior muscle of the brachium, the **biceps brachii**. **Triceps brachii**, meaning – you guessed it – three heads, is the antagonist to the biceps located on the posterior of the brachium. The biceps is responsible for flexion of the elbow joint, conversely, the triceps extends the elbow joint.

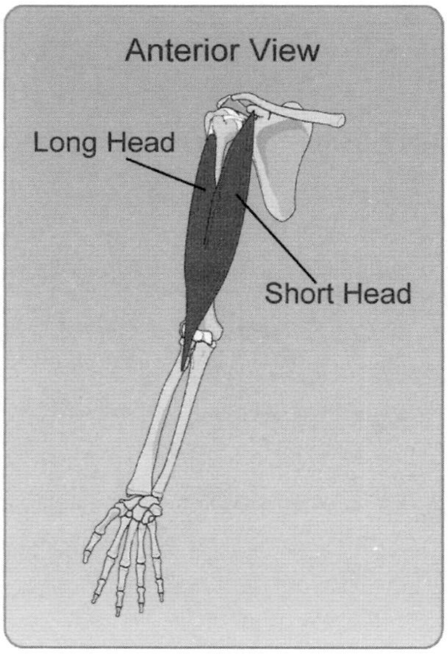

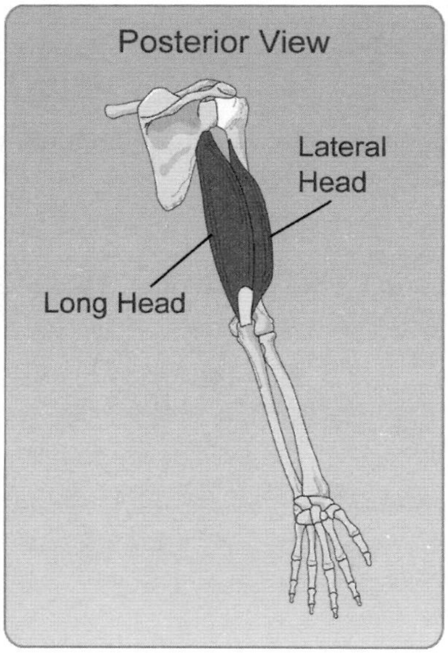

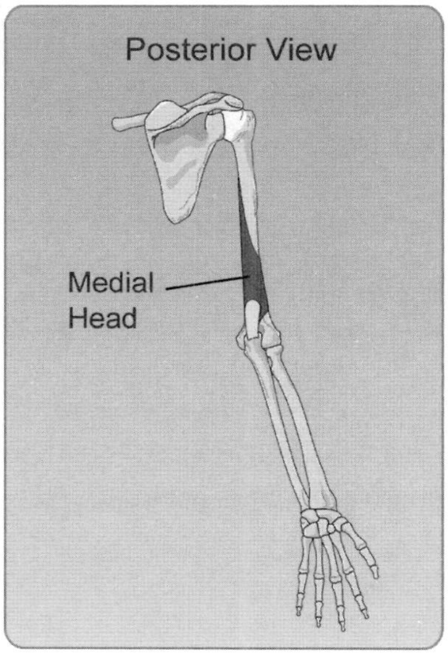

Muscles of the Antebrachium and Hand

There are three main types of muscles in the antebrachium based on function: flexors, extensors, and rotators.

The flexors, in anatomical position (palms up), occur on the anterior of the forearm and act to flex the carpal joint and the digits. Think of flexors clenching your fist and bringing your fingers closer to your biceps. We will look at six flexors, named as follows: **flexor carpi ulnaris, flexor carpi radialis, flexor pollicis longus, flexor digitorum profundus (deep digital flexor), flexor digitorum superficialis (superficial digital flexor)**, and **palmaris longus**.

That is a mouthful! Luckily you do not need to memorize these muscles' individual locations for this course, but you will want to be able to recognize that they are antebrachial flexors. To help you do this, let's break down the clues in the names of these muscles. Four of the six begin with "flexor". Two contain "flexor carpi", this refers to flexing the carpal joint. Those same two give us a clue as to their location: "ulnaris" meaning it lies on the ulna; "radialis" meaning it lies on the radius. "Pollicis" refers to the pollex, the Latin word for thumb. The superficial digital flexor and the deep digital flexor are flexors of the digits, or fingers. "Palmaris" would suggest that it is associated with the palm side of the forearm.

Note the term flexor retinaculum. A retinaculum (plural: retinacula) is a structure that holds an organ or tissue in place. (In surgery, it is also used to describe an instrument that retracts tissues.) As with the aponeurosis, this is not a muscle. It is, however, a significant structure of the arm as it keeps the tendons of the antebrachium in place.

The extensors are antagonists to the flexors that lie on the posterior forearm. The tendons of these muscles are held in place by the extensor retinaculum on the back of the wrist. The muscles we will review are as follows: extensor carpi radialis longus, extensor carpi radialis brevis, extensor carpi ulnaris, extensor digitorum, extensor policis longus, extensor policis brevis.

Rotators are responsible for either pronation (medial rotation) or supination (lateral rotation) of the antebrachium. The rotators are named as follows: brachioradialis, pronator, supinator, pronator quadratus.

In the hand are three thenar muscles that act on the thumb and form the fleshy bulb at the base of the thumb. On the contralateral side of the palm lies a smaller fleshy bulb composed of the hypothenar muscles, these act on the little finger. There are also four intermediate muscles of the hand that lie in the space between the two groups previously mentioned. Worth noting here is the dexterity of the thumb due to the result of eight different muscles acting upon it.

I. FILL IN THE BLANK.

In the blanks provided below, refer to the figure and enter the term that corresponds to the following numbers. Use the word(s) in the box to fill in the blanks.

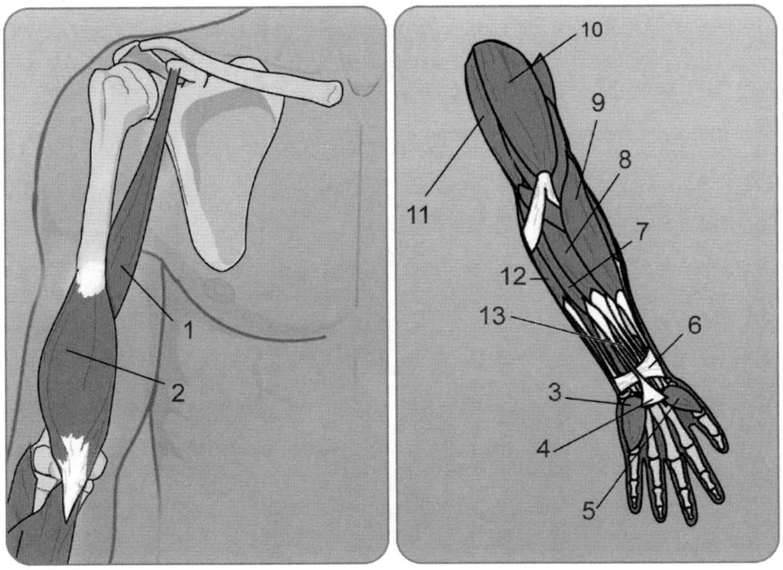

1. ____________
2. ____________
3. ____________
4. ____________
5. ____________
6. ____________
7. ____________
8. ____________
9. ____________
10. ____________
11. ____________
12. ____________
13. ____________

flexor retinaculum
brachioradialis
coracobrachialis
abductor pollicis brevis
flexor carpi ulnaris
hypothenar muscles
palmaris longus
brachialis
triceps
biceps brachii
palmar aponeurosis
flexor carpi radialis
flexor digitorum superficialis

ACTIONS OF ARM MUSCLES

The arm and hand muscles are most commonly seen in radiology (x-ray) reports, orthopedics (especially operative notes), and physical therapy, although, as with other terms, they might turn up virtually anywhere. It is important for you to begin to recognize the terms for the muscles associated with the hand that indicate position and movement, as well as more basic body location: supinate, pronate, flex, extend, digits, pollex, for example. The more you understand what you are reading, the more accurate and professional your work will eventually be. Lucky for you, you do **not** have to memorize exactly what each one of these muscles does.

The following are a few of the muscles of the antebrachium. A brief description is also provided.

anconeus: Located on the back of the humerus, it extends the forearm.

extensor digit minimi: A long narrow muscle located on the ulnar side of the extensor digitorum communis muscle. It assists in extension of the wrist and little finger.

extensor digitorum communis: Positioned in the center of the forearm along the posterior surface. Its tendon divides into four tendons beneath the extensor retinaculum, which attach to the distal tips of fingers one through four.

flexor digitorum profundus: Lies just underneath the flexor digitorum superficialis muscle. This muscle flexes the distal ends of the fingers (but not the thumb).

flexor pollicis longus: Positioned deep on the front of the radius. It attaches at the base of the thumb and flexes the thumb and makes grasping possible.

pronator teres: Positioned in upper middle part of the forearm. It arises from the epicondyle (a prominence or projection on a bone). It turns the hand downwards (called pronation) and flexes the elbow.

epicondyle: A prominence or projection on a bone.

pronator quadratus: Positioned deep and extends between the ulna and radius. It works with the other pronator muscle to rotate the palm of the hand down, as well as position the thumb medially.

supinator: Positioned around the upper portion of the radius. It works with the biceps to turn the palm upwards (called supination).

I. MULTIPLE CHOICE.
Choose the term which best describes the statement.

1. To extend the palm upwards.
   - ◯ suppinate
   - ◯ supinate
   - ◯ pronate
   - ◯ suepinate

2. The first digit of the hand (the thumb).
   - ◯ hallux
   - ◯ polex
   - ◯ pollex
   - ◯ carpals

3. Located behind the humerus and extends the forearm.
   - ◯ anconeus
   - ◯ anconius
   - ◯ anconeis
   - ◯ anconneus

4. Long narrow muscle which assists in extension of the wrist and little finger.
   - ◯ extensor digitus minimus
   - ◯ extensor digiti minimi
   - ◯ extensor digiti mimini
   - ◯ extensor digitus maximus

5. Another term for palmar.
   - ◯ tenar
   - ◯ theno
   - ◯ thenar
   - ◯ thennar

6. Descriptive muscle term meaning short.
   - ◯ longus
   - ◯ brevus
   - ◯ brives
   - ◯ brevis

7. Muscle attached to the humerus deep to the biceps.
   - ◯ coracobrachialis
   - ◯ coracobrachialus
   - ◯ coronobrachialis
   - ◯ chorobrachialis

8. A structure which holds an organ or a tissue in place.
   - ◯ aponeurosis
   - ◯ retinaculum
   - ◯ retinaculim
   - ◯ apponeurosis

9. The major muscle of the upper arm.
   - ◯ bicep
   - ◯ flexor carpi ulnaris
   - ◯ biceps
   - ◯ bicepps

10. A muscle which turns the palm of the hand downwards.
    - ◯ pronater teres
    - ◯ pronator teres
    - ◯ pronator terres
    - ◯ pronater teris

11. A muscle whose tendon divides into four different tendons.
    - ◯ extensor digitorum comminus
    - ◯ extensor digiti comminus
    - ◯ extensor digitorum communis
    - ◯ extensor digiti communis

12. Long slender arm muscle with a tendon which attaches to the palmar aponeurosis.
    - ◯ palmaris longus
    - ◯ palmaris brevis
    - ◯ palmarus longis
    - ◯ palmaris longis

13. Muscle located on the back of the arm.
    - ◯ tricep
    - ◯ thenar muscle
    - ◯ bicep
    - ◯ triceps

14. Muscle which flexes the fingers.
    - ◯ flesor digitorum profundis
    - ◯ flexor digitorum profundus
    - ◯ extensor digiti profundidi
    - ◯ flexor digotorum profundus

MUSCLES OF THE PELVIC GIRDLE AND UPPER LEG

The muscles of the pelvic floor support the anatomic structures of the pelvic cavity. The area inside the diamond-shaped outline is called the **perineum**. The anterior portion of the diamond is the **urogenital triangle**. It contains the ischiocavernosus and bulbospongiosus muscles associated with male and female anatomy. The coccygeus muscle lies behind the levator ani and, with that muscle, crosses the pelvic floor, like a hammock, providing support.

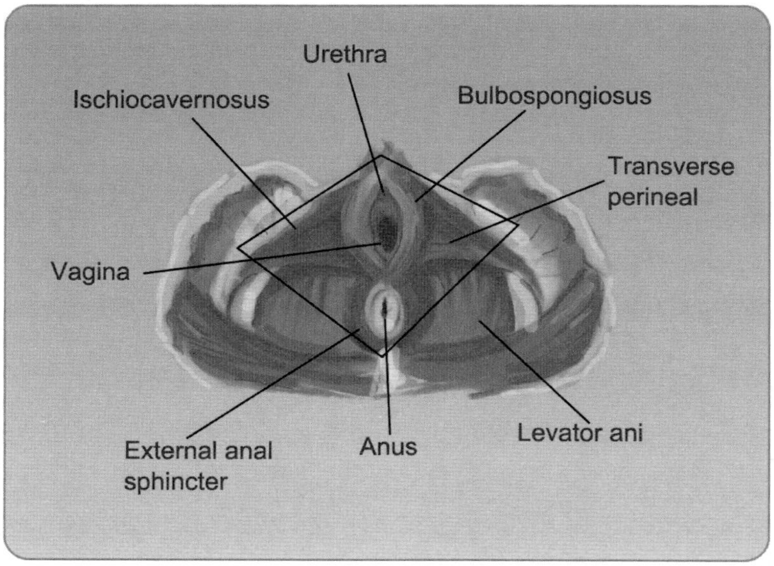

The deep muscles of the hip, as well as the ligaments of the pelvic girdle provide stability and strength to the hip joint and the lower back. The **iliopsoas muscles** are hip flexors, allowing flexion and internal rotation of the hip joint, as are the **adductor brevis, adductor longus**, and **gracilis** muscles.

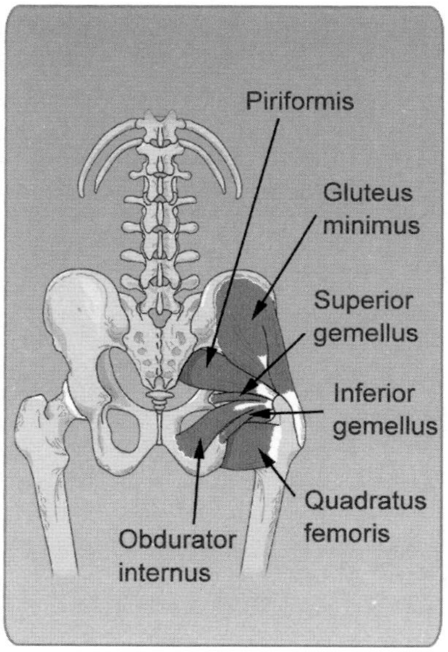

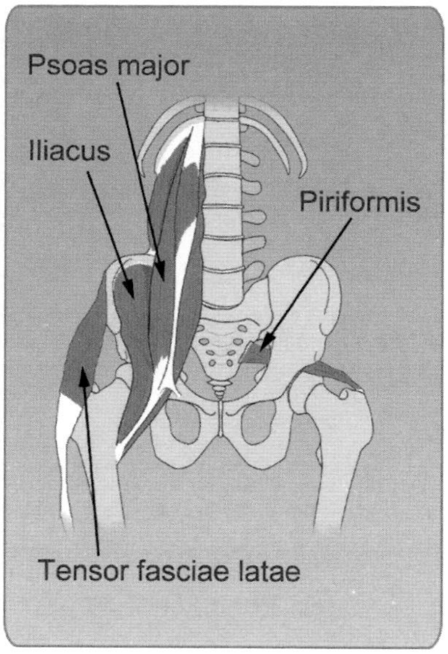

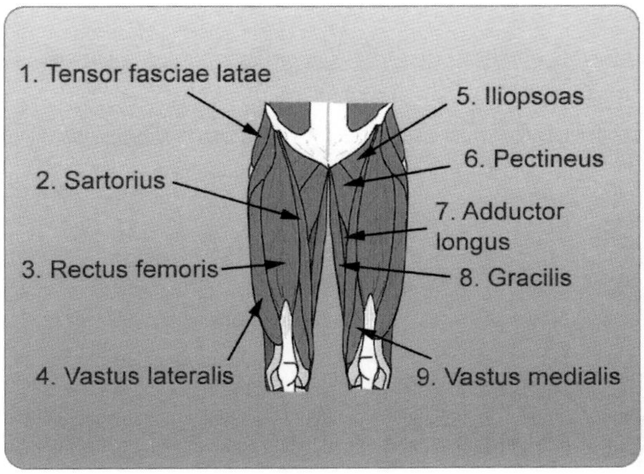

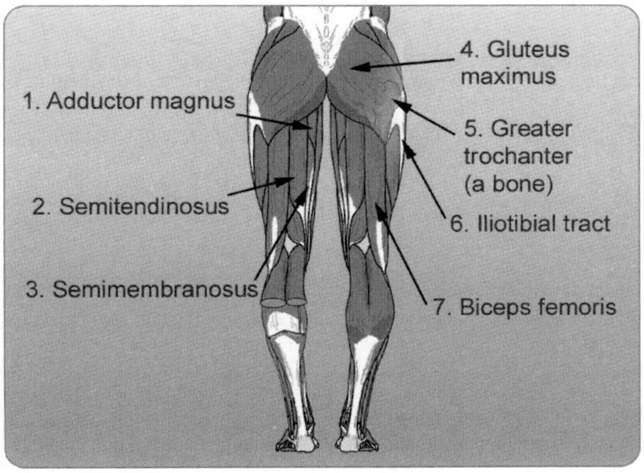

MUSCLES OF THE LEG

The femur is the longest and strongest bone in the body and, correspondingly, the muscles of the legs represent some of the longest and strongest muscles.

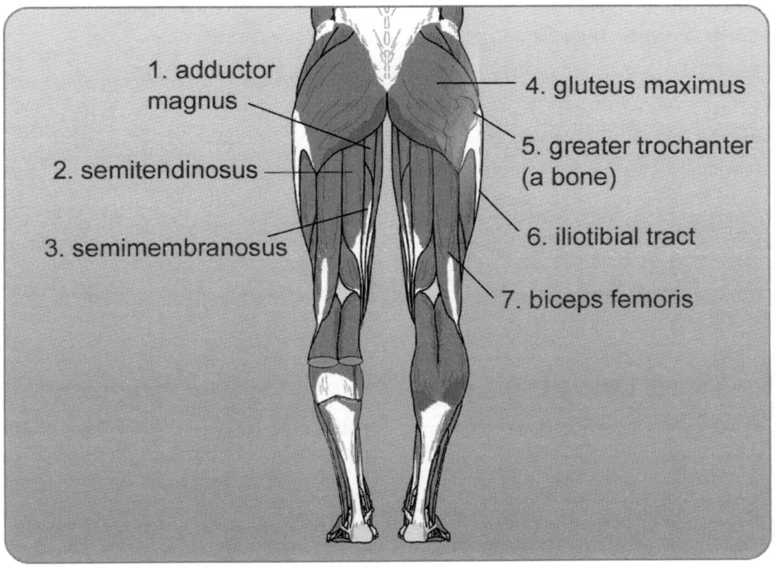

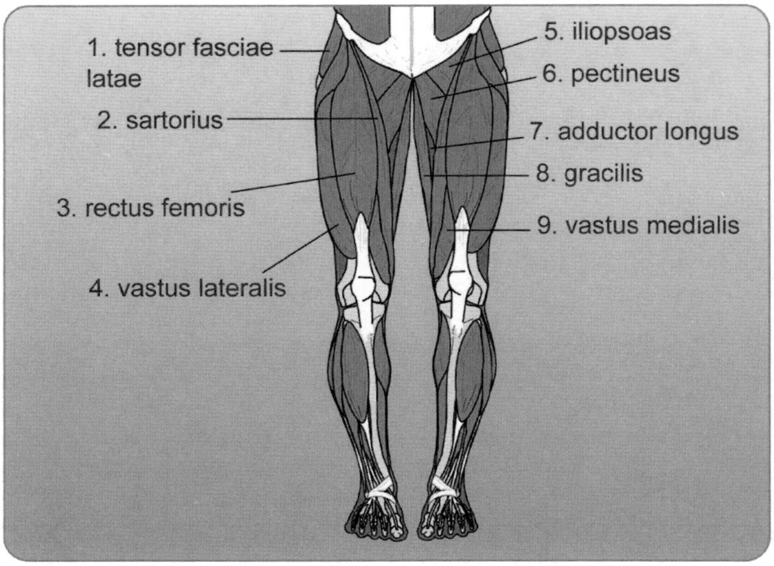

Glutes, quads, and hamstrings are the common terms used for the groups of muscles in the upper legs. Before we explore these groups we should note the **tensor fasciae latae**, as well as the **sartorius**. The tensor fasciae latae runs from the iliac crest two thirds of the way down the lateral aspect of the thigh. The muscle belly then terminates in a connection with the iliotibial band, a strong, fibrous band of connective tissue that continues inferiorly to insert on the lateral condyle of the tibia. The sartoius is the longest muscle in the human body. It crosses from the anterior portion of the iliac spine laterally to the medial portion of the body of the tibia.

The glutes, or gluteal muscles, are made up of four different muscles: **gluteus maximus**, the largest of the group and one of the strongest muscles in the body; **gluteus medius** and **gluteus minimus**, which lie deep to the gluteus maximus; and the tensor fasciae latae.

The “hamstrings” are three posterior leg muscles that act to flex the knee joint, bringing the heel toward the buttocks. Their names from lateral to medial are: **biceps femoris, semitendinosus**, and **semimembranosus**.

Quadriceps, or “quads”, lies on the anterior aspect of the thigh and is so named because of its four heads: **vastus lateralis, rectus femoris, vastus intermedius**, and **vastus medialus**.

I. **FILL IN THE BLANK.**

In the blanks provided below, refer to the image and enter the terms that correspond to the following numbers. Use the words in the box to fill in the blanks.

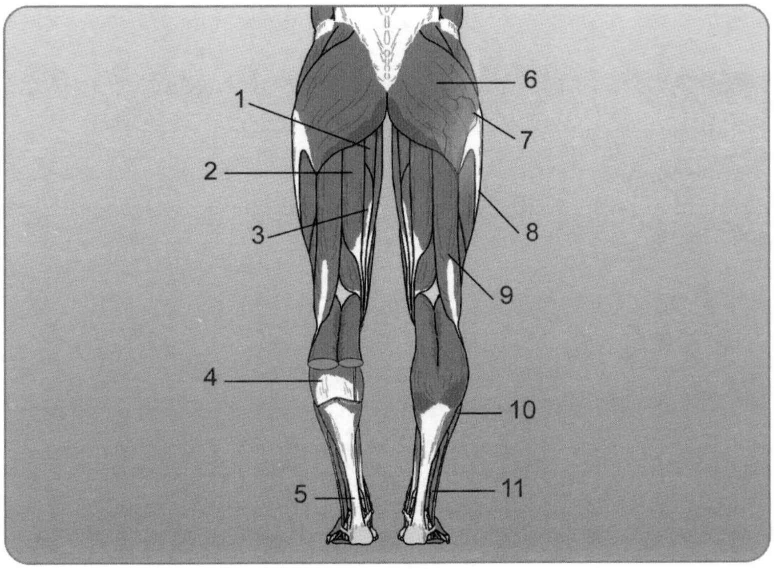

1. ____________________
2. ____________________
3. ____________________
4. ____________________
5. ____________________
6. ____________________
7. ____________________

iliotibial tract
semimembranosus
adductor magnus
gluteus maximus
semitendinosus
biceps femoris
greater trochanter

II. FILL IN THE BLANK.

In the blanks provided below, refer to the image and enter the terms that correspond to the following numbers. Use the words in the box to fill in the blanks.

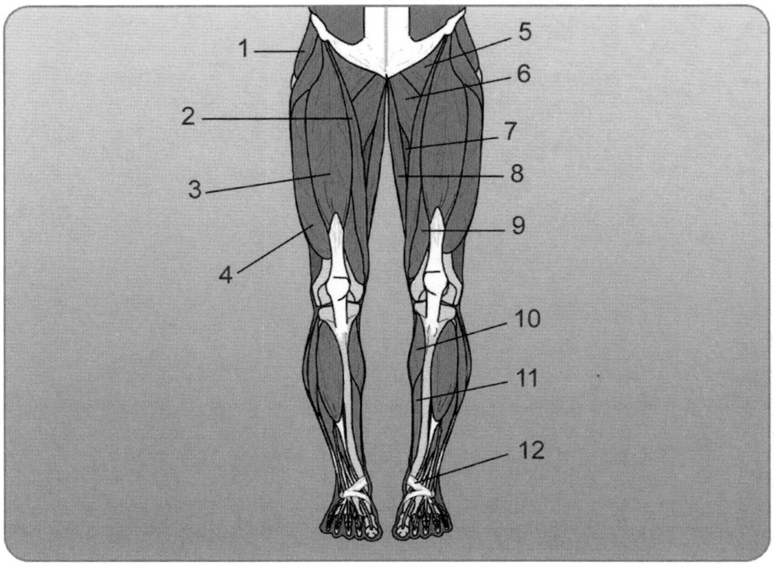

1. ____________________
2. ____________________
3. ____________________
4. ____________________
5. ____________________
6. ____________________
7. ____________________
8. ____________________
9. ____________________

adductor longus
sartorius
rectus femoris
vastus medialis
iliopsoas
pectineus
tensor fasciae latae
gracilis
vastus lateralis

MUSCLES OF THE LOWER LEG

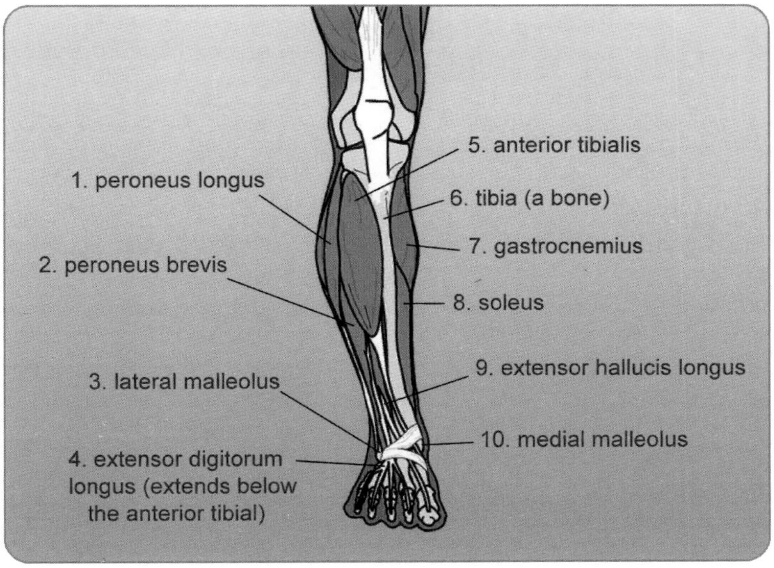

In medical notes, the legs are rarely referred to as "legs." They are instead called the lower extremities. (The arms are likewise called the upper extremities.) An extremity is simply the name for a limb. You should notice, as with the arm muscles, that there are several descriptive terms in the graphics which should be familiar by now, such as *longus, brevis, hallucis*, and *maximus*. Take just a moment to find any terms that you already know.

As with the muscle of the antebrachuim, the muscles of the lower leg are extensors and flexors (although they are not all named as such). These muscles are much larger than those in the forearm so they can accommodate the weight of the body during bipedal activities. Refer to the list below for the names and actions of the lower leg muscles.

Extensor digitorum longus muscle: Extends metatarsophalangeal joint of other toes.

Extensor hallucis longus muscle: Extends metatarsophalangeal joint of great toe.

Fibularis brevis muscle: Extends and everts foot (lifting the sole of the foot laterally).

Fibularis longus muscle: Extends and everts foot.

Flexor digitorum longus muscle: Plantar flexes foot.

Flexor hallucis longus muscle: Plantar flexes foot.

Gastrocnemius muscle: Flexes leg, plantar flexes foot.

Peroneus brevis muscle: Extends and everts foot.

Peroneus longus muscle: Extends and everts foot.

Popliteus muscle: Flexes and rotates leg medially.

Soleus muscle: Plantar flexes foot.

Tibialis anterior muscle: Dorsiflexes and inverts foot (lifting the sole of the foot medially).

Tibialis posterior muscle: Plantar flexes foot, inverts foot.

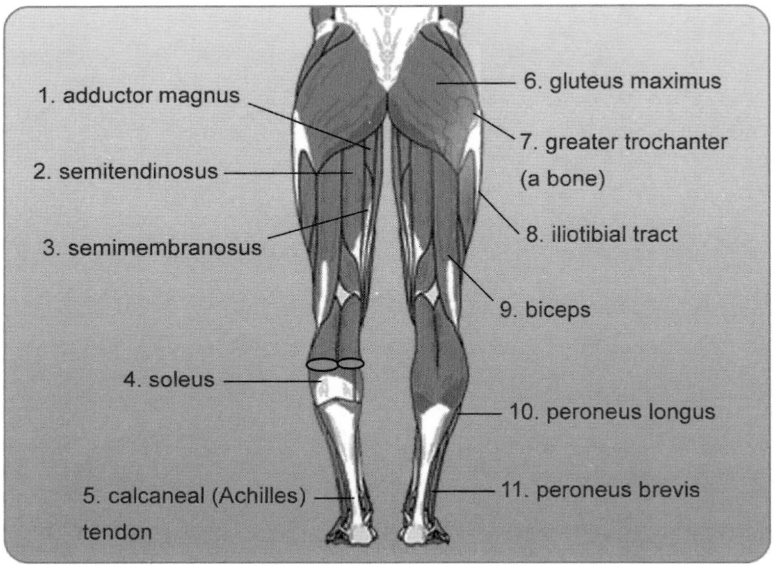

There are also a few terms listed on this image (and subsequent images) that are not muscles, although they are vital to the musculoskeletal system – especially the lower extremities. Notice the **calcaneal or Achilles tendon**. The Achilles is the thickest and strongest tendon in the body. You have already learned that tendons are fibrous cords to which muscle is attached.

If you are into mythology, you may know that the Achilles tendon is named for the Greek fighter Achilles. He was immortal and invulnerable except for the spot on his heel where he was held as he was dipped into the river water that turns mortals into gods. It was this area that was pierced by an arrow during the Trojan War, and this wound caused his death.

The **extensor retinaculum** is not a muscle but covers and holds in place the muscles and tendons of the front of the foot. The intrinsic muscles of the foot are listed below. Again, you will not be required for this course to memorize all the muscle names and locations; however, you should be able to recognize the muscle name and the general area of the body where it occurs.

Abductor hallucis muscle: Abducts great toe.

Adductor hallucis muscle: Adducts great toe.

Extensor digitorum brevis muscle: Extends toes.

Extensor hallucis brevis muscle: Extends great toe.

Flexor digitorum brevis muscle: Extends toes.

Flexor hallucis brevis muscle: Flexes metatarsophalangeal joint of great toe.

Quadratus plantae muscle: Flexes toes.

I. **FILL IN THE BLANK.**

In the blanks provided below, refer to the image and enter the terms that correspond to the following numbers. Use the words in the box to fill in the blanks.

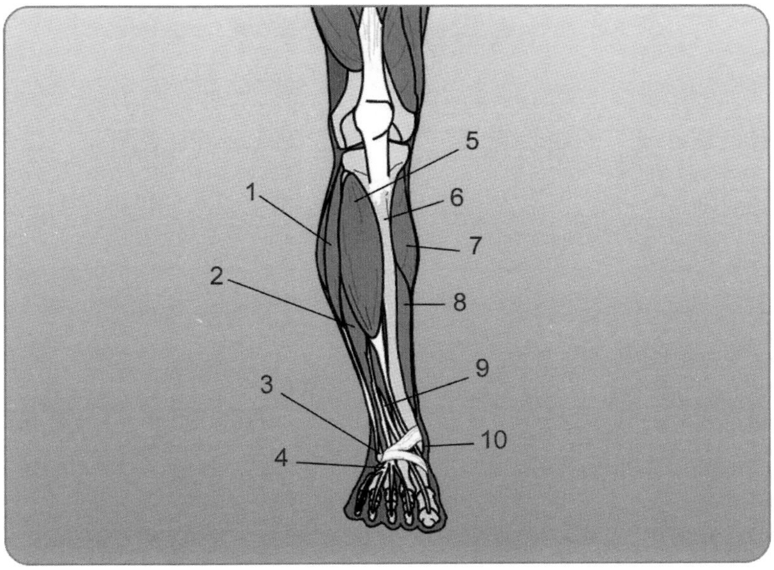

1. ____________
2. ____________
3. ____________
4. ____________
5. ____________
6. ____________
7. ____________
8. ____________
9. ____________
10. ____________

extensor digitorum longus
gastrocnemius
peroneus longus
medial malleolus
lateral malleolus
extensor hallucis longus
anterior tibialis
soleus
tibia
peroneus brevis

REVIEW: MUSCLE ANATOMY

As with any other part of the human anatomy, there are several things that can go wrong with these structures. Before you begin learning about pertinent disease processes, review all of the muscle groups that you have studied. Do the exercises on the following pages, and remember that the answers could be from any of the figures found in the muscle lessons.

I. FILL IN THE BLANK.

Determine which part of the body the muscle or term is part of (back, arm, leg, neck, torso, face).

1. ________________ mentalis
2. ________________ flexor carpi ulnaris
3. ________________ gluteus maximus
4. ________________ buccinator
5. ________________ sternocleidomastoid
6. ________________ temporalis
7. ________________ biceps
8. ________________ latissimus dorsi
9. ________________ orbicularis oris
10. ________________ risorius
11. ________________ anconeus
12. ________________ palmaris longus
13. ________________ trapezius
14. ________________ platysma
15. ________________ digastric
16. ________________ brachioradialis
17. ________________ supinator
18. ________________ corrugator
19. ________________ teres major
20. ________________ peroneus longus
21. ________________ gracilis
22. ________________ nasalis
23. ________________ lateral malleolus
24. ________________ brachialis
25. ________________ labii inferioris
26. ________________ medial pterygoid
27. ________________ soleus
28. ________________ masseter
29. ________________ adductor magnus
30. ________________ serratus anterior
31. ________________ omohyoid
32. ________________ pronator teres
33. ________________ tensor fasciae latae
34. ________________ iliopsoas
35. ________________ greater zygomatic
36. ________________ anterior tibia
37. ________________ greater trochanter
38. ________________ supraspinatus
39. ________________ depressor anguli oris
40. ________________ external oblique
41. ________________ extensor digiti minimi
42. ________________ lumbar aponeurosis
43. ________________ gastrocnemius

II. MULTIPLE CHOICE.
Choose the best answer.

1. The forearm muscle that pronates the hand.
   - ◯ anconeus
   - ◯ pronater dupli
   - ◯ pronator teres
   - ◯ biceps

2. A muscle that has two heads.
   - ◯ triceps
   - ◯ tricep
   - ◯ bicep
   - ◯ biceps

3. The muscle that makes pouting possible.
   - ◯ mentalis
   - ◯ lateral pterygoid
   - ◯ linea obliquus
   - ◯ frownicus

4. The major muscle of the rear end.
   - ◯ gluteus largus
   - ◯ gluteus minimus
   - ◯ gluteus maximus
   - ◯ posteroanterior

5. A long narrow muscle that assists in extending the wrist and little finger.
   - ◯ extensor digiti minimus
   - ◯ extensor digiti minimi
   - ◯ brevis
   - ◯ flexorum digiti minimi

6. The long muscle responsible for movement of the big toe.
   - ◯ extensor hallucis longus
   - ◯ extensor hallucis brevis
   - ◯ external oblique
   - ◯ mentalis

7. Previously called the dorsolumbar fascia.
   - ◯ brevis
   - ◯ lumbar aponeurosis
   - ◯ flexor retinaculum
   - ◯ occipitalis

8. Shaped like a rhomboid.
   - ◯ romboideus
   - ◯ rhomboidius
   - ◯ rhombodeus
   - ◯ rhomboideus

9. The major superficial muscle of the shoulder.
   - ◯ deltoid
   - ◯ occipitalis
   - ◯ gluteus maximus
   - ◯ biceps

10. Muscles responsible for chewing, located on the mandible.
    - ◯ lateral and medial pterygoid
    - ◯ medial pterigoid
    - ◯ lateral pterigoid
    - ◯ medial and lateral pterigoid

11. Bony prominence on the side of the ankle joint.
    - ◯ superior malleolus
    - ◯ lateral malleolus
    - ◯ greater trochanter
    - ◯ Achilles tendon

12. The muscle above the lips that is responsible for lifting.
    - ◯ platysma
    - ◯ costovertebral
    - ◯ levator labii superioris
    - ◯ biceps femoris

13. A muscle with three heads.
    - ◯ biceps
    - ◯ bicep
    - ◯ tricep
    - ◯ triceps

14. Abdominal muscle.
    - ◯ external oblique
    - ◯ external abdominis
    - ◯ Achilles tendon
    - ◯ linea oblique

15. Muscle surrounding the mouth.
   - ◯ orbicularis oris
   - ◯ costovertebral
   - ◯ boca muscalis
   - ◯ gracillus

16. Tendon named for a Greek hero.
   - ◯ Hercules tendon
   - ◯ Achilles tendon
   - ◯ Archimedes tendon
   - ◯ Zeus tendon

17. Process on the outer thigh to which several muscles are attached.
   - ◯ lesser trochanter
   - ◯ gluteus maximus
   - ◯ greater trochanter
   - ◯ gluteus minimus

18. Above and to the side.
   - ◯ distolateral
   - ◯ lateroventricular
   - ◯ inferolateral
   - ◯ superolateral

19. Muscle of the back of the leg.
   - ◯ gluteus maximus
   - ◯ semimembranosus
   - ◯ gluteus minimus
   - ◯ propioception

20. The term for perception of the stimuli.
   - ◯ mentalis
   - ◯ gracilis
   - ◯ proprioception
   - ◯ proprietor

21. The muscle that extends diagonally across the forearm and inserts onto the base of the second and third metacarpal bones.
   - ◯ flexor carpi radialis
   - ◯ flexor biceps radialis
   - ◯ biceps femoris
   - ◯ linea oblique

22. This is the most superficial of the medial thigh muscles.
- ◯ levator labii superioris
- ◯ gracilis
- ◯ longus
- ◯ brevis

23. This muscle can extend, laterally rotate, and adduct the thigh, as well as flex the knee.
- ◯ biceps femoris
- ◯ triceps femoris
- ◯ biceps brevis
- ◯ triceps brevis

24. Not the largest or the smallest of the gluteal muscles.
- ◯ gluteus medius
- ◯ gluteus maximus
- ◯ gluteus chica
- ◯ gluteus minimus

25. Term meaning short.
- ◯ brevus
- ◯ brevis
- ◯ longus
- ◯ longis

26. The system to which muscles belong.
- ◯ muculoskeletal system
- ◯ musculoskelletal system
- ◯ circulatory system
- ◯ musculoskeletal system

27. From back to front.
- ◯ posteroanterior
- ◯ spinofrontalis
- ◯ ventrolateral
- ◯ costovertebral

UNIT 5

The Joints

THE JOINTS - INTRODUCTION

A joint is an area where two or more bones come together. This contact point creates an important relationship with respect to the body's ability to move. If any of the bones in a joint do not function properly, the joint will not be able to operate as a unit (not all joints, however, are made for movement). There are three main classifications of joints: fibrous joints (non-moveable), cartilaginous joints (somewhat moveable), and synovial joints (very moveable). These main classifications are further subdivided based on structure and function. We will describe each type and give examples of each.

Fibrous Joints

The bones of fibrous joints are connected by fibrous connective tissue. Fibrous joints lack a joint capsule and in general do not allow movement. There are two subtypes of fibrous joints: sutures and syndesmosis.

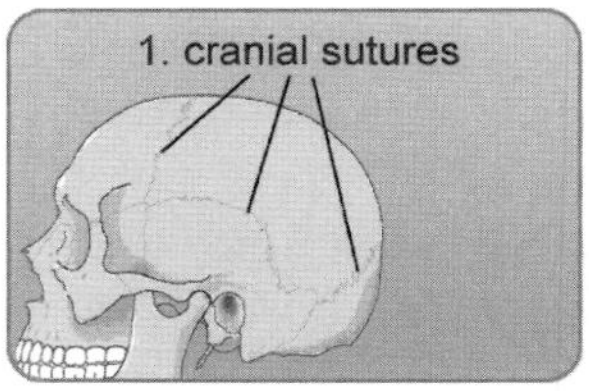

Sutures: These are the connections between the flat bones of the skull.

Syndesmoses: These are fibrous joints with a relatively large amount of fibrous connective tissue between the bones. Two examples are the radio-ulnar syndesmosis and the tibiofibular syndesmosis.

Cartilaginous Joints

The bones of cartilaginous joints are connected by cartilage. They allow little to no movement. There are two subtypes classified based on the types of cartilage they contain: synchondroses (contain hyaline cartilage) and symphyses (contain fibrocartilage).

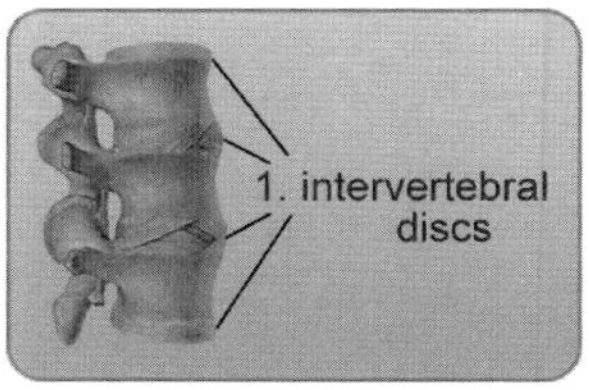

Synchondroses: Joints containing hyaline cartilage between skeletal components. Examples are: costochondral joints, a small insertion of hyaline cartilage between the anterior termination of the ribs and the costal cartilage; epiphyseal cartilage, commonly referred to as the growth plate, a line of hyaline cartilage occurring between the epiphysis and diaphysis of a growing long bone.

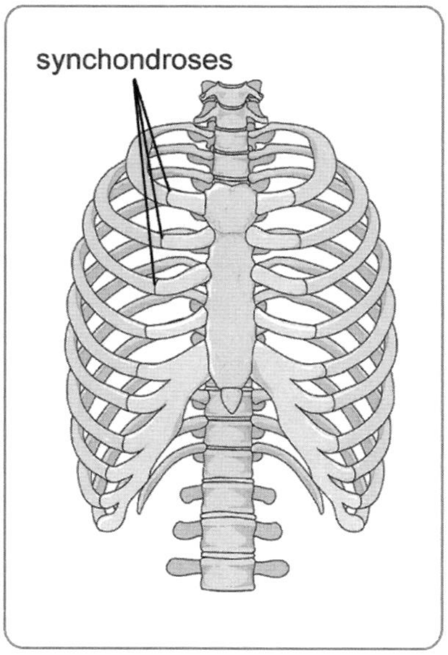

Symphyses: The skeletal components of these joints are joined by fibrocartilage. Examples include: intervertebral symphyses, these are the intervertebral discs; the pubic symphysis, joins the anterior bones of the os coxae.

Synovial Joints

There are four types of synovial joints: plane, uniaxial, biaxial, and multiaxial. A synovial joint has a joint cavity that is kept lubricated by synovial fluid. The looser the joint, the more unstable and susceptible it is to injury or other damage. The body compensates for the weakness in synovial joints with ligaments, tendons, and muscle overlays. In this way, joints can be strengthened and supported to a much higher degree, yet still be capable of functioning freely.

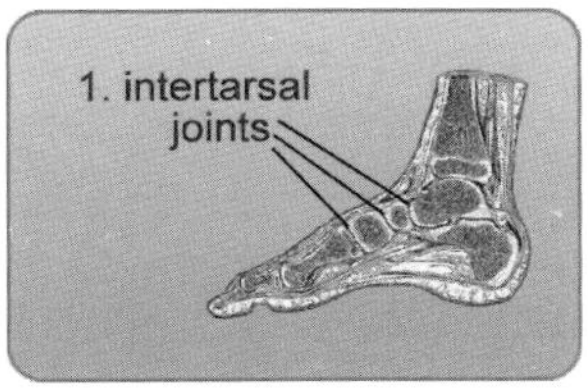

Plane joints are joints that glide where the flat ends of bones connect. Examples of plane joints are the intercarpal and intertarsal joints.

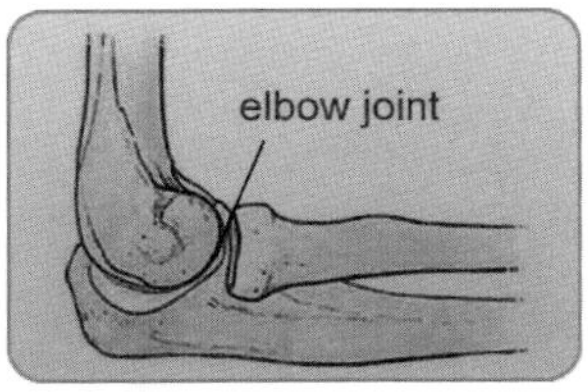

Uniaxial joints allow movement around one axis only. Examples of uniaxial joints are the elbow joint and the interphalangeal joint.

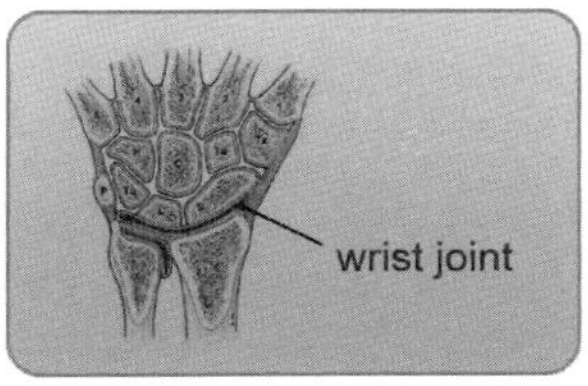

Biaxial joints allow movement around two axes. Examples of biaxial joints are the knee joint, the temporomandibular (jaw) joint, and the radiocarpal (wrist) joint.

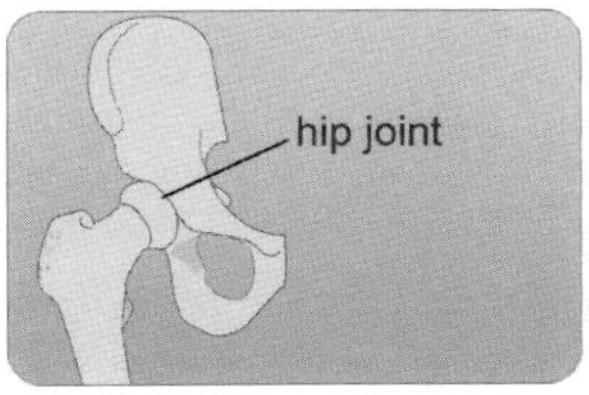

Multiaxial joints allow movement around three axes. Examples of multiaxial joints are the ball and socket joint found in the hip and shoulder, as well as the carpometacarpal joint of the thumb between the trapezium (base of thumb) and the first metacarpal. Ball-and-socket joints are the most freely moveable joints in the body.

I. TRUE/FALSE.
Mark the following true or false.

1. A biaxial joint is a type of synovial joint
   - ◯ true
   - ◯ false

2. Fibrous joints, in general, do not move.
   - ◯ true
   - ◯ false

3. Synviol joints have no cavities and are somewhat moveable.
   - ◯ true
   - ◯ false

4. The elbow is an example of a uniaxial joint.
   - ◯ true
   - ◯ false

5. A cranial suture is an example of cartilaginous joints.
   - ◯ true
   - ◯ false

II. FILL IN THE BLANK.

Using the word/word parts in the box, fill in the blanks.

1. A multiaxial joint has a joint cavity kept lubricated by ________________ fluid.
2. The two types of fibrous joints are ________________.
3. Synchondrosis and symphysis are examples of ________________ joints.
4. The knee joint is an example of a ________________ joint.
5. The body compensates for potential weakness in synovial joints with ________________ tendons and muscle overlays.

suture and syndesmosis
cartilaginous
ligaments
synovial
biaxial

JOINT MOVEMENT

Along with the many different types of joints in the body, there are many different ways in which joints move. These are often noted in the physical examination of patients with aches, pains, and difficulty with movement.

Take a moment to try each of these joint movements. What are you doing when you pick up a gallon of milk? What about when you reach for an item from a high shelf?

flexion: Bending to decrease the angle between two bones. Think of this as "flexing" the biceps.

extension: Unbending to increase the angle between two bones. Think of this as extending, as in reaching your arm as far as you can (virtually eliminating the angle between the humerus and the radius/ulna).

abduction: Moving a body part away from the midline.

adduction: Moving a body part toward the midline. (Think of this as adding a body part back to the body.)

circumduction: Movement of a body part in a circle, which can include all the above joint movements as well.

I. MATCHING.
Match the correct term to the definition.

1. ____ extension
2. ____ flexion
3. ____ abduction
4. ____ adduction
5. ____ circumduction

A. circling
B. bending
C. moving away from midline
D. adding a part back to the body
E. unbending

II. FILL IN THE BLANK.
Use the word(s) in the box to fill in the blanks.

circumduction
flexion
extension
abduction
adduction

1. Moving your hand into a fist is considered ________________.
2. From a sitting position, unbend the knee and bring one foot up to the level of the knee. This is ________________.
3. A great back stretch would be bending from the waist toward the right, and circling all the way around. This is called ________________.
4. ________________ would be used in raising your arm.
5. ________________ would be used in folding your arms.

III. FILL IN THE BLANK.
Enter the bolded terms in the space provided.

1. **rotation** ________________ Movement of a body part or parts around its axis (movement from side to side with the lower body stationary).
2. **supine** ________________ The position of the body when lying face up, including hands being palm up and feet bent upwards.
3. **prone** ________________ The position of the body when lying face down, including the hands being palm down and the feet bent downwards.

4. **dorsiflexion** ________________ Movement of the foot that brings the top of the foot closer to the leg.
5. **plantar flexion** ________________ Movement of the foot that brings the heel closer to the posterior part of the leg, the toe pointed farther away from the leg. This is the opposite of dorsiflexion.

IV. MATCHING.

Match the correct term to the definition.

1. ___ dorsiflexion	A. lying face down
2. ___ plantar flexion	B. lying face up
3. ___ rotation	C. pointing the toe
4. ___ supine	D. flexing the toe
5. ___ prone	E. around an axis

V. FILL IN THE BLANK.

Use the word(s) in the box to fill in the blanks.

plantar
flexion
supine
prone
rotation
dorsiflexion

1. Lying face down, as necessary for back surgery, is considered ________________.
2. ________________ is movement around an axis or stationary point.
3. In a chorus line, dancers must always use ________________.
4. In karate, in order to avoid breaking the toes, an athlete must use ________________.
5. Surgery on the chest cavity would require the patient to be placed in ________________.

VI. MULTIPLE CHOICE.
Choose the best answer.

1. Dorsiflexion is:
   - ◯ Movement of the foot that brings the heel closer to the posterior part of the leg.
   - ◯ Movement of a body part in a circle.
   - ◯ Movement of a body part on its axis.
   - ◯ Movement of the foot that brings the top of the foot closer to the leg.

2. Synovial joints _____.
   - ◯ rarely move
   - ◯ move with ease
   - ◯ never move
   - ◯ only move from the hips

3. Bending to decrease the angle between bones is called _____.
   - ◯ extension
   - ◯ abduction
   - ◯ flexion
   - ◯ plantar flexion

4. Circumduction is _____.
   - ◯ movement on the axis
   - ◯ movement in a circle
   - ◯ movement towards the midline
   - ◯ unbending to increase the angle between two bones

5. The position of the body when lying face down, including the hands being palm down and the feet bent downwards, is called _____.
   - ◯ rested
   - ◯ prone
   - ◯ flat
   - ◯ supine

6. An area where two bones meet is called a _____.
   - ◯ suture
   - ◯ joint
   - ◯ synovial
   - ◯ facet

7. The three types of joints are _____.
   - ◯ fibrous, fractured, synovial
   - ◯ synovial, cartilaginous, simple
   - ◯ fibrous, cartilaginous, synovial
   - ◯ syndesmosis, cartilaginous, fibrous

8. Plane joints are _____.
   - ◯ cartilaginous joints
   - ◯ fibrous joints
   - ◯ synovial joints
   - ◯ symphysis joints

9. Joints that allow movement around three axes are called _____.
   - ◯ uniaxial
   - ◯ triaxial
   - ◯ biaxial
   - ◯ multiaxial

10. Cartilaginous joints are _____.
    - ◯ freely moveable
    - ◯ somewhat moveable
    - ◯ generally not moveable

ARTICULATIONS - LESSON 1

In most joints, the contacting surfaces of the bones are protected with layers of cartilage. Cartilage is a specialized fibrous connective tissue needed for both the development and growth of bones. Some of the terms in these lists are made up of one or more types of cartilage. Some of the terms listed below describe junctions of bone with cartilage, as well as the junctions of one piece or type of cartilage with another.

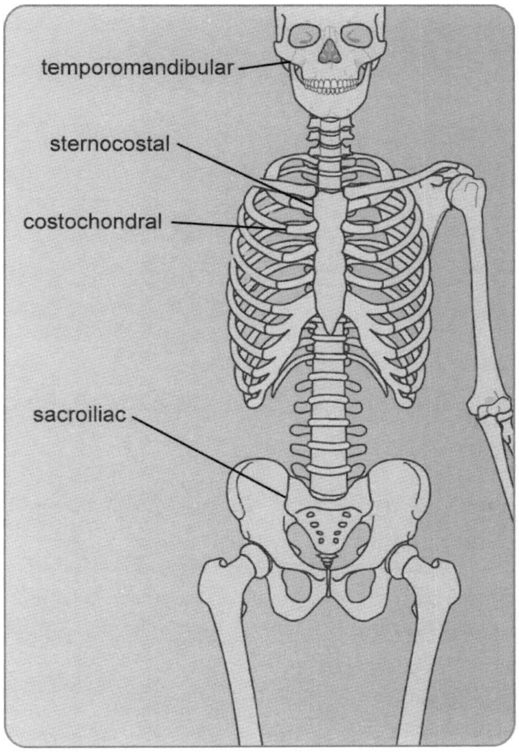

You will undoubtedly have recognized parts of familiar terms in this list. You should already be able to see your study of medical terminology coming in handy.

The following pages contain some lists of common articulations. These are terms you may frequently read in reports, and each is followed by the word "joint" or "junction." This is by no means a complete list.

Joints of the Axial Skeleton

- temporomandibular
- sternocostal
- costochondral
- sacroiliac

ARTICULATIONS - LESSON 2

Joints of the Vertebral Column

- atlanto-occipital – This joint allows you to nod your head. The superior surface of the atlas articulates with the bilateral occipital condyles to accommodate this movement.
- atlantoaxial
- costovertebral
- costotransverse
- intervertebral symphyses
- sacrococcygeal
- zygapophyseal joints (vertebral facet joints)
- lumbosacral

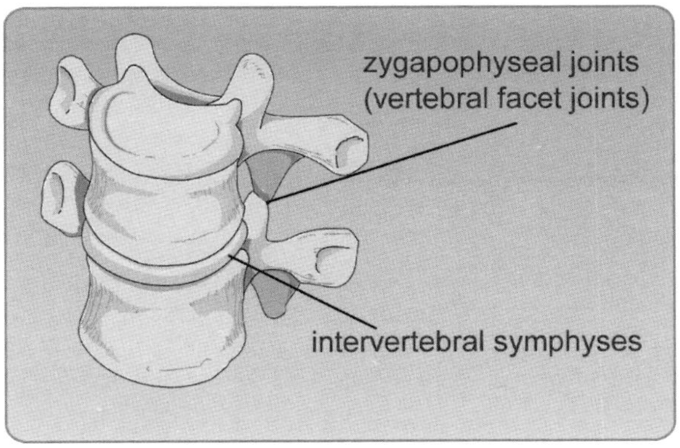

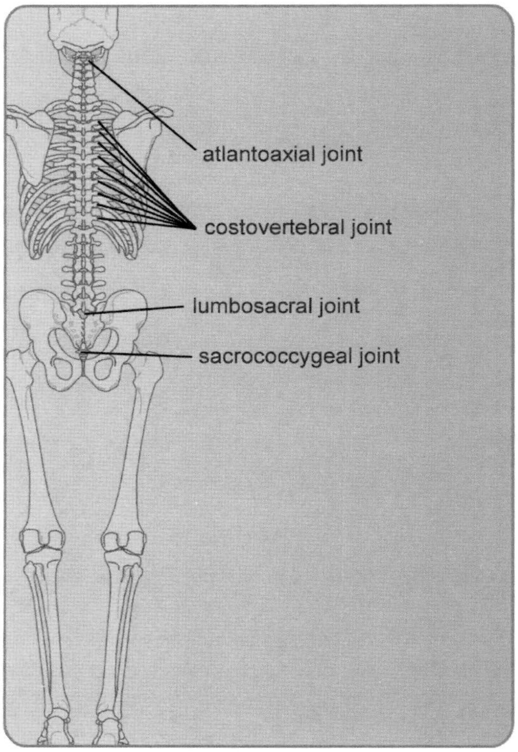

ARTICULATIONS – LESSON 3

Joints of the Appendicular Skeleton – Upper Extremity

- sternoclavicular
- acromioclavicular
- radio-ulnar symdesmosis

Articulations in the Shoulder Joint

- glenohumeral

Articulations in the Elbow Joint

- proximal radioulnar
- humeroradial
- humeroulnar

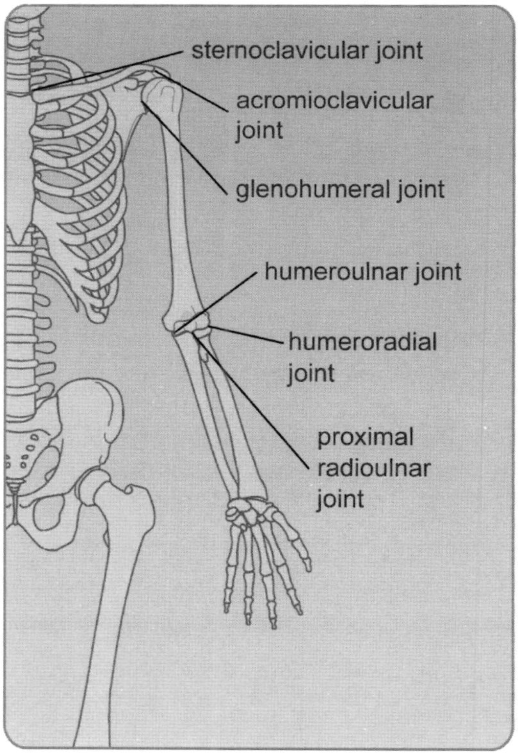

Articulations in the Carpal Joint (Wrist) and Hand

- radiocarpal
- distal radioulnar
- intercarpal – These include all the joints between the eight carpal bones.
- carpometacarpal
- metacarpophalangeal
- interphalangeal

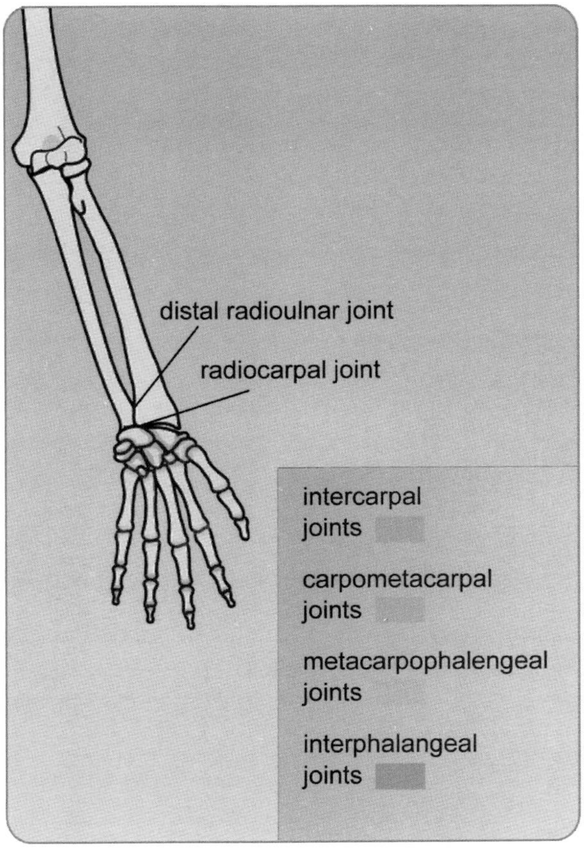

ARTICULATIONS – LESSON 4

Joints of the Appendicular Skeleton – Lower Extremity

- acetabulofemoral (hip)
- sacroiliac
- pubic symphysis
- tibiofibular
- tibiofibular syndesmosis

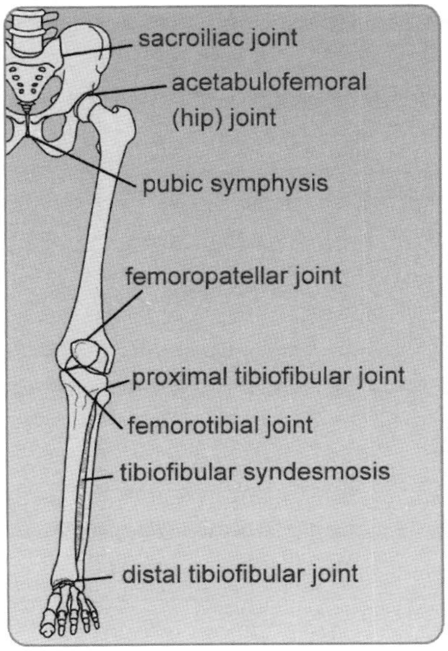

Articulations in the Genual Joint (Knee)

- femoropatellar
- femorotibial

Articulations in the Tarsal Joint (Ankle) and Foot

- talocrural
- intertarsal – These joints occur between the articular surfaces of adjoining tarsal bones and are named for each of the bones involved, for example: talocalcaneal, calcaneocuboid, cuneonavicular, cuboideonavicular, cuneocuboid, intercuneiform.
- tarsometatarsal
- metatarsophalangeal
- interphalangeal

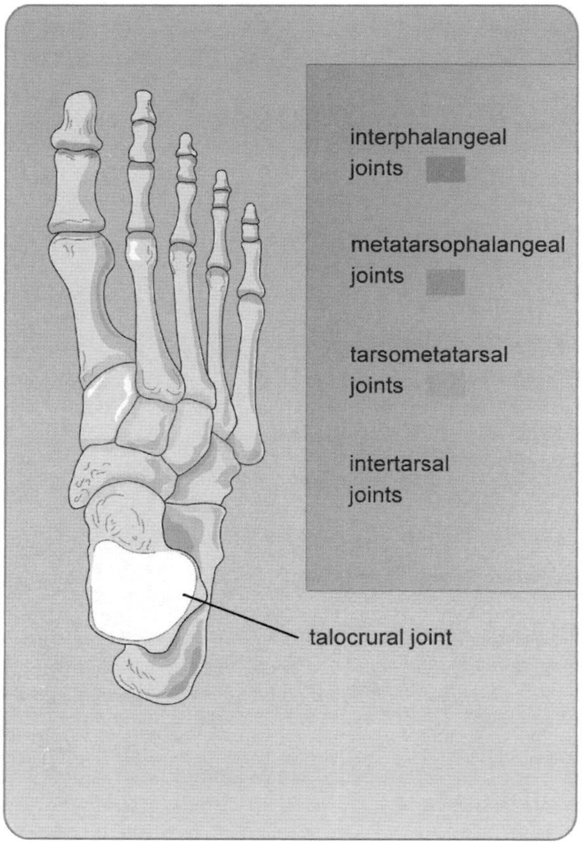

LIGAMENTS

Synovial joints are the most abundant joint type in the body and are designed for the heaviest wear and tear and the most movement. In order to accommodate their function, synovial joint structure is reinforced by strong bands of fibrous connective tissue called **ligaments**. Ligaments, which connect bone to bone, are often confused with tendons, which connect muscle to bone. In the next few pages you will become familiar with the names and locations of some of the ligaments in the body. You will not need to memorize them; however, it will be beneficial to recognize their names and locations within the body.

Most ligaments derive their names from the area where they are located, their shape, or the bones and/or structures near that area. For example, there is a carpal ligament in the wrist and a series of cervical ligaments in the neck, which are terms that, by now, should be somewhat familiar to you.

Because of the repetition that occurs in the naming of individual ligaments, there is no reason to map out and memorize each and every individual ligament in the body. Instead, we will deal specifically with two types of ligaments:

1. those that are susceptible to injury
2. those that are studied in common injuries and the terms related to them.

There are many ligaments that are not listed here. As you become more familiar with human anatomy, most of the ligaments will become familiar to you as well. You will be able to recognize the names as similar to the names of surrounding structures, shapes, and positions (such as anterior or lateral).

For more graphical depictions and detail on joints, ligaments and any of the structures discussed in this module click on the "Launch 3M Reference" link on the left hand side of your page. From the menu you can click on "Elsevier's Anatomy Plates" and select the body system you would like to explore. These anatomy images are very accurate and include a lot of detail that we will not learn in this module but they are a great reference to use through the remainder of the units of this course.

accessory ligament: Any ligament that strengthens or supports another ligament.

arcuate ligament: Means curved or bow-shaped ligaments; they are located in the spine and assist in maintaining the erect position. (Also called ligamenta flava [plural], and ligamentum flavum [singular].)

collateral ligament: There are several types of collateral ligaments, including fibular, radial, tibial, ulnar, etc. These are basically ligaments that are not direct, but are supporting ligaments.

coracoid ligament: Coracoid means like a raven's beak and is used to describe an area on the scapula. It is so named for its shape.

cruciate ligament: Cruciate means shaped like a cross. There are different types of cruciate ligaments, including anterior, posterior, and lateral. They appear in many places in human anatomy, such as the knees, fingers, and toes.

falciform ligament: Falciform means shaped like a sickle and appears near the sacral tuberosity as well as within the liver.

inguinal ligament: Inguinal is a term used to describe the groin area.

interosseous ligament: Interosseous means between bones and describes several different ligaments.

longitudinal ligament: Longitudinal simply means lengthwise. It is used to describe any ligament that runs lengthwise.

nuchal ligament: Nuchal means pertaining to the neck.

triquetral ligament: Triquetral means three cornered and appears in different places throughout the body. The prefix tri- should be familiar as meaning three.

I. MATCHING.
Match the correct term to the definition.

1. ____ cruciate		A. shaped like a cross
2. ____ arcuate		B. support
3. ____ accessory		C. indirect
4. ____ coracoid		D. like a raven's beak
5. ____ collateral		E. curved or bow-shaped ligament

II. FILL IN THE BLANK.

Use the word(s) in the box to fill in the blanks.

accessory
collateral
cruciate
coracoid
arcuate

1. An area of the scapula is shaped like a bird's beak. The ligament that surrounds it is called the ________________ ligament.
2. An ________________ ligament strengthens or supports another ligament.
3. A ________________ ligament is shaped like a cross.
4. Located on the spine, the ________________ ligament literally means "curved or bow-shaped ligament."
5. There are several types of ________________ ligaments that are made up of several bands and are not directly connected.

III. MATCHING.
Match the correct term to the definition.

1. ___ falciform
2. ___ nuchal
3. ___ interosseous
4. ___ triquetral
5. ___ inguinal
6. ___ longitudinal

A. the neck
B. lengthwise
C. sickle-shaped
D. groin area
E. three cornered
F. between bones

IV. FILL IN THE BLANK.

Use the word(s) in the box to fill in the blanks.

falciform
triquetral
longitudinal
inguinal
nuchal
interosseous

1. If a ligament runs along the length of a bone, it is usually called a ________________ ligament.
2. Within the liver, the ________________ ligament is shaped like a sickle.
3. Many ligaments, by virtue of their function to support and strengthen the skeletal system, run in between bones. These are called ________________ ligaments.
4. A ________________ ligament is found in the neck.

5. Three-cornered or ________________ ligaments are found throughout the body.
6. The ________________ ligament is found in the groin area.

LIGAMENT NAMES AND LOCATIONS - LESSON 1

Many of the ligaments of the body are depicted in the images included. Again, you are not required to memorize their names and locations; however, it will be beneficial to be able to recognize the names and have a general idea of the joint they are associated with. The following areas will be covered:

1. Vertebral Ligaments
2. Ligaments of the Upper Extremity
3. Ligaments of the Torso
4. Ligaments of the Lower Extremity
5. Ligaments of the Mandible

Vertebral Ligaments

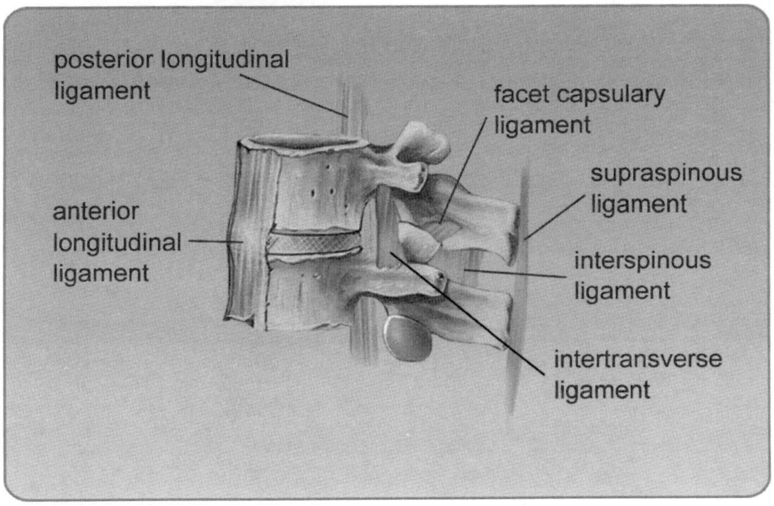

LIGAMENT NAMES AND LOCATIONS - LESSON 2

Below are ligaments found on articulations of the mandible with the rest of the skull as well as some ligaments of the torso. Don't worry about memorizing these, just read over them to gain some familiarity with the names and locations.

Ligaments of the Mandible

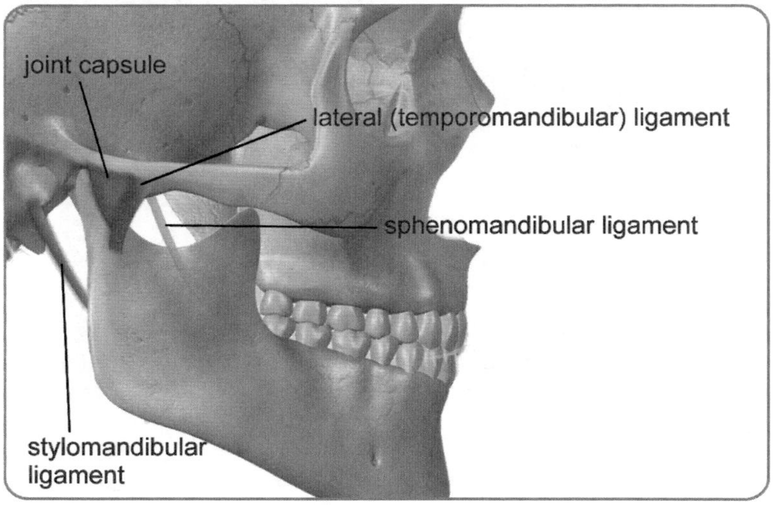

Ligaments of the Torso

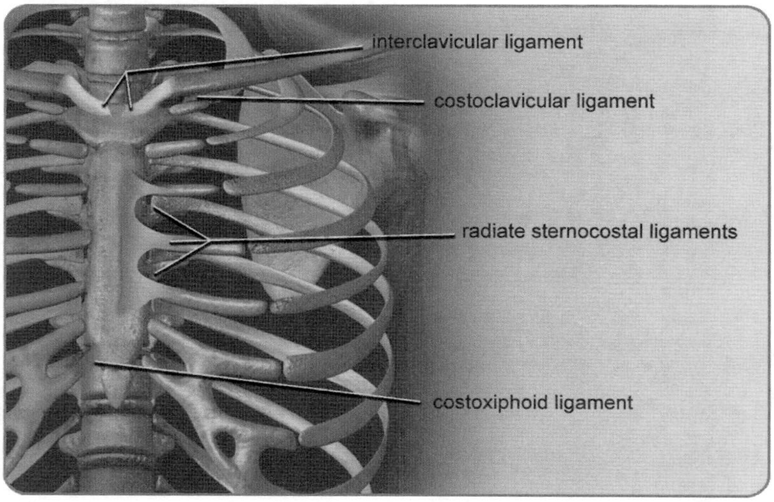

LIGAMENT NAMES AND LOCATIONS - LESSON 3

Study the images below to gain familiarity with ligaments found in the upper extremities including the shoulder girdle. Once again, don't be overly concerned with memorization, just general locations.

Ligaments of the Upper Extremity

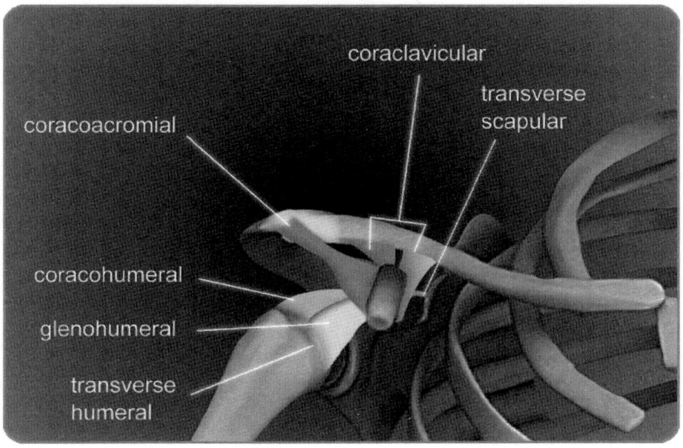

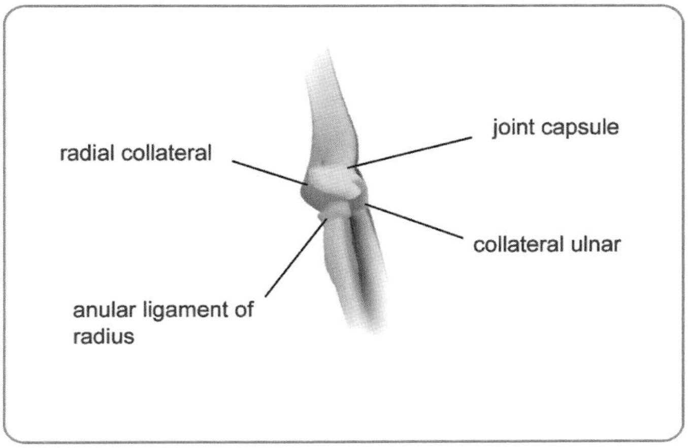

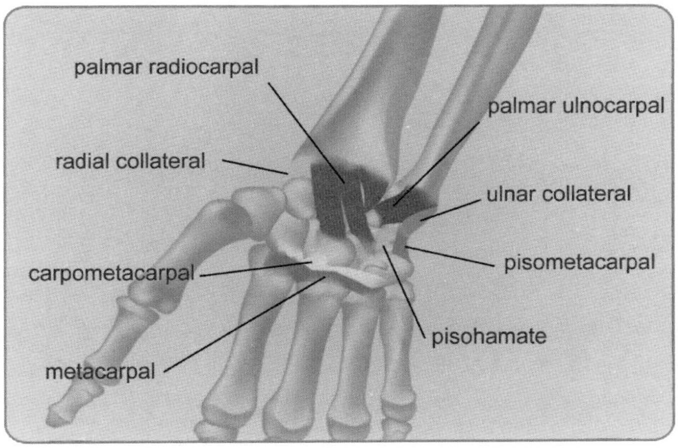

LIGAMENT NAMES AND LOCATIONS - LESSON 4

Ligaments of the lower extremity are shown below. As with the previous pages, study the images so you can be familiar with the names and general locations. The specific names and locations will not be tested on.

Ligaments of the Lower Extremity

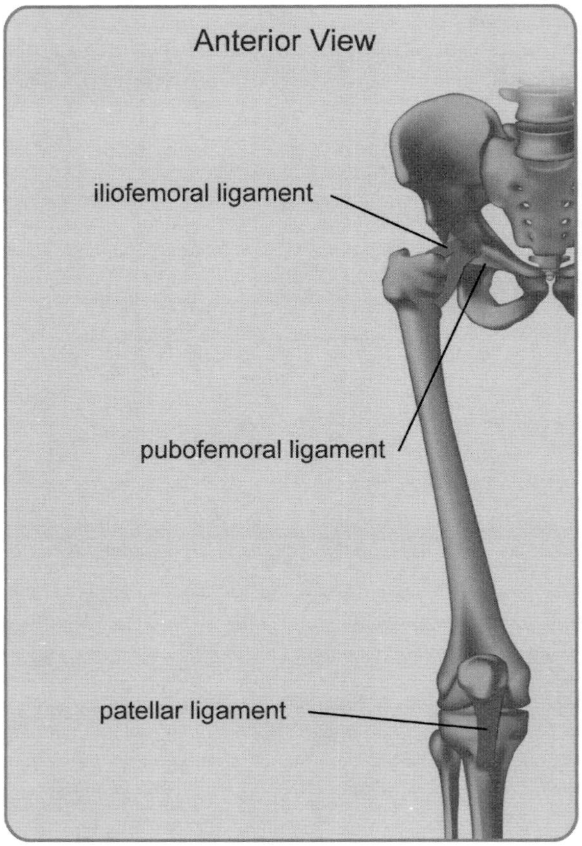

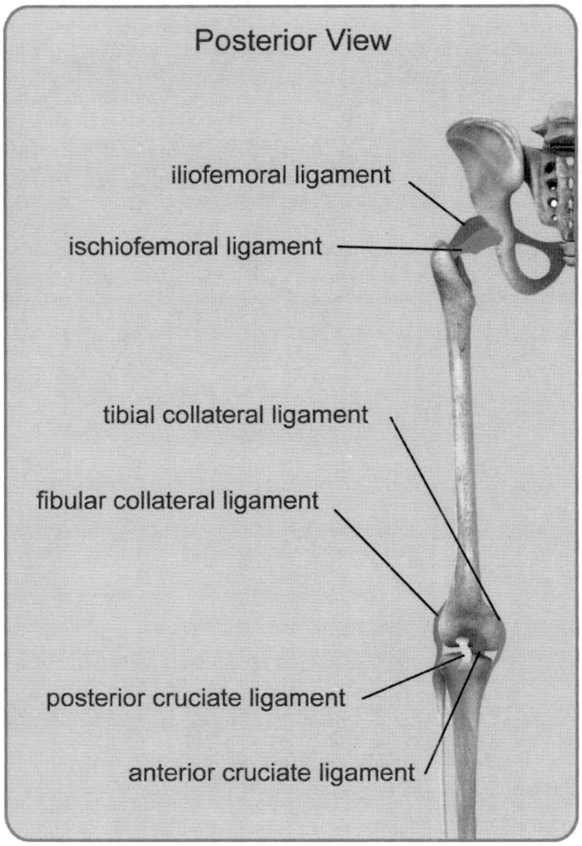

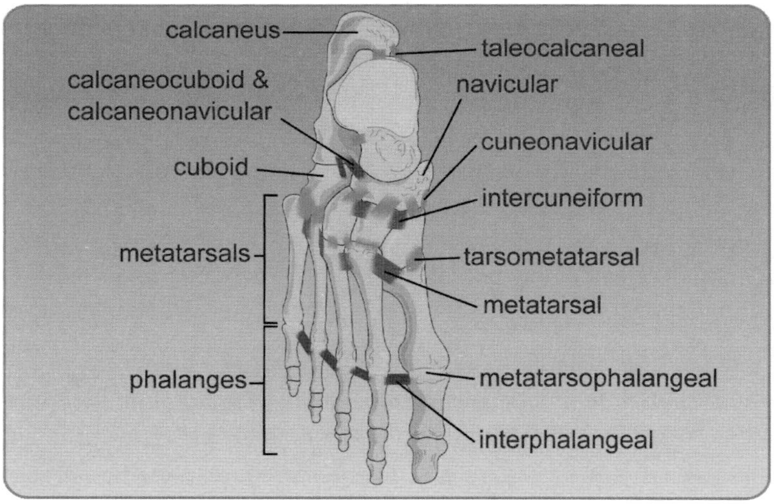

UNIT 6

The Circulatory System

THE CIRCULATORY SYSTEM - INTRODUCTION

The cardiovascular system (or circulatory system) is the system by which all vital components of life, namely blood, oxygen, nutrients, water, chemicals, and hormones, are distributed throughout the body. Additionally, this system is responsible for **homeostasis**, maintaining normalcy throughout the body and regulating temperature. Because the cardiovascular system works in concert with the vessels of the lymphatic system, we will also cover lymphatics in this module.

The major anatomical components covered in this module are:

1. blood
2. heart
3. arteries
4. veins
5. lymphatics

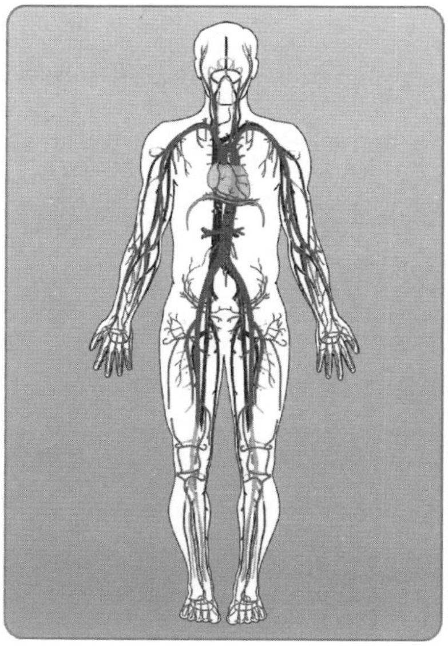

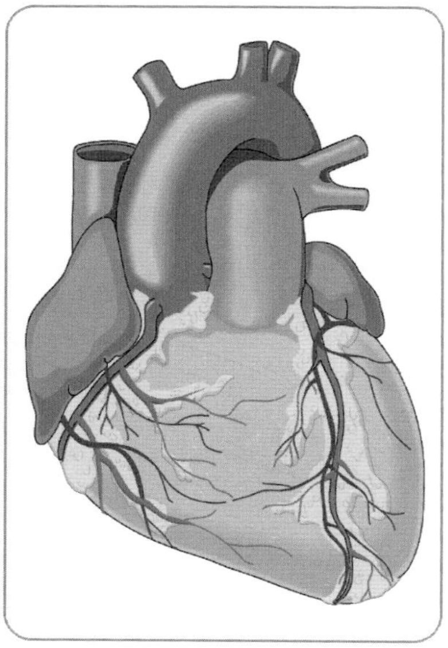

BLOOD

Blood moves throughout the body carrying with it all the major components of life. Blood is pumped by the heart to the various organs and tissues through a network of arteries and veins. Blood is actually a highly specialized fluid connective tissue.

The average person has approximately five liters of blood in the body, which comprises just less than 8% of his or her total body weight.

Blood is composed of a cellular portion and a fluid portion. The fluid portion is called plasma. The plasma constitutes about 55% of the blood volume, with 90% of its volume actually water and the remaining 10% containing the proteins, inorganic salts, metabolic wastes, respiratory gases, and other components.

The three basic cells that comprise the cellular portion of blood are:

- erythrocytes
- leukocytes
- thrombocytes

These cells are important keys for diagnosing disease and maintaining health, and so they are referred to often in medical reports. Erythrocytes, leukocytes, and thrombocytes are evaluated in a standard laboratory test called a CBC or complete blood count.

I. FILL IN THE BLANK.

Using the word/word parts in the box, fill in the blanks.

five
erythrocytes
plasma
CBC

1. The fluid portion of blood is called ________________ and constitutes about 55% of the blood volume.
2. An average person has ________________ liters of blood in the body.
3. A standard lab test for evaluating blood cells is called a ________________ or complete blood count.
4. The cellular portion of blood is composed of three basic cells: ________________ leukocytes, and thrombocytes.

ERYTHROCYTES, LEUKOCYTES, AND THROMBOCYTES

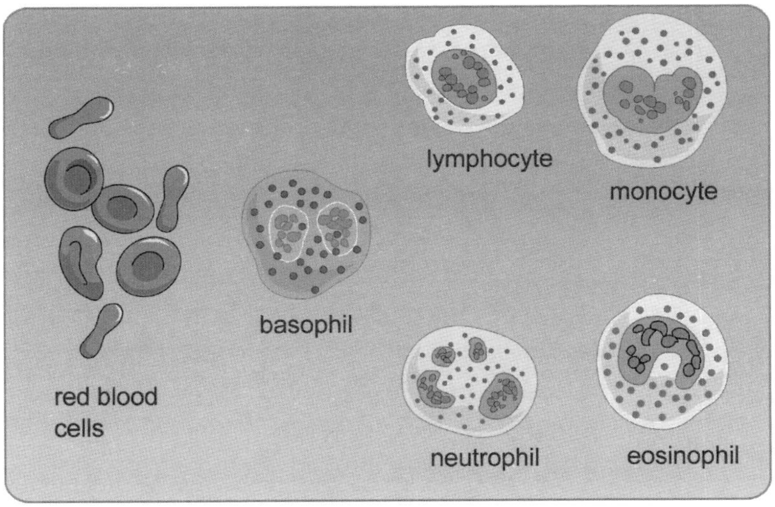

The first cellular components are the **erythrocytes** (or red blood cells, often referred to as RBCs). They constitute approximately 45% of the total blood volume. This percentage in the CBC is referred to as the **hematocrit**.

The oxygen-carrying pigment of the **erythrocytes** is called **hemoglobin**, and that value is also determined in a CBC. The amount of hemoglobin in the blood is dependent upon the amount of iron in the body. A low iron count can lead to anemia and poor tissue oxygenation.

Second are the **leukocytes** (or white blood cells, often referred to as WBCs). There are fewer white blood cells than red blood cells and their major function is to defend the body against infecting organisms and foreign agents. There are five main types of leukocytes that are divided into two basic categories:

granular

- neutrophils
- eosinophils
- basophils

agranular

- lymphocytes
- monocytes

These breakdowns are part of the CBC with a differential count. This report looks at white blood counts and is helpful in revealing specific diseases or infections within the body.

Finally, thrombocytes or platelets, as they are often called, are tiny bits of cytoplasm that have broken off from large cells in the bone marrow called megakaryocytes. Platelets play a major role in blood clotting and are a major component of the CBC. Medical reports often list the short forms for these words, such as *crit* for hematocrit, *segs* for segmented neutrophils, eos, basos, monos, lymphs, so you should be familiar with the terms and the common short forms.

We've placed a visual aid in the appendix on page 329.

I. MULTIPLE CHOICE.
Choose the best answer.

1. White blood cells are also called _____.
   - ◯ thrombocytes
   - ◯ hemoglobin
   - ◯ erythrocytes
   - ◯ leukocytes

2. Thrombocytes or platelets are bits of cytoplasm broken off from bone marrow cells called _____.
   - ◯ megakaryocytes
   - ◯ lymphocytes
   - ◯ neutrophils
   - ◯ erythrocytes

3. These blood cells constitute 45% of the total blood volume.
   - ◯ leukocytes
   - ◯ erythrocytes
   - ◯ thrombocytes
   - ◯ megakaryocytes

4. The major function of these cells is to defend the body against infection.
   - ◯ white blood cells
   - ◯ red blood cells
   - ◯ platelets
   - ◯ hematocrit

5. Hemoglobin serves what purpose?
   - ◯ to help blood clot
   - ◯ to fight off infection
   - ◯ to carry oxygen
   - ◯ to keep the blood from clotting

II. FILL IN THE BLANK.

Enter the correct short form for the medical word in the blank provided.

1. hematocrit________________
2. segmented neutrophils________________
3. basophils________________
4. eosinophils________________
5. lymphocytes________________

HEART

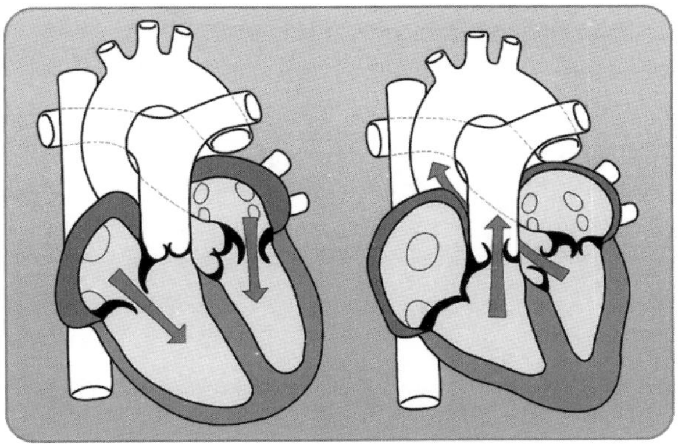

Blood travels through the body through a system of arteries and veins; this circulation is made possible by the heart.

The heart is a pump, or more specifically two pumps working simultaneously. The right ventricle pumps blood through the pulmonary trunk and into the lungs; the left ventricle pumps blood through the aorta and into the systemic arteries.

The actual contraction of the heart chambers is called **systole** and the relaxation is called **diastole**. These terms will be discussed in greater detail later. The measurement of time between contraction and relaxation is how blood pressure is determined.

At rest, the heart pumps approximately one gallon per minute to the 60,000,000,000,000 cells of the body. This increases to over five gallons per minute with activity. The heart is roughly the size of a clenched fist and weighs between 250-300 grams.

It is located in the chest or thoracic cavity, and is situated between the lungs in the mediastinum.

I. FILL IN THE BLANK.

Using the word/word parts in the box, fill in the blanks.

diastole
clenched fist
systole
pulmonary trunk
aorta

1. The heart is roughly the size of a _______________.
2. The right ventricle pumps blood through the _______________ and into the lungs.
3. The left ventricle pumps blood through the _______________ and into the systemic arteries.
4. The contraction of the heart chambers is called _______________.
5. The relaxation of the heart chambers is called _______________.

ANATOMY OF THE HEART

The heart is so essential to the function of the human body as to be the actual indicator of life. If an arm is removed or eyesight is completely impaired, the body still works. But if the heart stops pumping, all body systems cease to function. Because of its importance, an understanding of the heart, its components, and its structure is necessary. As you study the figure included, pay particular attention to the chambers of the heart (right and left atrium, right and left ventricles) and the valves they are associated with.

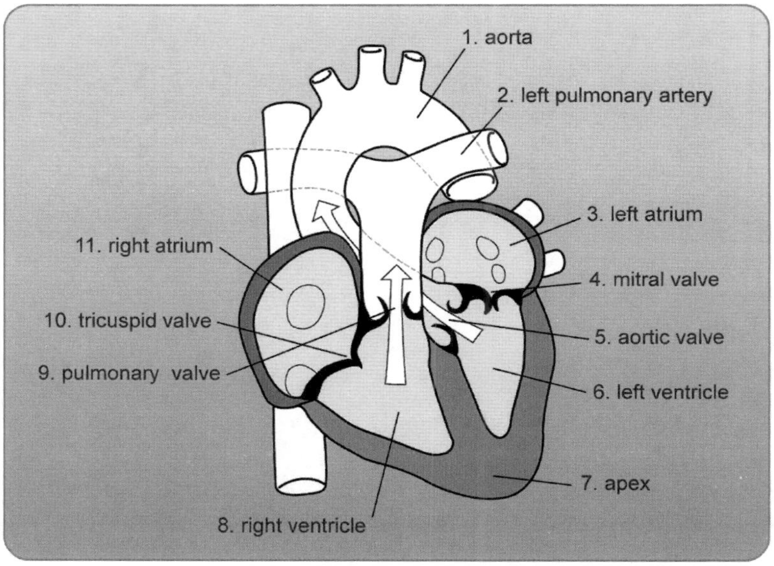

I. FILL IN THE BLANK.

In the blanks provided below, refer to the image and enter the term corresponding to the following numbers. Use the word(s) in the box to fill in the blanks.

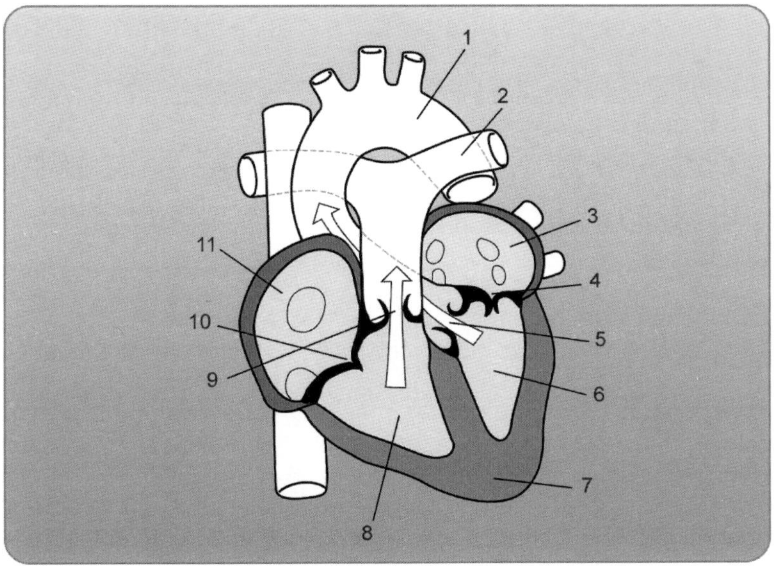

1. ________________
2. ________________
3. ________________
4. ________________
5. ________________
6. ________________
7. ________________
8. ________________
9. ________________
10. ________________
11. ________________

pulmonary valve
left atrium
apex
mitral valve
right ventricle
right atrium
left pulmonary artery
tricuspid valve
aortic valve
aorta
left ventricle

LAYERS OF THE HEART

The **pericardium** (meaning around the heart) is a triple-layered sac that encloses the heart. The outer layer, the fibrous pericardium, holds the heart in its proper anatomical position and prevents the heart from overfilling with blood. The serous pericardium is composed of two layers and is a closed sac sandwiched between the fibrous pericardium and the heart. Attached to the fibrous pericardium is the parietal layer of serous pericardium. Between the two layers of serous pericardium is a small cavity filled with lubricating fluid. The innermost layer of pericardium is the visceral layer of serous pericardium which is also referred to as **epicardium** where it comes in direct contact with the surface of the heart.

Highlights

The wall of the heart is composed of 3 layers:

1. epicardium
2. myocardium
3. endocardium

To simplify, the layers of pericardium are as follows from outermost to innermost layer: Fibrous pericardium→Parietal layer of serous pericardium→cavity with lubricating fluid→visceral layer of serous pericardium.

The wall of the heart itself is also composed of three different layers: epicardium (outer layer), **myocardium** (middle layer), which is made of muscles (myo-), and **endocardium** (inner layer).

I. TRUE/FALSE.
Mark the following true or false.

1. The serous pericardium holds the heart in position and prevents it from overfilling with blood.
   - ◯ true
   - ◯ false
2. The closed sac between the fibrous pericardium and the heart is the serous pericardium.
   - ◯ true
   - ◯ false
3. Pericardium means away from the heart.
   - ◯ true
   - ◯ false
4. The wall of the heart is made up of the epicardium, myocardium, and endocardium.
   - ◯ true
   - ◯ false
5. The parietal layer adheres to the inside surface of the fibrous pericardium.
   - ◯ true
   - ◯ false

HEART CHAMBERS AND VALVES

Inside the heart are four chambers: the **right and left atria** (plural of atrium) superiorly, and the **right and left ventricles** inferiorly. You have already learned something of the function of the right and left ventricles. While the ventricles pump blood into the arteries, the atria receive venous blood from the veins.

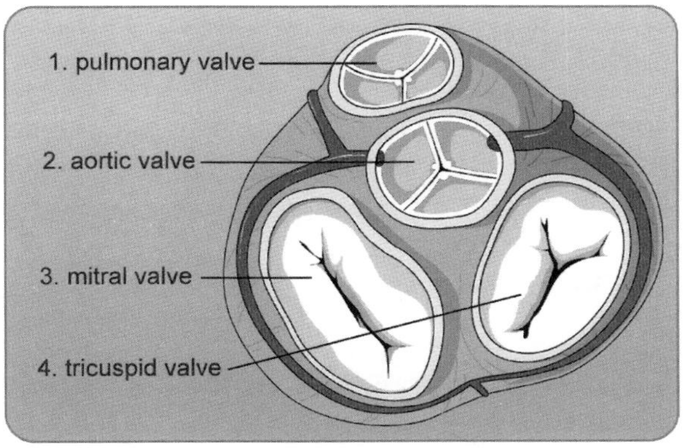

In addition, the heart contains valves that maintain the flow of blood in one direction. (Much like valves in plumbing, the valves of the heart shut out flow from any direction other than the proper one.)

The valves of the heart can be broken into two categories dependent on whether they exist between the atria and the ventricles or between the ventricles and carrying arteries.

Atrioventricular valves: Includes the **tricuspid valve** (located between the right atrium and right ventricle), and the **mitral** or **bicuspid valve** (located between the left atrium and left ventricle).

Semilunar valves: Includes the **aortic valve** (located between the left ventricle and aorta), and the **pulmonary valve** (located between the right ventricle and pulmonary artery).

I. **MULTIPLE CHOICE.**
Choose the best answer.

1. Which of the following is a chamber of the heart? (◯ right ventricle, ◯ semilunar valve)
2. The (◯ ventricles, ◯ atria) pump blood into the arteries.
3. One of the (◯ atrioventricular valves, ◯ semilunar valves) is located between the left ventricle and aorta.
4. The tricuspid valve is a(n) (◯ atrioventricular valve, ◯ semilunar valve).

CONTRACTION AND RHYTHM OF THE HEART

Diastole phase: Blood returning to the heart fills the atria, forcing the atrioventricular valves to hang limply open into the ventricles while the ventricles fill with blood. When the atria contract, more blood is forced into the ventricles.

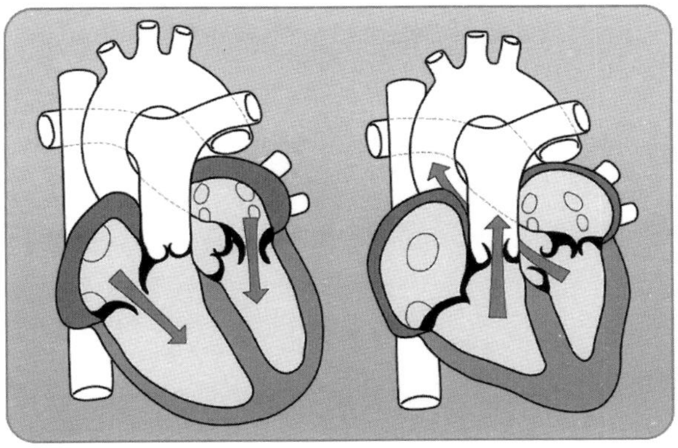

Systole phase: When the ventricles contract, blood is forced against the atrioventricular valves forcing them shut. As this pressure within the ventricles continues to rise, blood is forced up against the semilunar valves, forcing them to open and blood to rush into the arteries. When the ventricular contraction ends, blood flows back from the arteries filling the cusps of the semilunar valves, forcing them shut so that blood cannot flow back into the ventricles the wrong way.

The low pressure now in the ventricles allows the atrioventricular valves to hang open once more, and the cycle begins again. In a normal heartbeat, the atria contract at the same time that the ventricles relax. This sequence of contraction and relaxation of the heart chambers is termed the sinus rhythm.

Additional components of the heart will be illustrated on the following pages. The heart both receives and distributes blood directly through veins and arteries located within the heart. Blood is carried from veins and arteries and into subsidiary vessels throughout the body.

I. MATCHING.
Match the statement to the correct phase.

1. ____ Blood is forced up against the semilunar valves and blood rushes into the arteries.
2. ____ Blood flows back from the arteries and fills the cusps of the semilunar valves.
3. ____ Blood returns to the heart and fills the atria.
4. ____ The ventricles contract and blood forces the atrioventricular valves shut.
5. ____ The atrioventricular valves hang limply open into the ventricles while the ventricles fill with blood.

A. diastole phase
B. systole phase

ARTERIES AND VEINS

As noted, the heart's primary function is the delivery of the blood with its vital nutrients to every cell of the body. This is accomplished through the blood vessels, specifically the **arteries** and the **veins**.

The arteries transport blood away from the heart, and the veins transport blood towards the heart. The arteries feed into progressively smaller vessels and eventually into thousands of **capillaries**. This is where most of the action takes place. All exchanges of gases, nutrients, electrolytes, hormones, and other components actually occur through the capillary walls (which are only one cell thick). The blood flow through the venous system is opposite of that which occurs in the arterial system. In the venous system, blood flows from smaller vessels into progressively larger ones.

Because it is so important to keep the cardiovascular system healthy, its components and various functions are examined regularly as part of any general healthcare examination.

As a result, terms relating to the circulatory system are used often and in many different kinds of reports.

I. MATCHING.
Match the correct term to the definition.

1. ____ carries blood away from the heart
2. ____ carries blood toward the heart
3. ____ where gases, nutrients, etc. are exchanged
4. ____ its primary function is delivery of blood to every cell of the body

A. heart
B. veins
C. arteries
D. capillaries

CARDIOVASCULAR TERMINOLOGY

arteries: Transport blood away from the heart.

basophils: Granular leukocyte.

capillaries: Where exchange of gases, nutrients, electrolytes, hormones, and other components take place.

diastole: Relaxation of the heart chambers.

differential: Part of the complete blood count that includes the type of leukocytes in the blood.

eosinophils: Granular leukocyte.

erythrocytes: One of three basic cells that comprise the cellular portion of the blood (red blood cells).

hematocrit: Percentage of red blood cells in a complete blood count.

hemaglobin: Oxygen-carrying pigment of the erythrocytes.

leukocytes: Another name for white blood cells, their major function is to defend the body against infecting organisms.

lymphocytes: Agranular leukocyte.

mediastinum: Location of the heart.

monocytes: Agranular leukocyte.

neutrophils: Granular leukocyte.

plasma: Fluid portion of the blood.

platelets: Also called thrombocytes, they play a major role in blood clotting.

systole: Contraction of the heart chambers.

thrombocytes: Play a major role in blood clotting.

veins: Transport blood towards the heart.

ventricle: Pumps blood to specific parts of the body. The right ventricle pumps blood to the lungs, and the left ventricle pumps blood to the systemic arteries.

I. MULTIPLE CHOICE.
Choose the best answer.

1. Which of the following is not a granular type leukocyte.
   - ◯ neutrophils
   - ◯ plasma
   - ◯ eosinophils
   - ◯ basophils

2. The heart is located between the lungs in this.
   - ◯ mediastinum
   - ◯ plasma
   - ◯ capillaries
   - ◯ sternum

3. A contraction of the heart is called.
   - ◯ contraction
   - ◯ diastole
   - ◯ systole
   - ◯ asystole

4. The fluid portion of blood.
   - ◯ plasma
   - ◯ blood
   - ◯ leukocytes
   - ◯ platelets

5. Most of the action of the blood actually takes place within these.
   - ◯ platelets
   - ◯ capillaries
   - ◯ hemoglobins
   - ◯ hematocrits

6. Another name for thrombocytes.
   - ◯ platelets
   - ◯ monocytes
   - ◯ leukocytes
   - ◯ hemoglobin

7. Approximately 45% of the total blood volume.
   - ◯ hemoglobin
   - ◯ hematocrit
   - ◯ plasma
   - ◯ megakaryocytes

8. A count that looks at the leukocytes.
   - ◯ distant
   - ◯ differentiation
   - ◯ differential
   - ◯ systole

9. Relaxation of the heart.
   - ◯ systole
   - ◯ diastole
   - ◯ break
   - ◯ rest

10. A type of granular leukocytes.
   - ◯ eosinophils
   - ◯ capillary
   - ◯ osinophils
   - ◯ hemoglobin

11. Red blood cells.
   - ◯ diastole
   - ◯ erythrocytes
   - ◯ megakaryocytes
   - ◯ plasma

12. The oxygen-carrying pigment of the erythrocytes.
   - ◯ platelets
   - ◯ hematocrit
   - ◯ hemoglobin
   - ◯ systole

ARTERIES

The major artery of the heart through which all other arteries arise is called the **aorta**. On the other hand, all veins eventually come together to form the **superior** and **inferior vena cava**, which provide venous blood flow directly into the heart.

The major arteries and veins that lead into and away from the heart will also be illustrated on the following pages.

Naming of the arteries and veins is accomplished in much the same way as the naming of muscles. They are classified according to function and location in the body. You will notice many of the same terms that you have already learned in the chapter on muscles.

For example, near the brachialis muscle is the brachial artery. Also, most arteries have venous counterparts, and thus there are several names common to both the arterial and venous systems. Fortunately, as a general rule, it will not be necessary for you to identify whether the term refers to the vein or the artery.

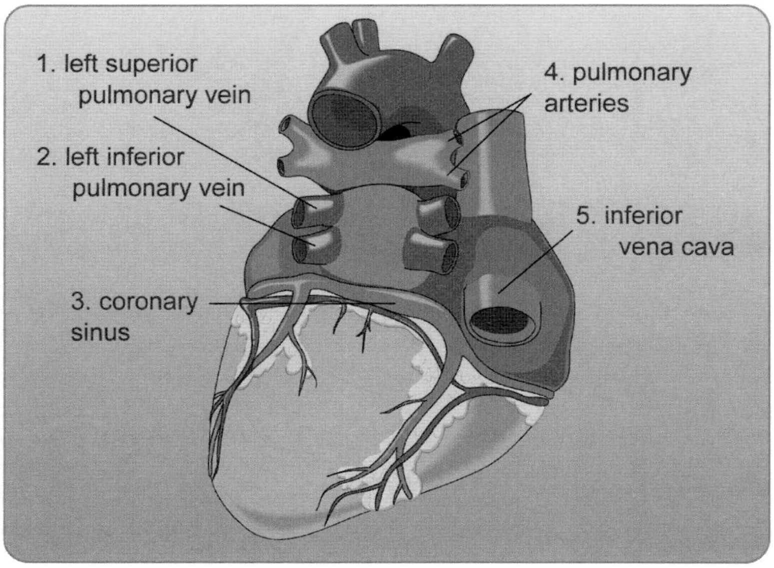

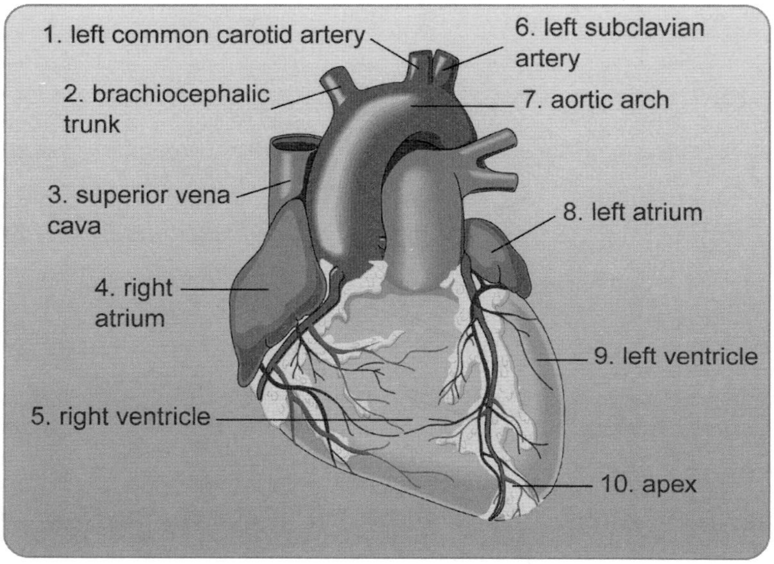

Generally, veins/arteries and structures of the heart are the same on both right and left, so not all of them have been delineated on the figure.

For example, on the opposite side of the first (left) figure there is a corresponding right superior pulmonary vein and right inferior pulmonary vein. Likewise, the pulmonary arteries can be designated right and left (left being opposite the ones labeled).

Another example is how the different vessels in the subclavian region are all labled "subclavian"—making a right subclavian artery, right subclavian vein, left subclavian artery, and left subclavian vein.

I. **FILL IN THE BLANK.**

Enter the correct word in the blank provided.

function
subclavian
the same
aorta

1. The major artery of the heart is called the ________________.
2. Arteries and veins are classified according to ________________ and location in the body.
3. An example of how different blood vessels can be similarly named are the vessels found on both the right and left ________________ region.
4. Veins and arteries are often ________________ on both right and left.

CONDUCTION MECHANISM OF THE HEART

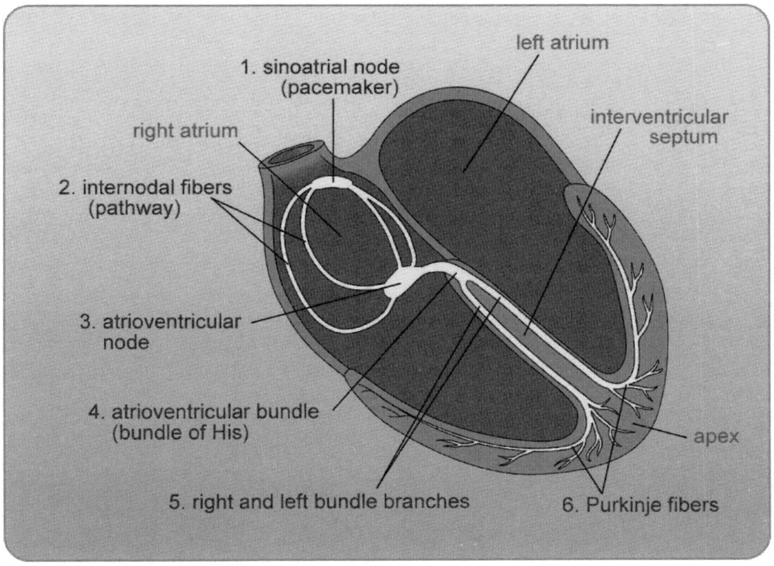

The myocardial fibers that make up the conduction system of the heart are modified cardiac muscle tissue. This means they do not contract like other cardiac muscle tissue. Instead they only allow generation of an action potential through the heart.

There are six components of the conduction system of the heart:

1. **sinoatrial node (pacemaker)** – origin of impulse/heartbeat
2. **internodal fibers (pathway)** – pathway through atria for electrical impulse
3. **atrioventricular node** – impulse delayed before sending to bundle of His
4. **atrioventricular bundle (bundle of His)** – runs through interventricular septum, then divides
5. **right and left bundle branches** – carry impulse into bundles of Purkinje fibers
6. **Purkinje fibers** – carry impulse towards apex of heart and into ventricles on either side

The initiation of each heartbeat begins at the **sinoatrial node** (pacemaker). The sinoatrial node is a mass of cells that lies in the wall of the right atrium, just inferior to the entrance of the superior vena cava. The basic heart rate is determined by the sinoatrial node and generally reaches 70–80 beats per minute.

Impulses from the sinoatrial node spread in a wave pattern along cardiac muscle and the internodal pathway to the atrioventricular node located in the inferior portion of the right atrium. Here the impulses are delayed for a millisecond before they race through the **atrioventricular bundle** (Bundle of His), which then runs through the interventricular septum.

At this point the signal continues through to the bundle branches that then divide with the signal going to both the right and left sides of the bundle branches. About halfway down the interventricular septum, the **bundle branches** (also known as crura or “legs”), become bundles of **Purkinje fibers**. These Purkinje fibers approach the apex of the heart and turn upwards (superiorly) into the walls of the ventricles on either side.

A fibrous skeleton exists between the atria and the ventricles. This fibrous skeleton is nonconductive and, therefore, prevents the impulses sent via the sinoatrial node from running directly through the atria and into the ventricles. This nonconductive barrier ensures proper contraction sequencing of the heart.

The slight delay of the impulse at the atrioventricular node allows just enough time for the atria to fill the ventricles adequately before ventricular contraction begins.

I. **MATCHING.**
In the blanks provided below, refer to the image and enter the letter for the corresponding term to the following numbers.

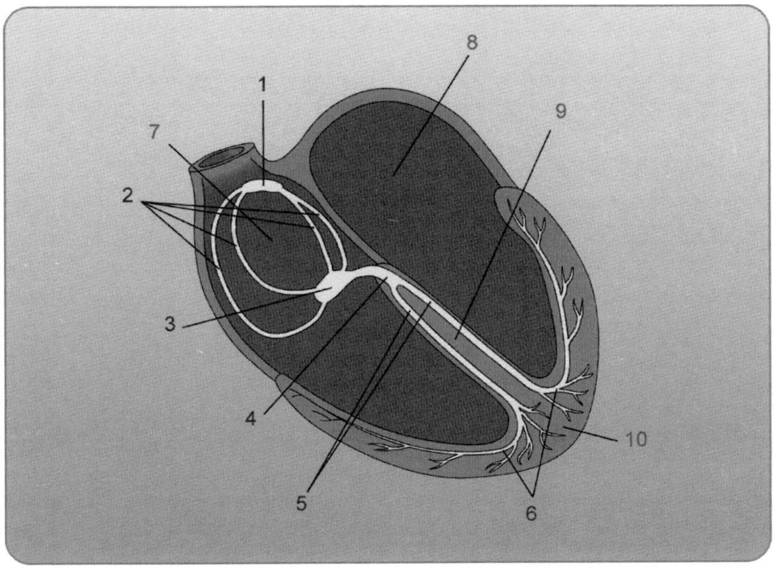

Conduction System:

1. ____
2. ____
3. ____
4. ____
5. ____
6. ____

Heart structures:

7. ____
8. ____
9. ____
10. ____

A. interventicular septum
B. atrioventricular node
C. internodal fibers (pathway)
D. right and left bundle branches
E. sinoatrial node (pacemaker)
F. Purkinje fibers
G. right atrium
H. apex
I. left atrium
J. atrioventricular bundle (bundle of His)

INTERNAL STRUCTURES OF THE HEART

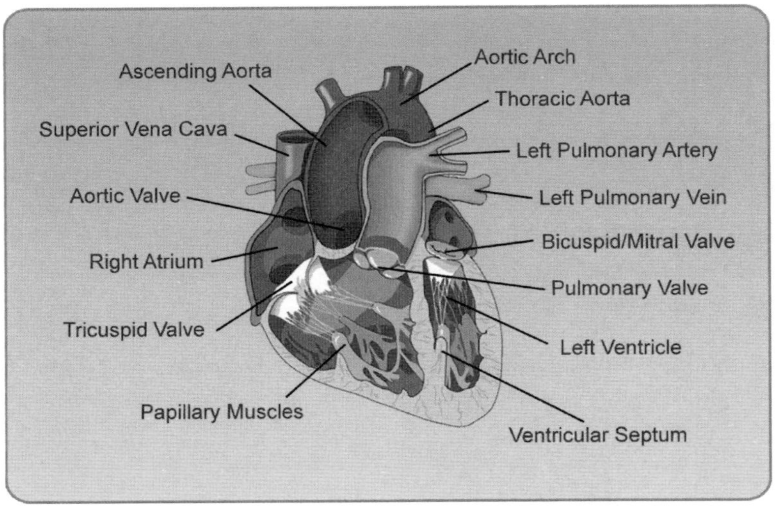

The right and left sides of the heart are divided by an internal wall of tissue called the **septum.** The area of the septum that divides the atria is called the atrial or inter-atrial septum. The area of the septum that divides the ventricles is called the ventricular or interventricular septum.

Within the vetnricles are the **papillary muscles**, which are connected to the cusps of the atrioventricular valves by cord-like tendons called the **cordae tendinea**. These help to prevent the prolapse of the valves so that they can continue to function properly.

BLOOD CIRCULATION

After the body's organs and tissues have used the oxygen in the blood, the vena cavae carry the oxygen-poor blood back to the right atrium of the heart. The **superior vena cava** carries oxygen-poor blood from the upper parts of your body, including your head, chest, arms, and neck. The **inferior vena cava** carries oxygen-poor blood from the lower parts of your body. The blood circulates through the right atrium to the right ventricle and exits the heart via the pulmonary artery, on its way to the lungs.

Highlights

The precise location of veins is much more variable from person to person than that of arteries.

The blood picks up oxygen from the lungs and returns the oxygen-rich blood to the heart via the **pulmonary veins**.

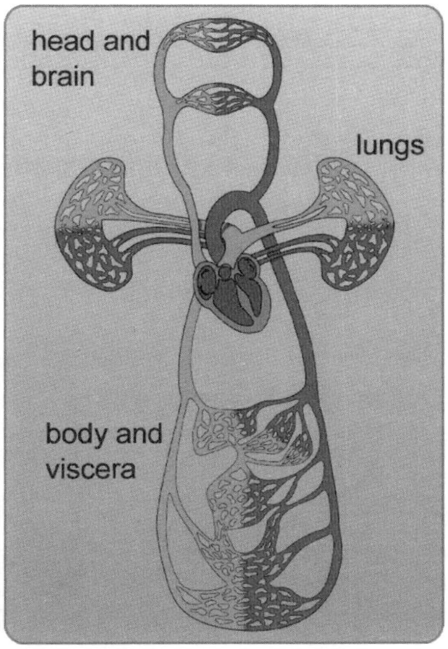

The oxygen-poor blood from the vena cava flows into the heart's right atrium and then on to the right ventricle. From the right ventricle, the blood is pumped through the pulmonary arteries (in blue in the center of the picture) to your lungs. There, through many small, thin blood vessels called capillaries, the blood picks up more oxygen.

The oxygen-rich blood passes from your lungs back to your heart through the pulmonary veins, into the left atrium. It then flows through the left ventricle and out the aorta to the rest of the body.

Oxygen-rich blood is forced into the large arteries from the heart. It then moves into successively smaller arteries, finally reaching their smallest branches, the **arterioles**, that feed into the capillary beds of body organs and tissues. Only the **capillaries** come into intimate contact with tissue cells and directly serve cellular needs, leaving oxygen nutrient proteins.

The normal cardiac circulation from the body, through the heart, and back to the body is: blood enters the right atrium > blood flows through tricuspid valve > blood enters right ventricle > blood flows through pulmonary valve > blood goes through the pulmonary artery to the lungs > blood enters left atrium > blood flows through mitral valve > blood enters left ventricle > blood flows through aortic valve > blood is distributed by the aorta to the body.

The largest artery in the body is the **aorta**, and the largest vein is the vena cava. A general "rule of thumb" to remember the difference between arteries and veins is that arteries carry blood away from the heart and veins carry blood to the heart. There is, however, an exception. **Portal veins** carry blood between capillary beds. For example, the hepatic portal vein takes blood from the capillary beds in the digestive tract and transports it to the capillary beds in the liver. From the liver the blood flows into the inferior vena cava and then back to the heart.

I. MATCHING.
Match the correct term to the definition.

1. ____ portal vein
2. ____ aorta
3. ____ vena cava

A. largest artery in the body
B. vein that does not directly connect to the vena cava
C. largest vein in the body

REVIEW: THE HEART

I. MATCHING.
In the blanks below, refer to the image and enter the letter for the corresponding term to the following numbers.

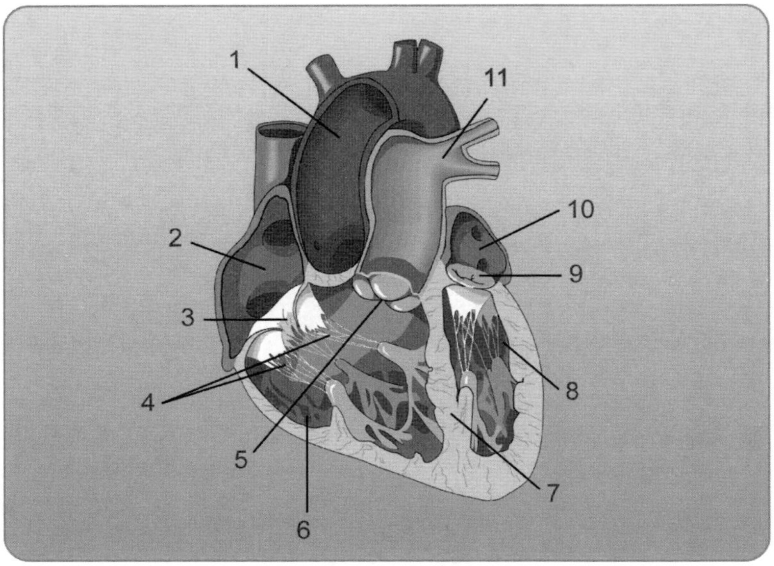

1. ____
2. ____
3. ____
4. ____
5. ____
6. ____
7. ____
8. ____
9. ____
10. ____
11. ____

A. pulmonary valve
B. left atrium
C. mitral valve
D. left ventricle
E. right atrium
F. left plumonary artery
G. tricuspid valve
H. aorta
I. chordae tendinae
J. ventricular septum
K. right ventricle

II. MATCHING.

Number the steps below as they occur during normal cardiac circulation from the body, beginning with deoxygenated blood returning to the heart.

1. ____
2. ____
3. ____
4. ____
5. ____
6. ____
7. ____
8. ____
9. ____
10. ____

A. blood is distributed by the aorta to the body
B. blood flows through tricuspid valve
C. blood enters right ventricle
D. blood flows through mitral valve
E. blood enters the right atrium
F. blood enters left ventricle
G. blood flows through pulmonary valve
H. blood goes through the pulmonary artery to the lungs
I. blood enters left atrium
J. blood flows through aortic valve

ARTERIES AND VEINS

You have been exposed to an abundance of information about the cardiovascular (circulatory) system, its attributes, and its functions. Do not allow yourself to be overwhelmed by all the information.

We will start with the arteries because this is where the blood begins its journey. Look for clues to help you learn the terms, such as nearby muscles or bones from which the names are derived.

We will start with an inspection of the aorta and go from the top of the body and work our way down. Be aware that the veins and arteries branch from the center outward, upward, and downward, and therefore the largest structures are those closest to the heart itself. This is discussed in greater detail later.

The terms that you will be learning in the rest of this section are by no means all of the arteries and veins in the body. However, you should have a much better idea of the major arteries, which are the ones most likely to be affected by procedures and operations and to show up on x-rays. Of course, the greater your exposure to and familiarity with the most commonly used terms, the easier it will be for you to search out the ones that are used only rarely.

ARTERIES OVERVIEW

The aorta is the largest artery of the body and the main conduit for circulating oxygen-rich blood to the rest of the body. All systemic arteries branch off this main *trunk*. Different sections of the aorta are named according to their location. The **ascending aorta** is the beginning of the aorta that arises from the left ventricle. The **aortic arch** is where the aorta turns 180 degrees downward, where it becomes known as the **descending aorta**. The **thoracic aorta** passes through the thoracic cavity and the part that is located in the abdominal cavity is called the **abdominal aorta**. As with the aorta, the arteries are named for their anatomical location, function, or organ that they supply.

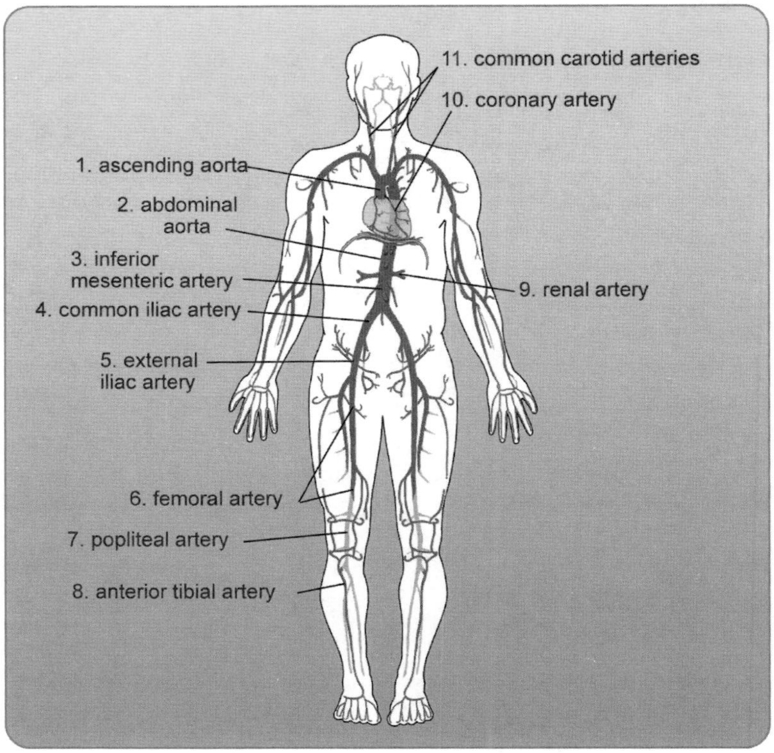

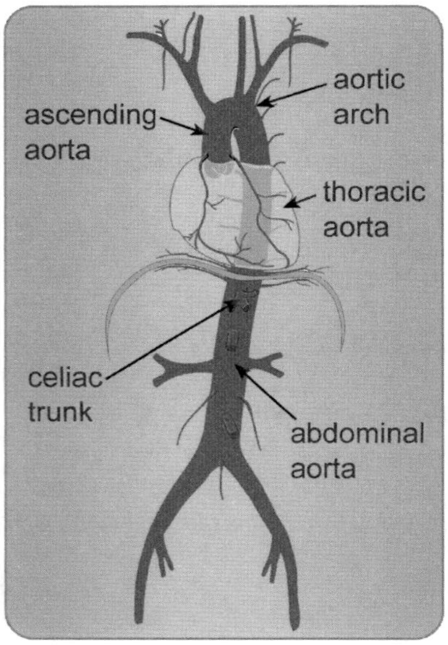

Three main vessels diverge superiorly from the aortic arch. From the patient's right to left they are the **brachiocephalic trunk**, the **left common carotid** and the **left subclavian** arteries. The brachiocephalic trunk quickly branches into the **right subclavian artery** and the **right common carotid artery**, which along with its counterpart the left common carotid supply oxygen rich blood to the brain, head and neck.

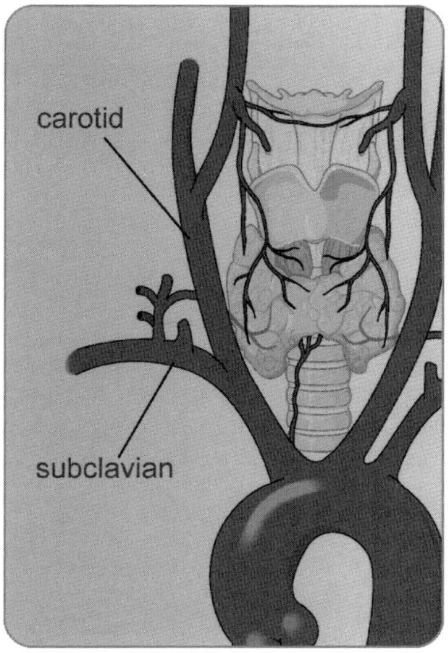

For more information about the arteries and the Circulatory System, visit: www.nhlbi.nih.gov.

I. MULTIPLE CHOICE.
Choose the best answer.

1. The part of the aorta that originates from the left ventricle is the _____.
   - ◯ descending aorta
   - ◯ ascending aorta
   - ◯ aortic arch
   - ◯ thoracic aorta

2. The carotid arteries branch directly from the _____.
   - ◯ descending aorta
   - ◯ ascending aorta
   - ◯ aortic arch
   - ◯ thoracic aorta

3. All system arteries branch from the _____.
   - ◯ Circle of Willis
   - ◯ abdominal aorta
   - ◯ descending aorta
   - ◯ aorta

ARTERIES OF THE BRAIN

The main arteries that provide blood to the brain (left and right common carotid) branch off the aortic arch. It would seem appropriate that the brain receives the most oxygen-rich blood, due to its need for a constant supply of adequate oxygen levels to maintain vital functions such as heart beat, respiration, etc. Similar to the cranial nerves, these arteries and their connection to the brain are very complex.

The Circle of Willis is named after Thomas Willis, who is also credited with coining the term *mellitus* as in diabetes mellitus.

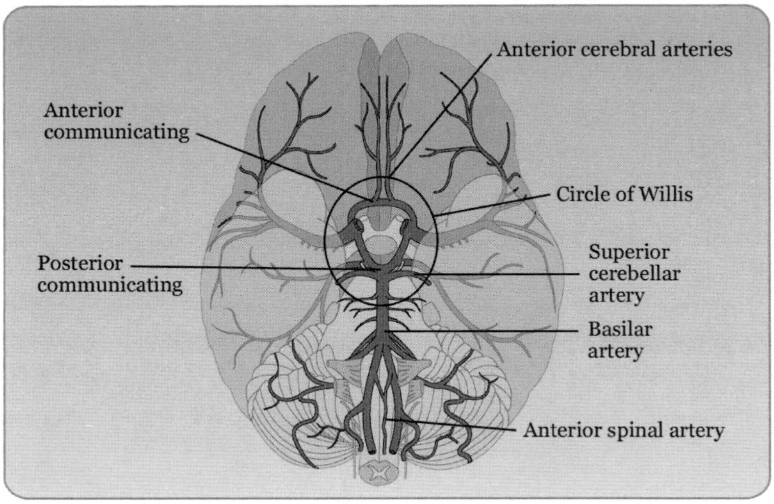

One unique structure in the vascular tissue of the brain is the **cerebral arterial circle (Circle of Willis)**, which is where the **internal carotid arteries** (shown on the next page) branch into smaller arteries that supply blood to over 80% of the cerebrum. This structure is important in that it provides alternate paths of blood circulation to the brain should one of the other arteries in the circle become occluded.

I. MULTIPLE CHOICE.
Choose the best answer.

1. Most of the blood to the cerebrum is supplied by the _____.
   - ◯ Circle of Willis
   - ◯ ascending aorta
   - ◯ descending aorta
   - ◯ aortic arch

2. The _____ provides an alternative blood flow in case of occlusion of one of the main intracranial arteries.
   - ◯ vertebral artery
   - ◯ Circle of Willis
   - ◯ anterior spinal artery
   - ◯ internal carotid artery

ARTERIES OF THE HEAD AND NECK

The arteries depicted have the important task of carrying oxygen to the brain. The human brain cannot go for more than a few minutes without proper blood flow before severe results occur.

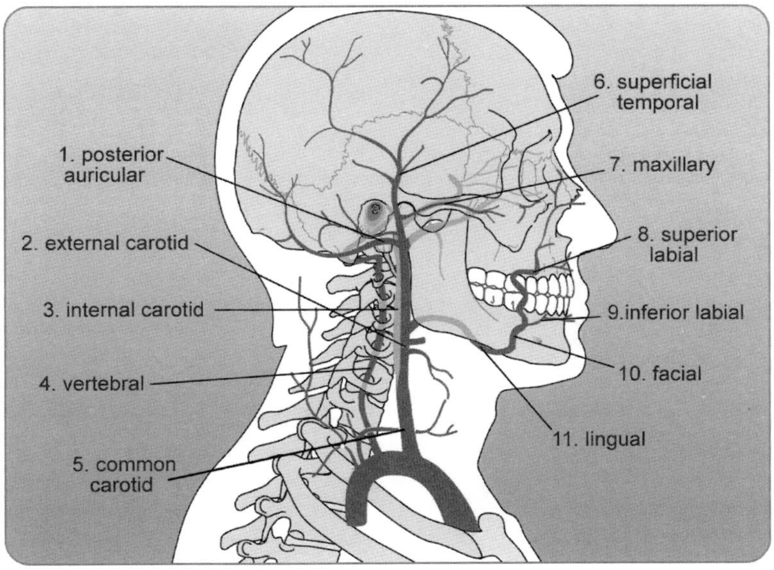

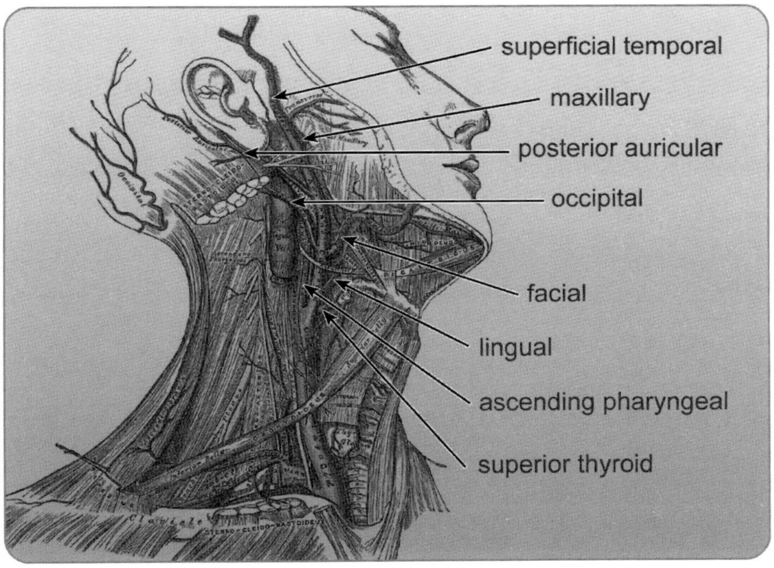

Most structures of the body that have an "inferior" have a corresponding "superior" that may not be listed. You should also take notice of terms such as *ophthalmic*, which means "pertaining to the eye" and *auricular*, which means "pertaining to the ear."

I. FILL IN THE BLANK.

In the blanks provided below, refer to the image and enter the term corresponding to the following numbers. Use the word(s) in the box to fill in the blanks.

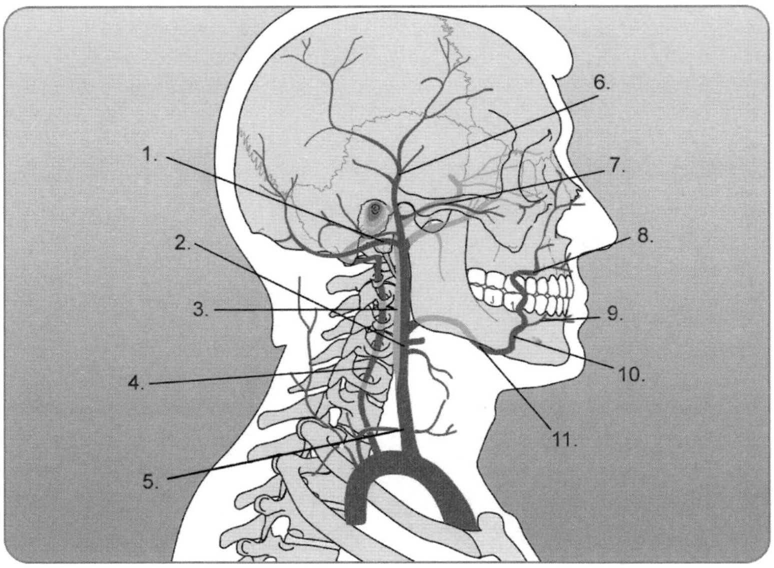

1. ________________
2. ________________
3. ________________
4. ________________
5. ________________
6. ________________
7. ________________
8. ________________
9. ________________
10. ________________
11. ________________

inferior labial
external carotid
lingual
superficial temporal
vertebral
facial
maxillary
posterior auricular
internal carotid
superior labial
common carotid

II. MULTIPLE CHOICE.
Choose the best answer.

1. A term meaning pertaining to the eye.
   - ◯ vetebral
   - ◯ ophthalmic
   - ◯ auricular
   - ◯ external

2. The artery that passes through the vertebrae.
   - ◯ vertebral
   - ◯ facial
   - ◯ femoric
   - ◯ spinal

3. The artery that runs in the front of the face.
   - ◯ mandibular
   - ◯ vertebral
   - ◯ facial
   - ◯ auricular

4. Arteries above and below the lips.
   - ◯ lipeal
   - ◯ labial
   - ◯ oral
   - ◯ ophthalmic

5. Means pertaining to the ear.
   - ◯ auricular
   - ◯ oriccle
   - ◯ stapedial
   - ◯ laryngeal

ARTERY LOCATIONS

As you work your way from the center down the body, you will see that the arteries divide into increasingly smaller branches. If you have ever seen figures or images of the arteries throughout the body, this is apparent. It becomes harder to distinguish individual arteries the smaller they get. For illustrative purposes, here is a figure depicting the major arteries of the body. Smaller and more minor ones are not pictured at all.

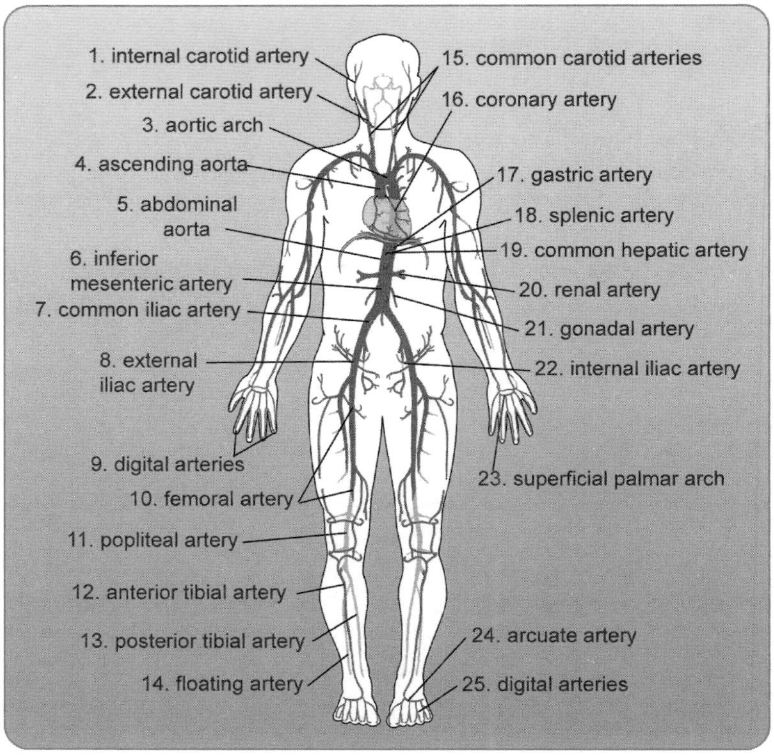

It will not be necessary for you to identify each and every artery pictured in the above image or the many more arteries too small to appear. In an effort to make this section of your training a little easier on the eyes and less cumbersome, the arteries have been broken out by general body area, and several exercises have been included to assist you in retaining the information.

ARTERIES OF THE UPPER BODY - ARMS AND SHOULDERS

The first major aortic branches that serve the upper arms are the right and left **subclavian arteries**. It is formed on the right from the brachiocephalic trunk, and on the left directly from the aortic arch. The subclavian arteries pass laterally and, as suggested by their name, inferior to the clavicle. Major branches of the subclavian artery prior to reaching the upper extremity are the **costocervical trunk**, **dorsal scapular artery** and the **internal thoracic artery**.

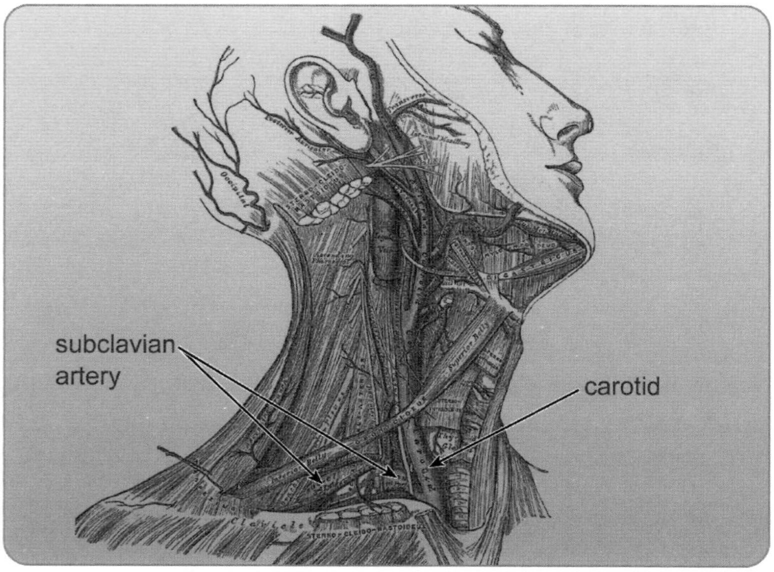

As the subclavian comes near the "armpit" it is called the axillary artery. Branches of the axillary artery include the **subscapular artery** as well as the **lateral thoracic artery**, which courses inferiorly to supply lateral structures of the chest and breast.

The **axillary artery** enters the upper extremity and branches into the **ulnar**, **radial** and **superficial palmar**. The ulnar artery branches into the anterior and posterior ulnar recurrent arteries as well as the **common interosseous artery**.

Note: not all vessels described are depicted in the images on this page. **Refer to your 3M Reference** on the left hand side of the page. Click on "Elsevier's Anatomy Plates", then "1 Circulatory System", then "Arteries of the Upper Limb."

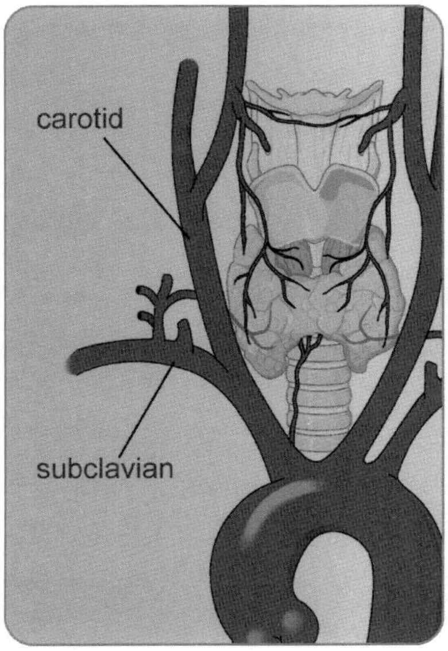

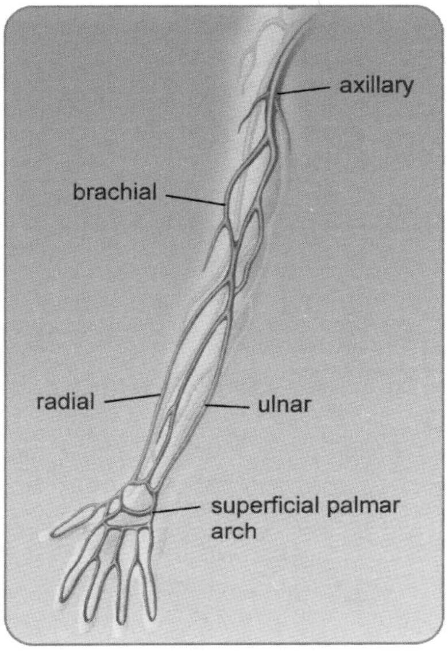

ARTERIES OF THE UPPER EXTREMITY - LESSON 1

axillary: Passes underneath the armpit, carries blood to the arm.

brachial: Enters the upper arm region.

deltoid branch: Supplies the deltoid muscle.

humeral circumflex: There is both a posterior and anterior humeral circumflex artery, wrapped around the humerus.

deep brachial: Both the deep brachial and superficial brachial arteries are branches of the brachial artery. They supply blood to the arm.

ulnar collateral: There are both superior and inferior ulnar collateral arteries. They are branches of the brachial artery. They supply blood to the triceps and elbow.

medial collateral: This is a branch of the deep brachial artery and also supplies the triceps muscle and elbow joint.

radial collateral: Also a branch of the deep brachial artery, the radial collateral supplies the brachioradialis and brachialis muscles.

ulnar recurrent: There are both posterior and anterior branches of the ulnar recurrent artery. These supply the elbow joint region.

radial recurrent: This is a branch of the radial artery which supplies the brachioradialis, brachialis, and elbow region.

interosseous: There are several interosseous arteries, including the common interosseous, posterior interosseous, anterior interosseous, and recurrent interosseous. They distribute blood to various places within the arm. The word means "between bones."

ARTERIES OF THE UPPER EXTREMITY - LESSON 2

radial: This is a fairly major artery off of the brachial artery. It supplies blood to the forearm, wrist, and hand.

ulnar: Also, a fairly major artery off of the brachial artery, which distributes blood to the forearm, wrist, and hand.

dorsal carpal branch of ulnar: The name describes a specific branch of the ulnar artery. You already are familiar with dorsal and carpal, so you should be able to figure out where the blood supply goes.

superficial palmar branch of radial: As with the one above, this name is self-descriptive.

palmar arch: There are both deep and superficial palmar arches, which supply the hand and specifically the palm.

metacarpals: There are both palmar and dorsal metacarpal arteries. These supply the metacarpals.

common palmar digitals: This artery and the following two arteries all supply the digits (fingers).

proper palmar digitals: Supplies the fingers.

dorsal digitals: Supplies the fingers.

princeps pollicis: This is the principal artery of the thumb.

radialis indicis: This is the radial artery of the index finger. It specifically supplies the index finger (first digit).

REVIEW: ARTERIES OF THE UPPER EXTREMITY

I. FILL IN THE BLANK.

Use the word(s) in the box to fill in the blanks.

common palmar digitals
ulnar recurrent
interosseous
brachial
princeps pollicis
deep brachial
humeral circumflex
metacarpal
palmar arch
radial

1. As the subclavian artery passes through different structures of the body, its name changes three times to become the axillary artery, ________________ artery, and the deltoid branch.
2. The ________________ is the artery that is wrapped around the humerus.
3. Both the ________________ and superficial brachial arteries are branches of the brachial artery. They supply blood to the arm.
4. There are both posterior and anterior branches of the ________________ artery. These supply the elbow joint region.
5. There are several ________________ arteries, including the common, posterior, anterior, and recurrent. They distribute blood to various places within the arm. The word means "between bones."
6. There is both a deep and superficial ________________ that supply the hand and specifically the palm.
7. There are both palmar and dorsal ________________ arteries. These supply the metacarpals.
8. The ________________ and the proper palmar digitals and dorsal digitals all supply the digits (fingers).
9. The ________________ is the principal artery of the thumb.
10. Two fairly major arteries that distribute blood to the forearm, wrist, and hand are the ulnar and ________________ arteries.

ARTERIES OF THE HEART

As with any muscle in the body, the heart needs oxygen-rich blood to function properly. There are arteries located on the external surface of the heart called the **coronary arteries** that supply oxygen to the heart. They are the first branches of the aorta. There are two main coronary arteries: the left and right. On the left the main artery further branches into the **left circumflex artery**, **left marginal artery**, and **left anterior descending artery**. The right main coronary artery further divides into the **right marginal branch**. There are many variances to additional branching, but these are the main coronary arteries found in most humans.

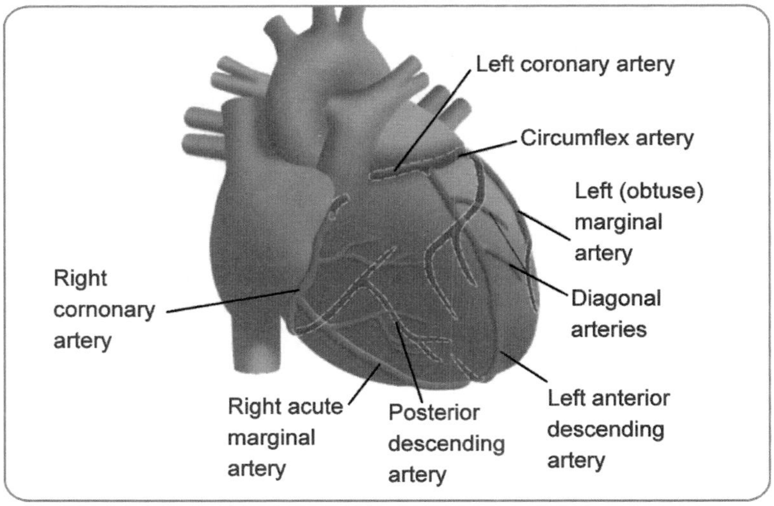

AORTA AND THORACIC ARTERIES

The aorta is the largest artery of the body and the main conduit for circulating oxygen-rich blood to the rest of the body. All systemic arteries branch off this main *trunk*. Different sections of the aorta are named according to their location. The **ascending aorta** is the beginning of the aorta that arises from the left ventricle. The **aortic arch** is where the aorta turns 180 degrees downward, where it becomes known as the **descending aorta**. The **thoracic aorta** passes through the thoracic cavity and the part that is located in the abdominal cavity is called the **abdominal aorta**. As with the aorta, the arteries are named for their anatomical location, function, or organ that they supply.

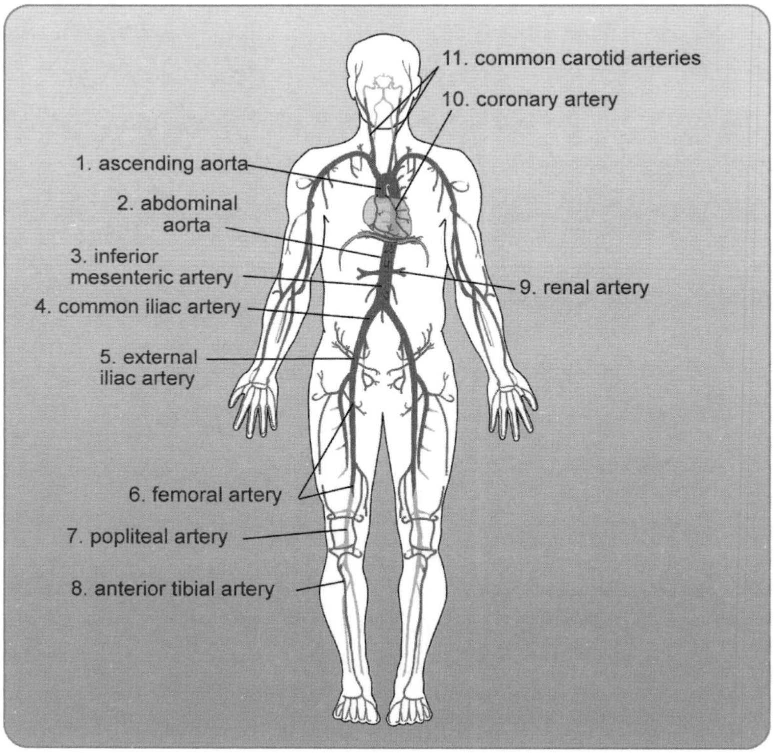

The thoracic aorta gives rise to some arteries vital to digestion and respiration. The **esophageal arteries** are a series of four or five vessels emerging from the front of the aorta to supply blood to the esophagus. The **bronchial arteries** also arise from the thoracic aorta to supply blood to the bronchi, bronchioles, visceral pleura and connective tissue of the lungs. The lower part of the thoracic aorta gives rise to the **superior phrenic artery**, which supplies the diaphragm.

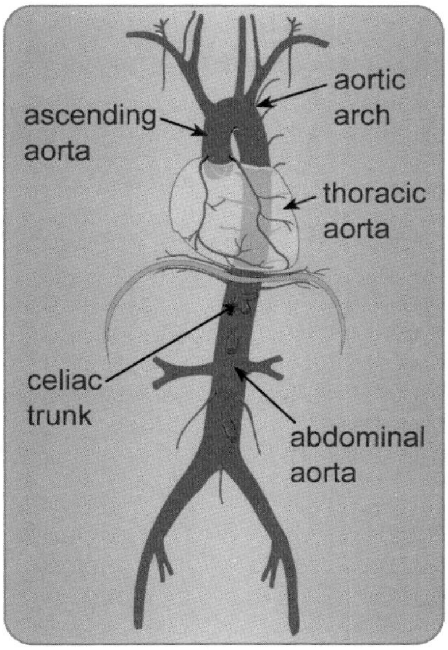

In addition to these arteries of the thorax you can view more detail by clicking on your 3M Reference on the left hand side of the page, then click on "Elsevier's Anatomy Plates", select "1 Circulatory System", then "Arteries of the thorax and axilla." Use this detailed plate to locate the following arteries of the thorax: **internal thoracic**, **superior epigastric**, **thoracoacromial**, **thoracodorsal**, and **intercostal**.

For more information about the arteries and the Circulatory System, visit: www.nhlbi.nih.gov.

I. MULTIPLE CHOICE.
Choose the best answer.

1. The part of the aorta that originates from the left ventricle is the _____.
   - ◯ descending aorta
   - ◯ ascending aorta
   - ◯ aortic arch
   - ◯ thoracic aorta

2. The carotid arteries branch directly from the _____.
   - ◯ descending aorta
   - ◯ ascending aorta
   - ◯ aortic arch
   - ◯ thoracic aorta

3. All system arteries branch from the _____.
   - ◯ Circle of Willis
   - ◯ abdominal aorta
   - ◯ descending aorta
   - ◯ aorta

ARTERIES OF THE LOWER BODY – ABDOMEN AND TRUNK

As the **abdominal aorta** descends, it divides further into the visceral and parietal branches. The *visceral branch* carries blood to the peritoneum, which covers the abdominal organs and the *parietal* to the peritoneum that covers the abdominal cavity.

The **visceral division** further divides into the **celiac**, **superior mesenteric**, **suprarenal**, **renal**, **gonadal**, and **inferior mesenteric arteries**.

The **parietal branches** are the **inferior phrenic**, **lumbar**, and **median sacral arteries**.

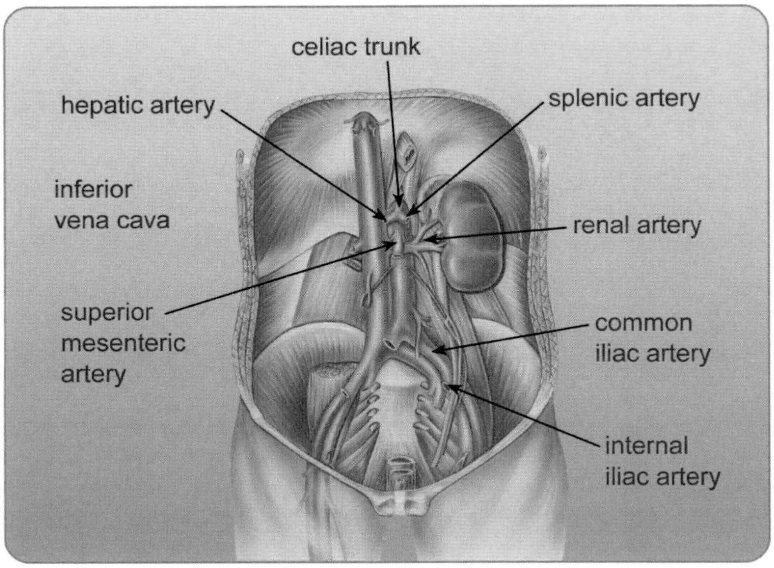

The **superior mesenteric artery** (SMA) supplies the intestine from the lower part of the duodenum through two-thirds of the transverse colon, as well as the pancreas.

The **inferior mesenteric artery** supplies the large intestine from the left splenic flexure to the upper part of the rectum.

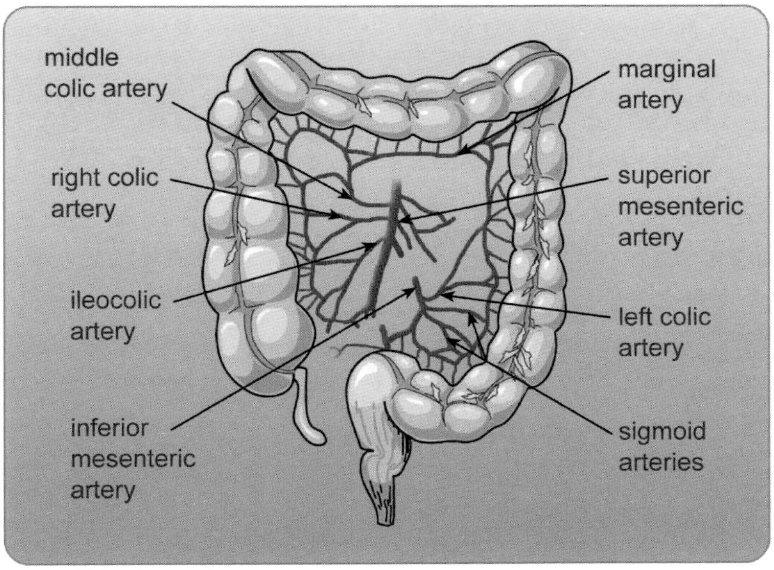

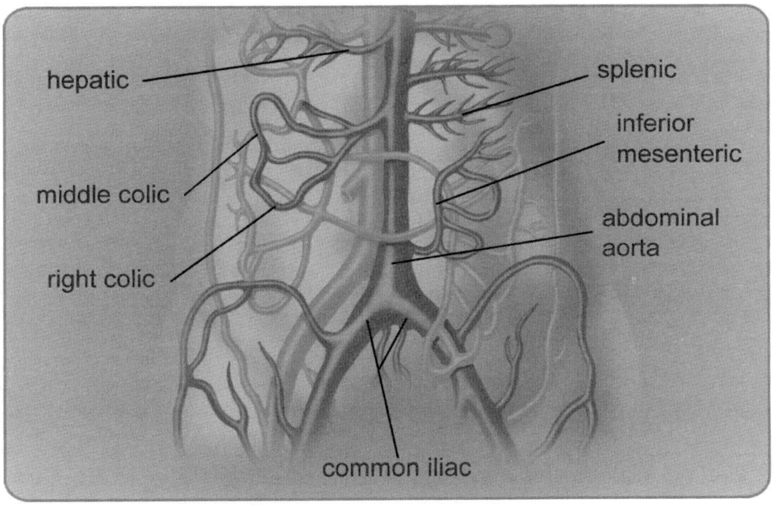

Using the images above and your 3M Reference Elsevier's Anatomy plates locate the following arteries:

- inferior suprarenal
- ileal
- ileocolic
- jejunal
- left and right gastric
- splenic
- common hepatic

ARTERIES OF THE LOWER BODY - LOWER EXTREMITIES

Just above the level of the sacrum, the aorta bifurcates into the **common iliac arteries** which further divide into the **external** and **internal iliac arteries**. The external iliac branches into the **femoral**, **popliteal**, **anterior tibial**, **posterior tibial**, and **plantar arch arteries**.

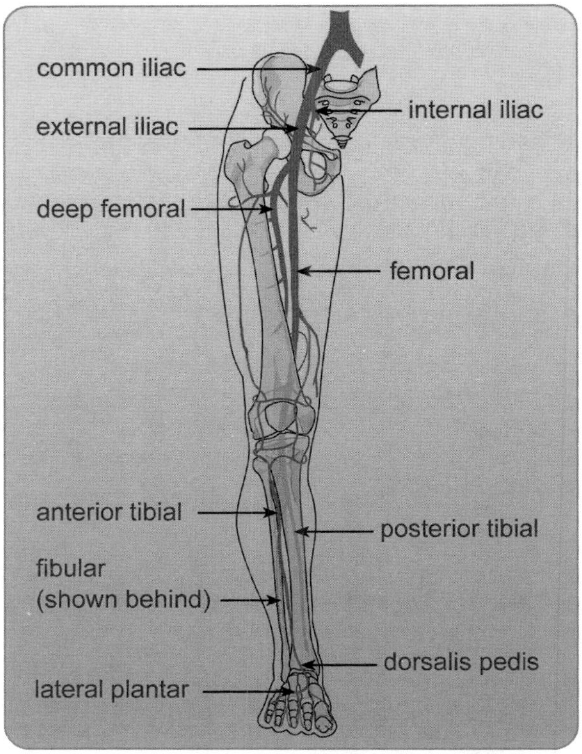

The internal iliac, formerly hypogastric, has both visceral and parietal branches, similar to the abdominal aorta. The visceral branches are the **middle rectal**, **vaginal** and **uterine**. The parietal branches are the **lateral sacral**, **superior gluteal**, **obturator**, **internal pudendal**, and **inferior gluteal**.

Thus, the external iliacs supply the legs and the internal iliacs supply the hips and pelvic region.

Use your 3M Reference Elsevier's Anatomy plates to locate the bolded arteries on this page, the following 2 terminology pages, as well as the **ileocolic**, **ileolumbar**, and **inferior epigastric**.

Remember, while you have been exposed to many new anatomical names, many of the arteries that we have identified have corresponding veins that share the same names!

The fibular artery is also known as the peroneal artery.

ARTERIES OF THE LOWER EXTREMITY - LESSON 1

common iliac arteries: The right and left common iliac arteries arise from the dorsal aorta in the posterior pelvic area. These pass down and divide into the internal and external iliac arteries.

internal iliac: This artery supplies the gluteal muscles and the organs of the pelvic region.

external iliac: This artery passes out of the pelvic cavity underneath the inguinal ligament. At this point, it becomes the femoral artery.

femoral: This is the major artery from which several other vessels arise. It is derived from the word "femur" for the femur bone in that area. There are several branches of the femoral artery that also are named for it: medial femoral circumflex, lateral femoral circumflex, common femoral, superficial femoral, deep femoral.

iliac circumflex: There is both a superficial and a deep iliac circumflex artery. These are near in proximity to the ilium bone.

gluteal: There are both superior and inferior gluteal arteries, which supply blood to the gluteal region.

sacral: There are both lateral and median sacral arteries. They supply the sacrum, coccyx, and rectum.

pudendal: There are both internal and external pudendal arteries. These were also covered in the arteries of the torso.

obturator: This arises off the internal iliac and supplies the pelvic muscles and hip joints.

perforating: There are three perforating arteries. These arise off the deep femoral artery and perforate (which means to pierce or bore through) the adductor magnus muscle to reach the back of the thigh. They supply the adductor, hamstring, gluteal muscles, and femur.

genicular: There are several genicular arteries, including the descending genicular, inferior lateral genicular, inferior medial genicular, middle genicular, superior lateral genicular, and superior medial genicular. The name is derived from the root word genu meaning "knee."

ARTERIES OF THE LOWER EXTREMITY - LESSON 2

popliteal: The femoral artery becomes the popliteal artery as it passes across the back of the knee. It is a large artery with several branches. It supplies the calf region.

sural: This artery arises off the popliteal and supplies the calf region.

tibial: There are anterior and posterior tibial arteries, as well as anterior tibial recurrent. The name is derived from the tibia bone.

fibular: The fibular artery comes off the posterior tibial artery and has several branches, including a fibular circumflex branch. It supplies the ankle and deep calf muscles.

peroneal: The term peroneal literally means pertaining to the fibula or outer side of the leg. It is very important not to confuse this term with perineal, which is derived from perineum and refers to the "region between the thighs." There is both a peroneal and a perforating peroneal artery.

malleolar: The term malleolus refers to a rounded protuberance, as you have learned previously. Usually when it is used in medical reports it is referring to the ankle. There is a medial malleolar branch, a lateral malleolar branch, a medial anterior malleolar artery and a lateral anterior malleolar artery. They all basically supply the region of the ankle joint.

dorsal of foot: This is a continuation of the anterior tibial artery. It distributes blood to the foot and toes. The pulsation of blood through this artery is called the dorsalis pedis pulse, and is often checked on examinations.

tarsal: There is a lateral tarsal artery and a medial tarsal artery. They distribute to the tarsus, which is the region between the foot and the leg.

plantar: There is a deep plantar artery, an external plantar artery, a lateral plantar artery, and medial plantar artery. These supply the sole of the foot.

arcuate: This arises off the dorsal artery of the foot and supplies the foot and toes. The term arcuate means literally "shaped like an arc" and you may see this term used elsewhere.

metatarsals: There are both dorsal and plantar metatarsal arteries. Both of these descriptive terms should be familiar to you. These arteries distribute blood to the toes.

VEINS OF THE CARDIOVASCULAR SYSTEM

The blood flow through the venous system is opposite of that which occurs in the arterial system. In the venous system, blood flows from smaller vessels (venules) into progressively larger ones. There are more veins than there are arteries, both deep and superficial. The superficial veins are those that are visible on most people closest to the surface of the skin (especially on the wrists). Some people's veins even protrude above the level of the skin. It is through these **superficial veins** that blood is drawn or intravenous injections are administered. The **deep veins** are close to the arteries and are generally similarly named.

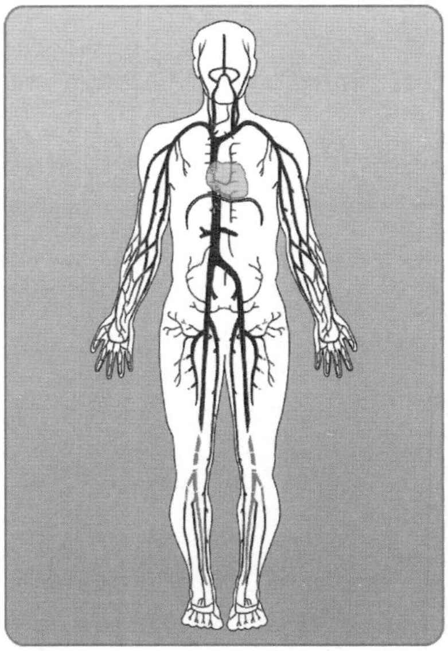

Venous Sinuses	
Venous Sinus	**Area Drained**
Superior Sagittal Sinus	Cerebral hemispheres
Inferior Sagittal Sinus	Medial surfaces of the cerebral hemispheres
Straight Sinus	Deep parts of cerebrum, cerebellum
Occipital Sinus	Cerebellum
Transverse Sinus	Brain
Cavernous Sinus	Orbit and brain
Superior and Inferior Petrosal Sinuses	All regions drained by cavernous sinus, orbit and brain
Sigmoid Sinus	Brain and meninges

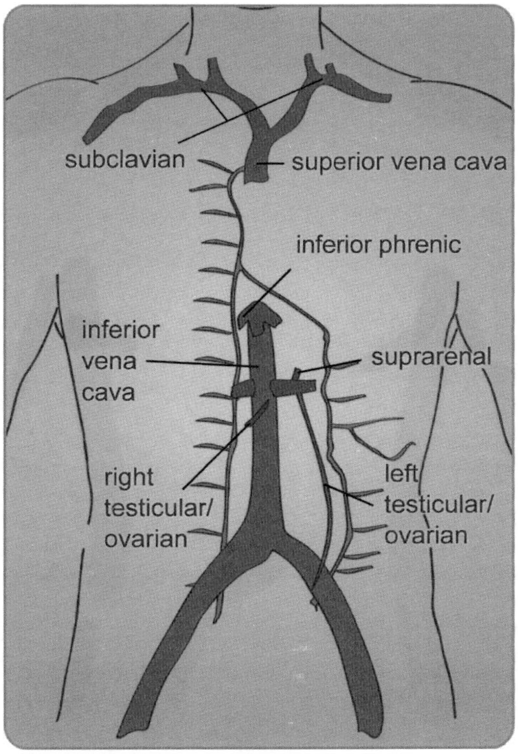

Blood flow of the veins is carried toward the heart. Eventually, all veins of the body, except for the pulmonary veins, converge into two major vessels that empty into the right atrium. These are the **superior vena cava** and the **inferior vena cava**. Deoxygenated blood from the head, neck, upper extremities, and thoracic cavity (excluding the lungs) drains into the superior vena cava. The inferior vena cava transports deoxygenated blood from the lower extremities and abdomen.

The veins are more numerous than the arteries and their anatomy differs among individuals. For instance, the median cubital vein is not present in all humans.

I. MULTIPLE CHOICE.
Choose the best answer.

1. The veins begin with the _____ and eventually flow into the vena cavae.
   - ◯ arterioles
   - ◯ capillaries
   - ◯ venules
   - ◯ venioles

2. The veins that lie closest to the body's surface are called _____.
   - ◯ venules
   - ◯ superficial veins
   - ◯ venioles
   - ◯ dermal veins

3. Veins in the cranium formed from the dura mater are called _____.
   - ◯ capillaries
   - ◯ sinuses
   - ◯ venules

4. The superior vena cava delivers deoxygenated blood to the heart from the _____.
   - ◯ neck, head and lungs
   - ◯ head, arms and lungs
   - ◯ head, arms and thoracic cavity
   - ◯ head, arms, and thoracic cavity (except the lungs)

5. The inferior phrenic vein flows into the _____.
   - ◯ superior vena cava
   - ◯ inferior venous sinus
   - ◯ inferior vena cava
   - ◯ superior venous sinus

VEINS OF THE UPPER BODY

We begin our discussion of the veins with a look at the veins of the head and neck. As you can see from the image below, the veins running through the head and neck have familiar-sounding names. Take some time to study the image and table below, then complete the exercise to help you remember what you learn.

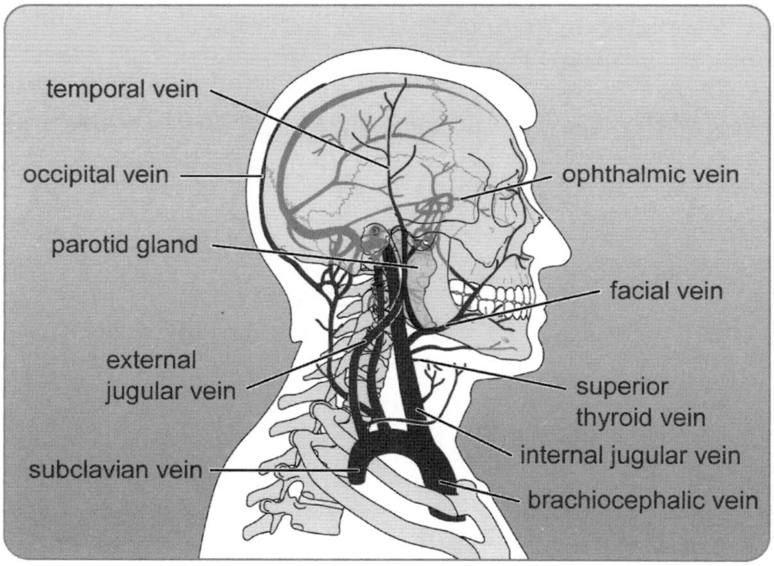

The **superficial veins** of the same area drain into the **external jugular vein**, then to the **subclavian vein**, **brachiocephalic vein** and into the superior vena cava.

Another difference between veins and arteries is the formation of venous sinuses in the cranium. The **venous sinuses** collect blood and cerebrospinal fluid then drain into the superior vena cava. (These are not the same as the sinuses in the bones of the skull.)

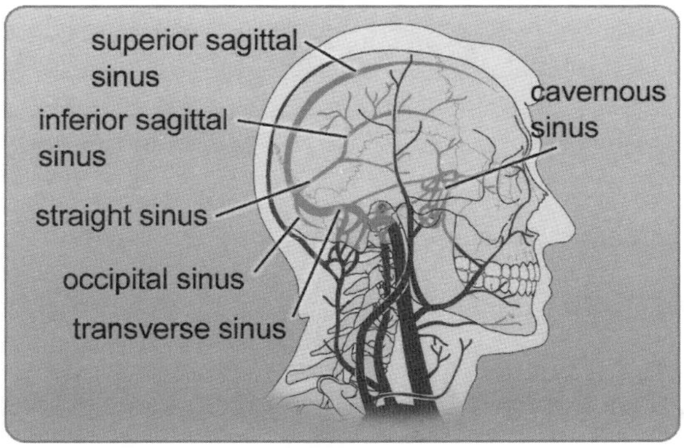

Venous Sinus	Area drained
Superior Sagittal Sinus	Cererbral hemispheres
Inferior Sagittal Sinus	Medial surfaces of the cerebral hemispheres
Straight Sinus	Inferior thyroid vein
Vein, Intracranial	Deep parts of cerebrum, cerebellum
Straight Sinus	Inferior thyroid vein
Occiptal Sinus	Cerebellum
Transverse Sinus	Brain
Cavernous Sinus	Orbit and brain
Superior and Inferior Petrosal Sinuses	All regions drained by cavernous sinus, orbit and brain
Sigmoid Sinus	Brain and meninges

The **hemiazygos vein** drains the blood from the left interior posterior wall of the thorax and abdomen, esophagus and mediastinum. The hemiazygos vein then drains into the **azygos vein** which also drains blood from the right posterior wall of the thorax and abdomen, esophagus, bronchi, pericardium, and mediastinum. The left suprarenal vein and left testicular (or ovarian) vein drain into the left renal vein.

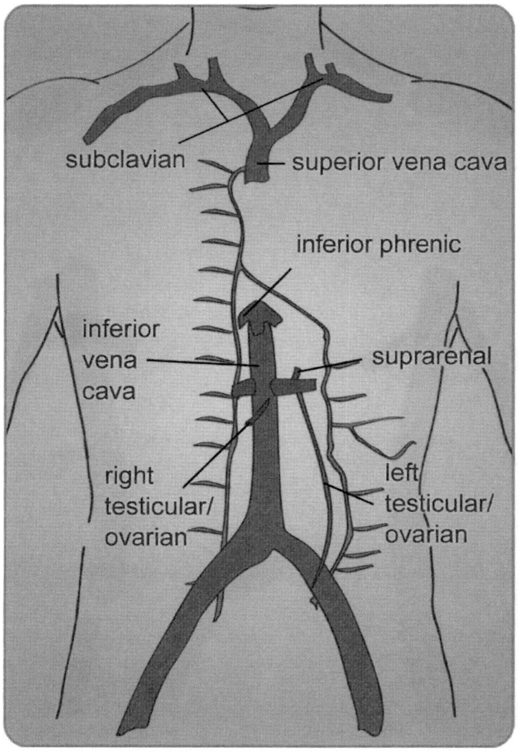

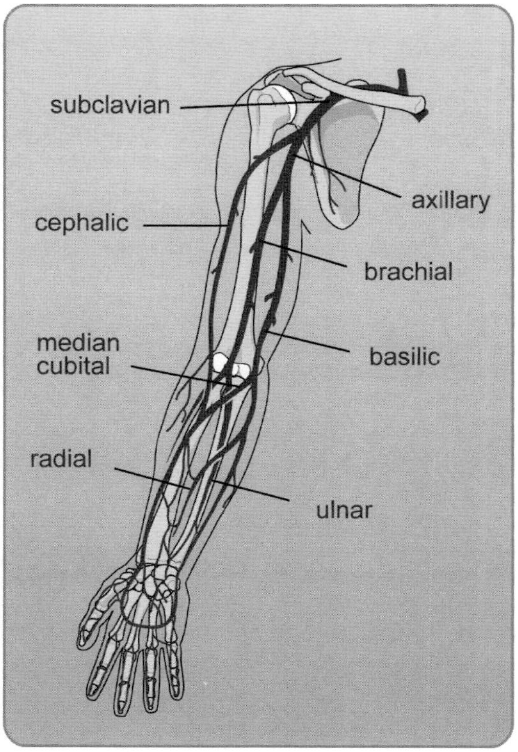

The veins of the upper extremity empty into the subclavian vein, to the brachiocephalic vein and then to the superior vena cava.

There are three veins in the extremity which do not have an arterial counterpart: the **median cubital vein** which drains the arm and hand; the **basilic vein** which drains the medial and lower arm; and the **cephalic vein** which drains the lateral and lower arm and hand.

Use the images on this page or the Elsevier's Anatomy plates in your 3M Reference to identify the following veins:

Head and neck:

- Facial
- superior thyroid
- great cerebral
- maxillary
- supraorbital

Upper extremity and hand:

- cephalic
- accessory cephalic
- dorsal metacarpal
- radial
- ulnar
- basilic

VEINS OF THE LOWER BODY

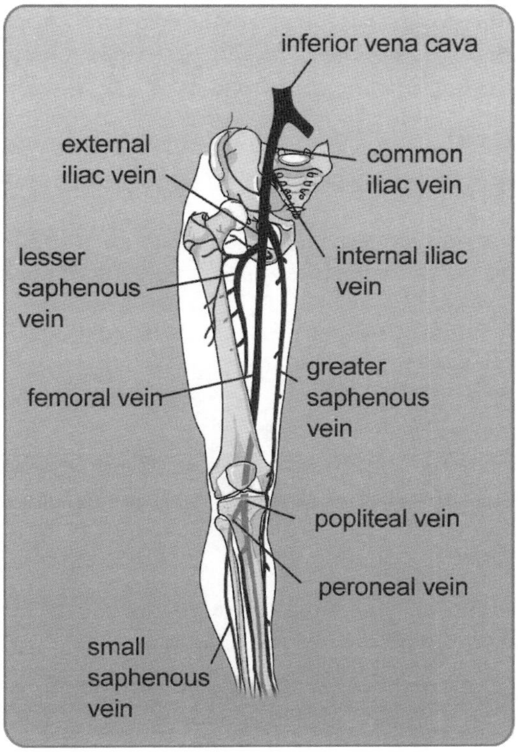

Most veins of the lower body and extremities are named similar to their arterial counterpart, and drain blood from the same body part or region. However, one major exception, as was briefly discussed in the circulatory system, is the **hepatic portal vein**.

The digestive veins that contribute to the hepatic portal vein are the **right** and **left gastric veins**, **superior mesenteric vein**, **splenic vein**, and **inferior mesenteric vein**. The blood in the hepatic portal vein goes through a network of smaller vessels called **sinusoids**, which filter out bacteria, old red blood cells and similar substances to complete some of the main functions of the liver. The cleaned blood then leaves the liver via the **hepatic veins**, which drain directly into the inferior vena cava.

Use the images on this page or the Elsevier's Anatomy plates in your 3M Reference to identify the following veins of the lower body:

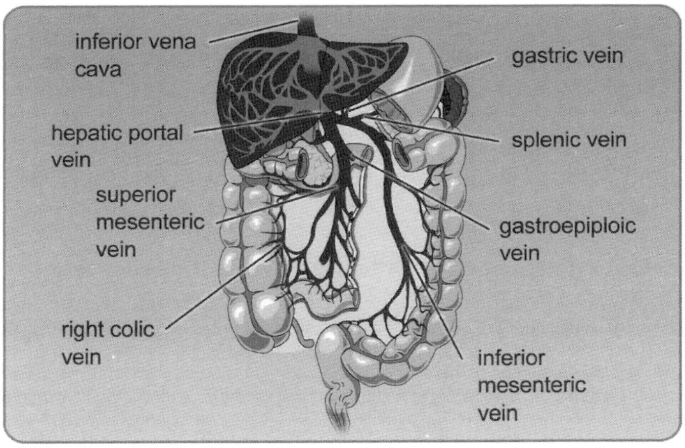

- gastroepiploic
- right colic
- external and internal pudendal
- obturator
- gluteal veins
- internal iliac
- external iliac
- great saphenous
- lesser saphenous
- femoral
- popliteal
- dorsal metatarsal

VEIN TERMINOLOGY

internal jugular: This vein is extremely important to the venous system because all blood from the brain and deep areas of the face and neck are drained into it. There are two jugular veins, and they pass down the neck beside the common carotid arteries. They empty into the subclavian veins.

brachiocephalic: These are also called innominate veins. This is where the subclavian and internal jugular veins come together. There are two of these, and they merge together to form the superior vena cava.

external jugular: The blood from the top of the head, part of the face, and the superficial neck region drains into these veins. They also empty into the subclavian veins.

diploic: There are several diploic veins, including the frontal diploic vein, occipital diploic vein, anterior temporal diploic vein, and posterior temporal diploic vein. These comprise the veins of the skull.

supratrochlear: These two veins begin high in the forehead and descend to the root of the nose. Root of the nose is the upper least protruding portion of the external nose situated between the two orbits.

retromandibular: This is formed in the parotid gland by a union of the maxillary vein and the superficial temporal vein. It means "behind the mandible."

basilic: This is a major superficial vein of the upper extremity. It passes on the ulnar side of the forearm and eventually forms the axillary vein.

cephalic: In addition to the cephalic vein, there are accessory cephalic and median cephalic veins. The cephalic vein is the other main superficial vein of the arm.

median cubital: This is a large branch of the cephalic vein that goes over the cubital fossa and joins with the basilic vein.

median antebrachial: A vein which arises from the palmar venous plexus and passes up the forearm. The term plexus means literally "a network or tangle." It is a general term for a network of lymphatic vessels, nerves, or veins.

azygos: In addition to the azygos vein, there is a left azygos and a lesser superior azygos vein. The azygos vein extends superiorly along the abdominal and thoracic walls on the right side of the vertebral column. At the level of T4 it joins directly with the superior vena cava.

hemiazygos: This is a tributary of the azygos vein.

saphenous: The small saphenous and the great saphenous veins are the superficial veins of the lower extremity. They are also called the greater saphenous and lesser saphenous veins. The greater saphenous is the longest vein of the body, and is often harvested to repair vessels of the heart.

REVIEW: VEINS

I. FILL IN THE BLANK.

Use the word(s) in the box to fill in the blanks.

retromandibular
median cubital
saphenous
external jugular
internal jugular
cephalic
median antebrachial
supratrochlear
hemiazygos
brachiocephalic
azygos
diploic
basilic

1. The ________________ vein is extremely important to the venous system because all blood from the brain and deep areas of the face and neck are drained into it. There are two of them, one on either side of the neck.
2. The greater and lesser ________________ veins are the superficial veins of the lower extremity. The greater one is the longest vein of the body, and is often harvested to repair vessels of the heart.
3. This is where the subclavian and internal jugular veins come together. There are two of these, and they merge together to form the superior vena cava ________________.
4. The blood from the top of the head, part of the face, and the superficial neck region drain into the ________________ veins. They also empty into the subclavian veins.
5. The ________________ veins comprise the veins of the skull.
6. The two ________________ veins begin high in the forehead and descend to the root of the nose.
7. The ________________ vein is formed in the parotid gland by a union of the maxillary vein and the superficial temporal vein. It means "behind the mandible."
8. The ________________ is a major superficial vein of the upper extremity. It passes on the ulnar side of the forearm and eventually forms the axillary vein.
9. The ________________ vein is the other main superficial vein of the arm.
10. The ________________ vein is a large branch of the cephalic vein that goes over the cubital fossa and joins with the basilic vein.

11. The ________________ vein that arises from the palmar venous plexus and passes up the forearm.

12. The ________________ is a tributary of the azygos vein.

13. The ________________ vein extends superiorly along the abdominal and thoracic walls on the right side of the vertebral column. At the level of T4 it joins directly with the superior vena cava.

II. MULTIPLE CHOICE.
Choose the best answer.

1. "A network or tangle."
   - ◯ bunch
   - ◯ mess
   - ◯ plexus
   - ◯ gathering

2. The longest vein in the body.
   - ◯ lesser saphenous
   - ◯ greater saphenous
   - ◯ great quadriceps
   - ◯ great biceps

3. All veins eventually converge into two vessels. One of them is _____.
   - ◯ para vena cava
   - ◯ lower vena cava
   - ◯ inguinal vena cava
   - ◯ inferior vena cava

THE LYMPHATIC SYSTEM - LESSON 1

Lymph is a fluid that is composed of blood plasma minus certain macroproteins. The lymphatic system is part of the circulatory system because the lymphatic vessels drain fluid from interstitial tissues and return it to the blood, in a fashion similar to the veins. One crucial function of the lymph is that it drains excess fluids which gather in tissues, thereby preventing an abnormal accumulation of tissue fluid called **edema**. Lymph vessels have valves, similar to veins, which help to keep lymph flowing in one direction. The motion of the skeletal muscles and the diaphragm also help move lymph through the body.

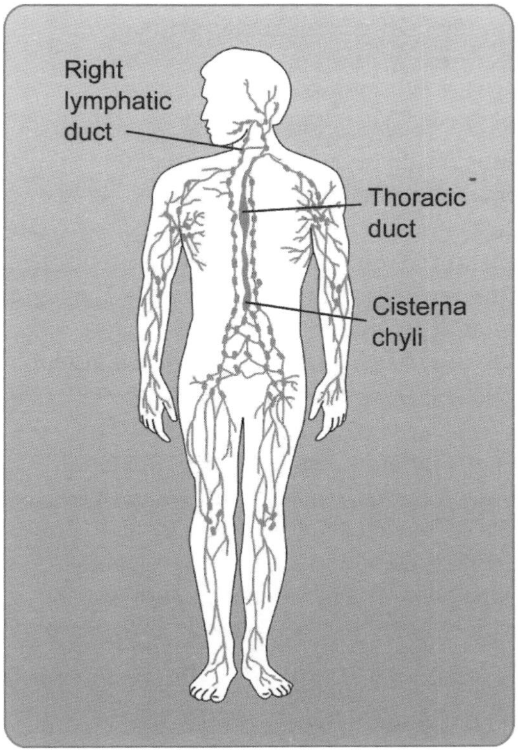

Unlike the cardiovascular system, the lymphatic system is not a closed system; the lymph vessels arise from the intercellular spaces of the body's soft tissue, forming **lymphatic capillaries**. The capillaries then branch into larger lymphatic vessels, drain into regional **lymphatic trunks (5)** and eventually drain into the main lymphatic ducts: the **right lymphatic duct** and the **thoracic duct**. The thoracic duct receives lymph from the body except for the right upper quadrant. Lymph from the right upper quadrant empties into the right lymphatic duct. Both main ducts empty into the subclavian veins and the lymph then becomes part of the blood plasma and enters the heart via the upper vena cava.

Along with lymph and the lymphatic vessels, the lymphatic system contains **lymph tissue**, composed of a special type of reticular tissue made up of lymphocytes and other cells of the immune system. The lymph nodes are collections of lymphoid tissue found throughout the body.

Lymph nodes are small, bean shaped organs that lie along the network of lymphatic vessels. Lymph nodes serve as a maturation center for lymphocytes as well as a location for mature lymphocytes that actively product antibodies. Swelling of lymph nodes is a clinically significant sign of infection. There are around 200 lymph nodes in the human body with a wide distribution.

Refer to the Elsevier's Anatomy plates in your 3M reference to locate the following lymph nodes:

- Apical (subclavicular) lymph node
- Brachial lymph node
- Celiac lymph node
- Cervical lymph node
- Common iliac (subaortic) lymph node
- Cubital lymph node
- Hepatic lymph node
- Inferior mesenteric lymph node
- Infraclavicular lymph node
- Intercostal lymph node
- Jugular lymph node
- Mastoid (postauricular) lymph node
- Obturator lymph node
- Superior mesenteric lymph node

THE LYMPHATIC SYSTEM - LESSON 2

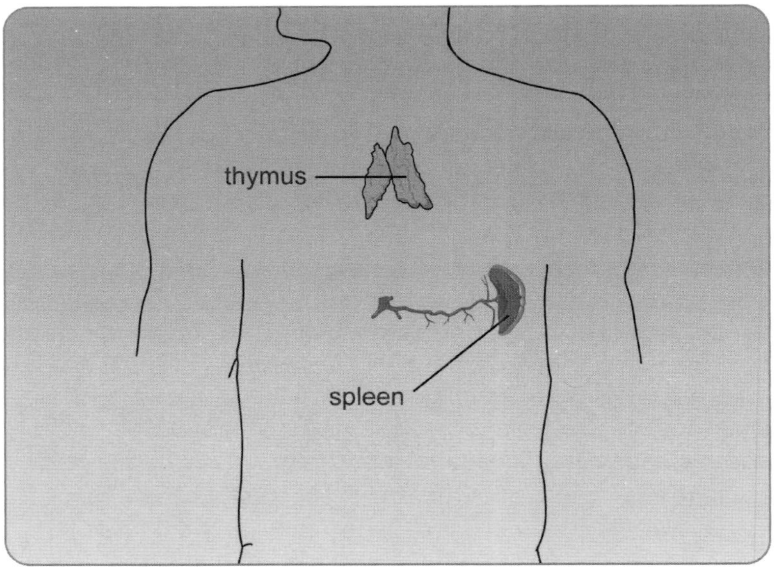

The thymus, tonsils, spleen and bone marrow are also a part of the lymphatic system. The **thymus gland**, located in the mediastinum, produces lymphocytes before birth, and hormones called **thymosin** after birth. Thymosin hormones are responsible for lymphocytes developing into T cells which are important for the immune function. The **tonsils** (discussed in the Gastrointestinal unit) are masses of lymphoid tissue in the nose **(pharyngeal tonsils)**, throat **(palatine tonsils)** and tongue **(lingual tonsils)** protect against exterior bacteria that may enter the body via the mouth or nose. The **spleen** destroys microorganisms in the blood, activates monocytes and lymphocytes, removes worn out red blood cells, and serves as a blood reservoir. **Bone marrow** produces the blood cells that become a part of the lymphatic system.

I. MATCHING.
Match the correct term to the definition.

1. ___ responsible for maturing lymphocytes into T cells
2. ___ protection from external bacteria
3. ___ destroys microorganisms in the blood
4. ___ produces blood cells that become part of the immune system

A. bone marrow
B. spleen
C. thymus
D. tonsils

REVIEW: THE LYMPHATIC SYSTEM

I. **MULTIPLE CHOICE.**
Choose the best answer.

1. The lymph system is made up of the lymph, lymphatic vessels and _____.
   - ◯ lymphoid tissue
   - ◯ nodules of epithelial tissue
   - ◯ the thyroid gland
   - ◯ the splenic flexure

2. The lymphatic structure which receives most of the lymph from the body is the _____.
   - ◯ left jugular trunk
   - ◯ left subclavian trunk
   - ◯ thoracic duct
   - ◯ right lymphatic duct

3. Lymph flows back into the heart via the _____.
   - ◯ inferior vena cava
   - ◯ subclavian vein
   - ◯ right jugular vein
   - ◯ superior vena cava

UNIT 7

The Nervous System

THE NERVOUS SYSTEM - INTRODUCTION

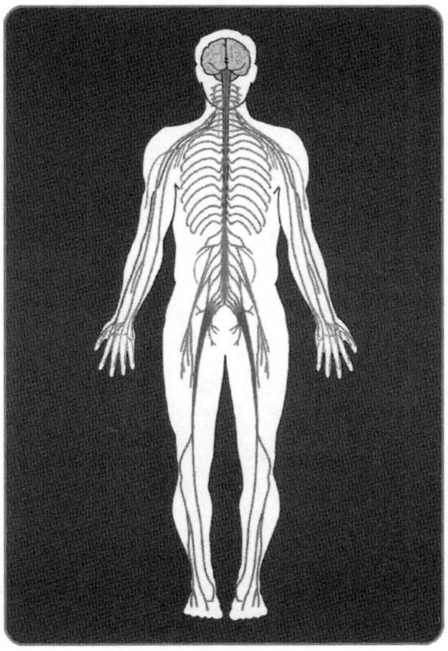

The nervous system is responsible for every activity, both voluntary and involuntary, including muscle contractions to initiate all motions, the involuntary or autonomic processes of heart contraction, blood movement, sweating, digestion, and reactions to stimuli.

The nervous system also assimilates and processes all experiences of life in the mental functions of memory, learning, reasoning, judgment, language, comprehension, and emotion. The nervous system consists of a vast and intricate network of nerve cells (neurons) and fibers that extend throughout the body.

Neurons are the basic units of the nervous system and are unique in the way they pass impulses to and from other nervous system structures. Similar to the conduction of electricity outside the body, the neurons depend on the presence of conductive materials, such as positive and negative ions, to carry out their functions. Additionally there are essential fluids, such as cerebrospinal fluid, that are critical to the body's ability to communicate and interpret impulses from within and outside the body.

The nervous system consists of two "subsystems." The **central nervous system** contains the brain and spinal cord. The **peripheral nervous system** is made up of the nervous structures, leading "to" (**afferent**) and "from" (**efferent**) the brain and spinal cord. Our study of nervous system anatomy will concentrate on the major anatomical structures of both subsystems.

NERVOUS TISSUE AND NEURONS

The entire nervous system is made up mostly of nervous tissue, which in turn is made up of two types of cells: neurons and glial (or supporting) cells.

The human body contains billions of **neurons** (nerve cells) whose main function is to conduct electrical impulses to and from the nervous system. As noted above, neurons are classified according to structure and function as either sensory (afferent) or motor (efferent). These cells are specialized to react to physical and chemical changes occurring in their surroundings.

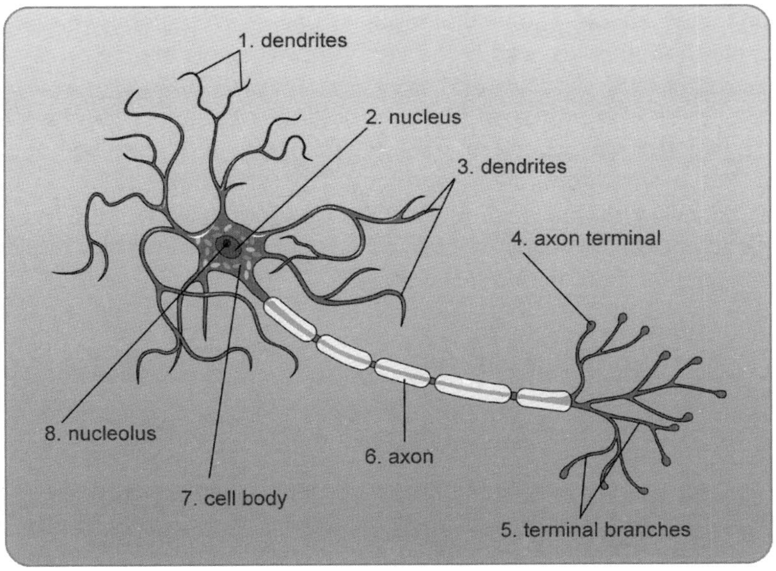

Neurons have an extreme longevity (of more than 100 years) and require plenty of oxygen and glucose to survive and function properly. Neurons can only survive for a few minutes without oxygen.

Neurons are unable to replicate themselves. The neurons present at birth have to serve the human body throughout its entire life.

Neurons, like other cells, contain a nucleus. But because of their unique functions, neurons are unable to replicate themselves as other cells can. Therefore, the neurons present at birth have to serve the human body throughout its life.

Other nerve cells that are important in the nervous system are called **glial cells**. These are supportive cells that form a connective tissue component in the nervous system. These cells also provide the framework within the organs of the nervous system.

When a glial cell, or many glial cells, surrounds a portion of the neuron to provide support, it creates a fatty white material called **myelin**.

In most neurons, the nucleus is spherical and clear, and the center of the nucleus contains a dark nucleolus. Surrounding the nucleus is cytoplasm, which contains important cellular materials vital to the longevity of the neuron. Arm-like processes extend from the cell body of neurons. There are two of these arm-like processes called dendrites and axons.

Dendrites look like tree branches and function as receptors for signals and conduct electrical signals towards the nerve cell body. **Axons** are thin, chain-like extensions with a uniform appearance. They are the impulse generators and conductors that transmit nerve impulses away from the nerve cell body.

A nerve is composed of many axons (nerve fibers) that are arranged in parallel bundles and are wrapped in connective tissue. Each axon within a nerve is surrounded by **Schwann cells** that are then wrapped in a layer of endoneurium. Groups of axons are grouped into bundles called nerve **fascicles** by the perineurium, a connective tissue. The whole nerve is finally surrounded by a tough fibrous sheath called the epineurium. Within the nerve are also blood vessels that supply the axons and Schwann cells.

Most nerves are composed of both motor and sensory neurons and are called mixed nerves. Specialized nerves, specifically some of the cranial nerves, are composed of either sensory neurons only (sensory nerves) or motor neurons only (motor nerves). A nerve is visible to the naked eye and has the appearance of a cord. All nerve impulses and signals are sent by way of the neuron. The site at which neurons communicate or transmit electrical impulses is called a **synapse**. This is a cell junction or intersection in which one neuron transmits its signal to another.

afferent: Signals picked up by sensory receptors throughout the body and are sent via nerve fibers of the peripheral nervous system to the central nervous system.

nervous tissue: Makes up almost the entire nervous system.

somatic: Consists of the structures that lie outside the ventral body cavity.

efferent: Signals sent away from the central nervous system via nerve fibers.

visceral: Consists of the structures that lie within the ventral body cavity.

glial: Type of cell located in the nervous system that surrounds a portion of the neuron to provide support.

myelin: Fatty white material.

supporting cells: Cells that form a connective tissue component in the nervous system.

nucleus: Group of nerve cells located within the central nervous system.

nucleolus: Center of the nucleus.

cytoplasm: Contains important cellular materials vital to the longevity of the neuron.

dendrites: Function as receptors for signals and conduct electrical signals towards the nerve cell.

axons: Impulse generators and conductors that transmit nerve impulses away from the nerve cell body.

mixed nerves: Nerves composed of both motor and sensory neurons.

ventral body cavity: Body cavity that contains the heart, lungs, intestines, and kidneys.

somatic sensory: Senses whose receptors are widespread throughout the outer parts of the body.

visceral sensory: Include temperature, pain, and stretching of the visceral organs or parts of the body.

somatic motor: Supply of nervous energy to all of the muscles of the skeleton minus the pharyngeal arch muscles.

visceral motor: Supply of nervous energy to the glands, cardiac muscle, and smooth muscle.

synapse: The site at which neurons communicate or transmit electrical impulses.

I. FILL IN THE BLANK.

In the blanks provided below, refer to the image and enter the term corresponding to the following numbers. Use the word(s) in the box to fill in the blanks.

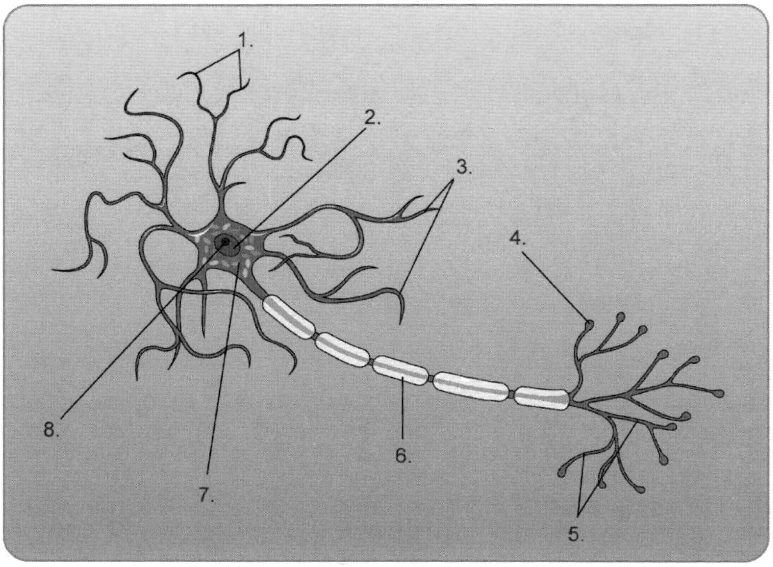

1. ________________
2. ________________
3. ________________
4. ________________
5. ________________
6. ________________
7. ________________
8. ________________

terminal branches
dendrites
nucleolus
axon terminal
cell body
nucleus
axon
dendrites

II. MULTIPLE CHOICE.
Choose the best answer.

1. The neuronal stimuli that affect the ventral body cavity organs.
   - ◯ somatic sensory
   - ◯ visceral sensory
   - ◯ somatic motor
   - ◯ visceral efferent

2. The body region that consists of structures that lie outside the ventral body cavity.
   - ◯ visceral
   - ◯ somatic
   - ◯ ventral
   - ◯ general

3. The two subdivisions of sensory input.
   - ◯ somatic sensory and visceral sensory
   - ◯ somatic motor and visceral motor
   - ◯ somatic sensory and visceral motor
   - ◯ visceral sensory and somatic motor

4. The visceral body region consists of structures that lie here.
   - ◯ outside the ventral body cavity
   - ◯ within the visceral body cavity
   - ◯ within the somatic body cavity
   - ◯ within the ventral body cavity

5. Signals that are sent to the central nervous system.
   - ◯ efferent
   - ◯ motor
   - ◯ afferent
   - ◯ neurons

6. The entire nervous system is made up of mostly _____.
   - ◯ neurons
   - ◯ nerve roots
   - ◯ nervous tissue
   - ◯ supporting cells

7. Neurons have the extreme longevity of at least this amount of time.
   - ◯ 75 years
   - ◯ 100 years
   - ◯ 65 years
   - ◯ 85 years

8. Every neuron contains only one of these.
   - ◯ glial cell
   - ◯ supporting cell
   - ◯ nucleus
   - ◯ dendrite

9. The tree-like branch of a neuron.
   - ◯ axon
   - ◯ cytoplasm
   - ◯ synapse
   - ◯ dendrite

10. Thin chain-like extensions of the neuron.
    - ◯ dendrite
    - ◯ axon
    - ◯ cytoplasm
    - ◯ nucleolus

11. Nerves that are composed of both motor and sensory neurons.
    - ◯ special neurons
    - ◯ general neurons
    - ◯ mixed nerves
    - ◯ multiple neurons

THE BRAIN

The human brain is divided into six major regions:

1. cerebrum
2. cerebellum
3. diencephalon
4. mesencephalon (midbrain)
5. pons
6. medulla oblongata

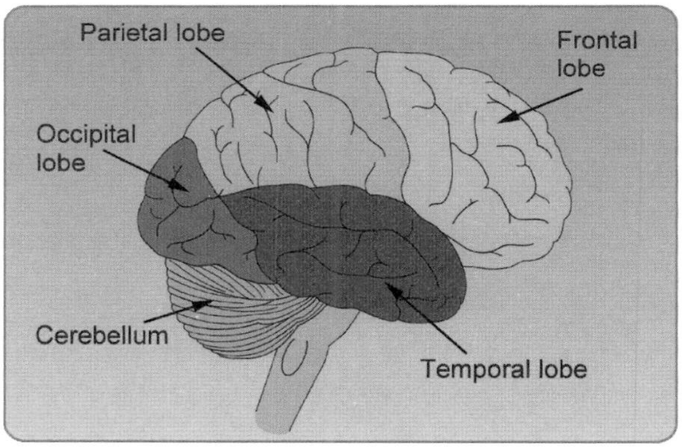

Cerebrum

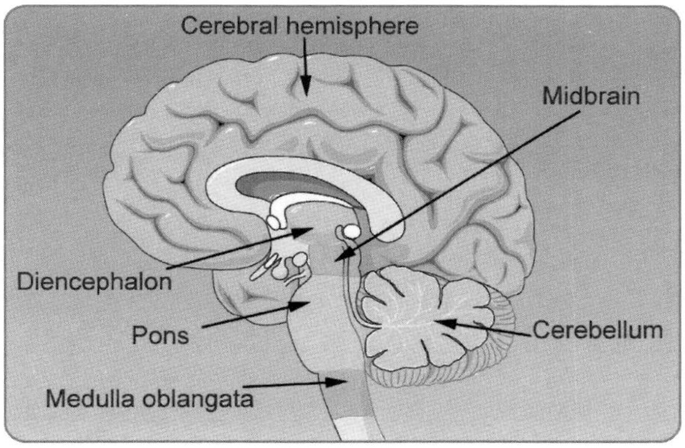

The **cerebrum** is the largest and most obvious portion of the brain. It accounts for approximately 80% of the brain's mass. It is divided into two equal hemispheres: right and left. Each hemisphere is then divided into four lobes, named for the skull bones that overlie them.

The lobes are divided by deep grooves called **fissures**. The surface of the cerebrum, or the cerebral cortex, is deeply convoluted, like a walnut. The raised areas are called **gyri**, and the grooves in between them are called **sulci**. The cerebrum is responsible for higher mental functions, including reasoning and memory.

Cerebellum

The **cerebellum** is located below and behind the cerebrum. It looks like a smaller version of the brain, sometimes called the "little brain." It is responsible for coordinating muscle movement and maintaining posture.

The undersurface, or ventral portion of the brain, is made up of the next four major brain sections. They are (in order from front to back): the diencephalon, the midbrain or mesencephalon, the pons, and the medulla oblongata.

Diencephalon

The **diencephalon** contains vital activity centers, including the thalamus, hypothalamus, optic chiasm, and pituitary gland. All impulses entering the cerebrum, except for the sense of smell, are relayed through cells in the thalamus. The **basal ganglia** are clusters of nerve cells that surround the thalamus and are responsible for initiating movement. Autonomic activities, such as sight and sound, are regulated by the **hypothalamus**. A part of the hypothalamus, the optic chiasma is the point where the optic nerves cross.

Mammillary bodies of the hypothalamus are concerned with smell. The infundibulum of the pituitary gland also originates here.

Mesencephalon

The **midbrain,** mesencephalon, contains structures associated with visual reflexes and hearing.

Pons

The **pons** functions as a relay center within the brain.

Medulla Oblongata

The **medulla oblongata** is continuous, with the spinal cord posterior and the pons anterior. It works as a relay center for the impulses to and from the spinal cord and is the nervous center that controls the heart, respiration, and vasomotor reactions. The pons and medulla oblongata together are called the **brain stem**.

For a detailed look at the structures of the diencephalon and the brainstem check out the "Brainstem and diencephalon" depictions under the Nervous System section in the Elsevier's Anatomy plates in your 3M Reference.

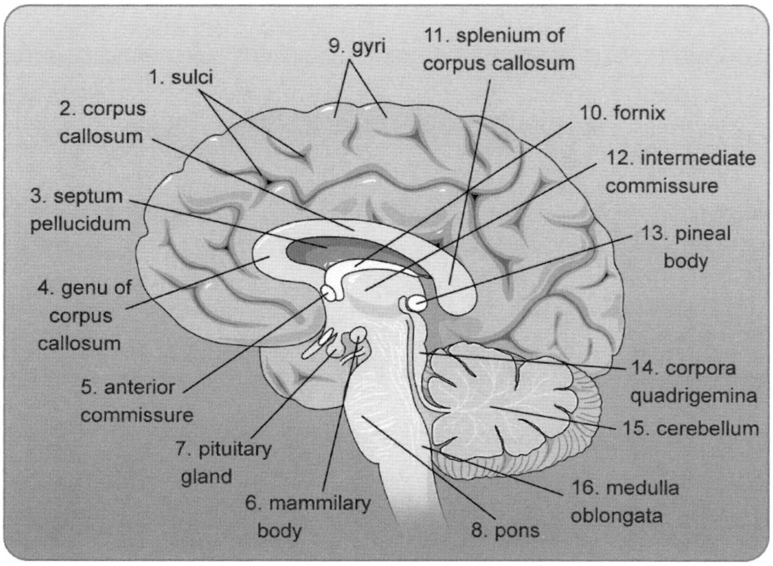

MENINGES AND CEREBROSPINAL FLUID

Meninges is a term given to the three membranes that protect the brain and spinal cord.

There are sinuses in the brain to collect blood and cerebrospinal fluid that are channeled to the veins.

The **dura mater** is the outermost membrane layer. It contacts the bones of the cranium. Underneath this is a mesh of connective tissue, thinner and more delicate than the other two layers, called the **arachnoid**. The innermost membrane that lies on the surface of the brain is the **pia mater**, which is similar in makeup to the dura mater. It is a dense and highly vascular sheet of connective fibers. In the spinal canal the pia mater goes through the arachnoid and attaches directly to the dura mater via denticulate ligaments, providing more stability to the spinal cord in this area.

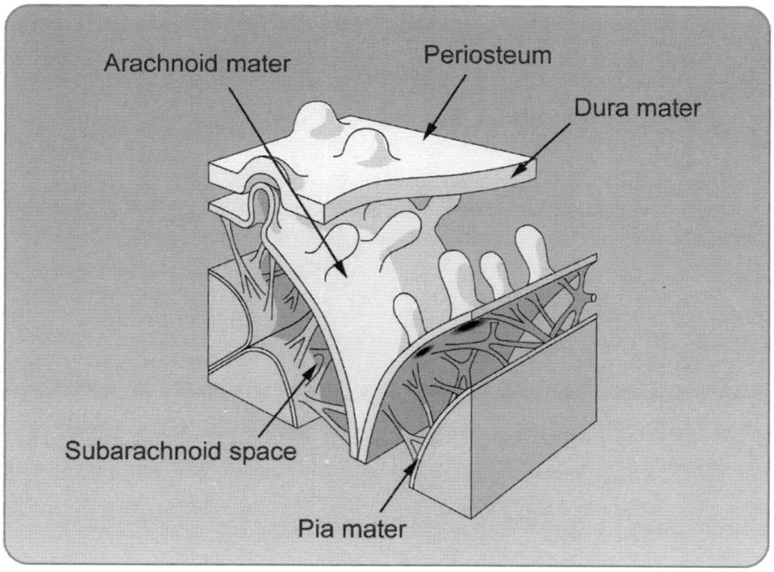

The meninges have several spaces between and around them, serving various functions. The three spaces that are referenced most often in medical conditions are:

1. The **epidural space** is between the dura mater and vertebral canal lining. It contains fat and other connective tissues. Most often this space is where injections are performed for pain relief or anesthesia during procedures, such as delivery.
2. The **subdural space** is the space between the dura mater and the arachnoid. It contains lubricating fluid.
3. The **subarachnoid space** is between the pia mater and the arachnoid. It contains cerebrospinal fluid. Hemorrhage into this space may be documented as part of an injury or ruptured aneurysm.

The blood vessels of the pia mater fold in and are covered by a thin layer of cells that then project into the third, fourth, and lateral ventricles of the brain. These projections are called the **choroid plexus** and are covered with ependymal cells that produce cerebrospinal fluid. Cerebrospinal fluid, or CSF, then circulates through the **cerebral ventricles** and the **cerebral aqueduct** (aqueduct of Sylvius). The cerebral ventricles allow flow of CSF through the internal, hollow areas of the brain. They are continuous with the vertebral central canal, allowing transmission of CSF down the spinal cord.

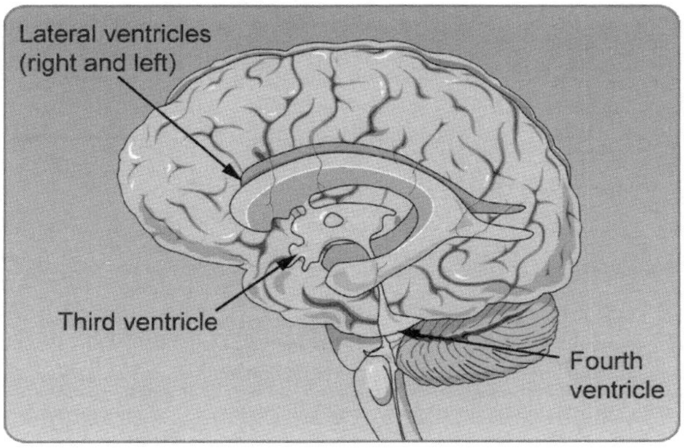

Cerebrospinal fluid provides cushion for the central nervous system structures and also allows the brain to monitor the internal status of certain elements, such as CO_2 levels. Analysis of the cerebrospinal fluid can be used to diagnose various abnormal conditions.

BRAIN TERMINOLOGY

The description of the brain thus far is basically a gross description. If you were to look at a brain, for the most part, this is what you would be able to visualize and identify. The terms are primarily general terms related to the overall structure of the brain. The brain is, however, extremely intricate and complex, befitting an organ responsible for so many vital and varied processes. It will not be necessary for you to understand everything about the inner workings of the brain—after all, no one does. However, there are additional terms related to the brain that you will undoubtedly encounter, particularly in specialties dealing with brain function.

neuron: Transmits instructions to and receives information from every minute part of every human system.

cerebrum: Responsible for higher mental functions including reasoning and memory.

fissure: Deep grooves in the lobes of the cerebrum.

gyri: Raised areas of the cerebrum.

sulci: Grooves in between the gyri.

cerebellum: Responsible for coordinating muscle movement and maintaining posture.

diencephalon: Contains vital activity centers to include the thalamus, hypothalamus, optic chiasm, and pituitary gland.

mesencephalon: Contains structures associated with visual reflexes and hearing.

pons: Functions as a relay center within the brain.

medulla oblangata: Relay center for the impulses to and from the spinal cord, and is the nervous center which controls the heart, respiration, and vasomotor reactions.

optic chiasm: Point where the optic nerves cross.

meninges: Three membranes that protect the brain and spinal cord.

dura mater: Outermost membrane layer that contacts the bones of the cranium.

arachnoid: Mesh of connective tissue.

pia mater: Innermost membrane that lies on the surface of the brain.

choroid plexux: Responsible for generating cerebrospinal fluid that circulates through the hollow areas of the brain and spinal cord.

cerebrospinal fluid: Functions primarily to transport nutrients and as a shock absorber.

splenium of corpus callosum: The posterior rounded end of the corpus callosum; it conveys visual information.

commissure: A site of union of common parts.

corpus callosum: An arched mass of white matter found in the depths of the longitudinal fissure.

corpora quadrigemina: Part of the mesencephalon.

THE SPINAL CORD

The **spinal cord** carries signals to and from the brain and the rest of the body. It also serves as the reflex center for spinal reflexes. The spinal cord is located within the foramen of the vertebrae, called the **spinal canal**. Sections of the spinal canal are named after the regions of the vertebra with which they interact. In the lumbar portion of the spinal canal, the cord splits into various nerves. These nerves remain bundled until the end of the spinal canal, the **conus medullaris**, and are called the **cauda equina**. Some of the filaments of the meninges (covering for the spinal cord) continue into the sacrum and are called the **filum terminale**.

Highlights

The spinal canal ends in the L1-L2 region.

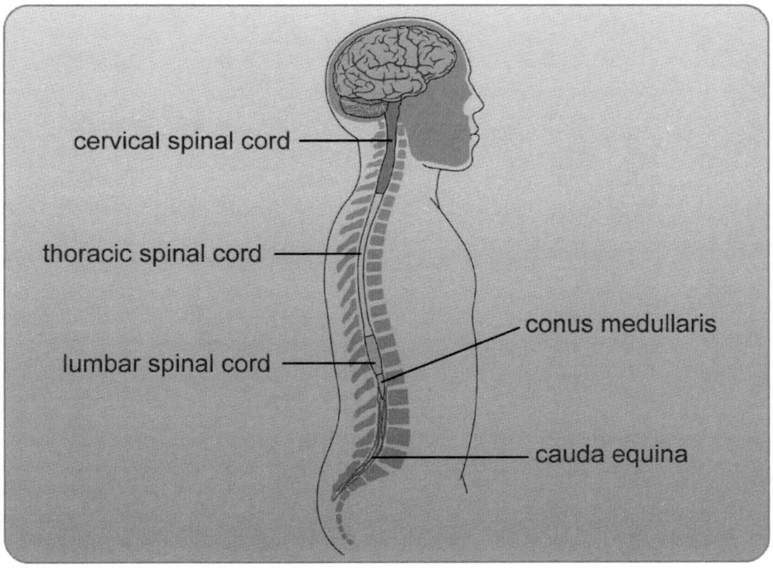

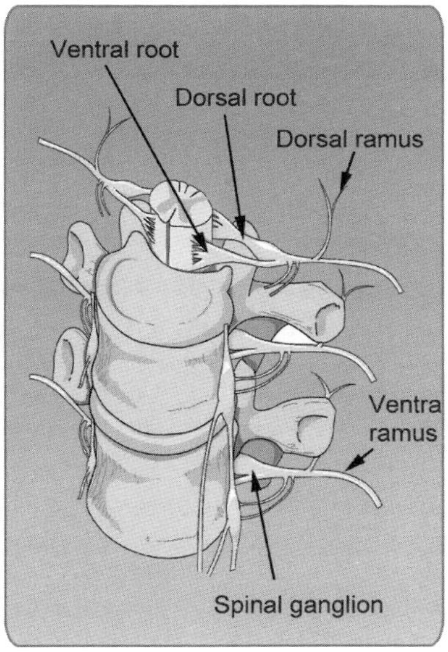

There are two grooves running down anterior and posterior to the spinal cord, almost dividing it into two sections. The deepest groove is on the anterior side and is one way to tell the front from the back in a cross section, such as the one shown here. Two nerve roots exit the spinal cord on each side. Each root has a ventral (anterior) and dorsal (posterior) portion. The **ventral root** carries information to the motor nerves and away from the spinal cord. The **dorsal root** carries sensory information toward the spinal cord.

REVIEW: NERVOUS SYSTEM ANATOMY

I. MULTIPLE CHOICE.
Choose the best answer.

1. The raised portions of the cerebral surface.
   - ◯ meninges
   - ◯ sulci
   - ◯ gyri
   - ◯ fissures

2. Functions as a relay center within the brain.
   - ◯ pons
   - ◯ choroid plexus
   - ◯ pia mater
   - ◯ medulla oblongata

3. A general term meaning nerve cell.
   - ◯ nerve
   - ◯ gyri
   - ◯ neuron
   - ◯ fornix

4. The three membranes that protect the brain and spinal cord.
   - ◯ triplex
   - ◯ meninges
   - ◯ septum
   - ◯ medulla

5. Accounts for 80% of the brain's mass.
   - ◯ cerebrum
   - ◯ skull
   - ◯ cortex
   - ◯ sulci

6. Projections into the brain ventricles that produce cerebrospinal fluid.
   - ◯ choroid plexus
   - ◯ fornix
   - ◯ arachnoid
   - ◯ medulla oblongata

7. Deep grooves which divide the lobes of the cerebral hemisphere.
   - ◯ fractures
   - ◯ gyri
   - ◯ genu
   - ◯ fissures

8. The posterior rounded end of the corpus callosum; it conveys visual information.
   - ◯ splenium of corpus callosum
   - ◯ splinium of corpus callosum
   - ◯ spalenium of corpus callosum
   - ◯ spleniem of corpus callosum

9. Together with the pons makes up the brain stem.
   - ◯ cerebrum
   - ◯ cortex
   - ◯ medulla oblongata
   - ◯ spinal cord

10. Contains structures associated with visual reflexes and hearing.
    - ◯ crevice
    - ◯ septum
    - ◯ cortex
    - ◯ mesencephalon

11. Grooves between the gyri.
   - ◯ cortex
   - ◯ sulci
   - ◯ fissures
   - ◯ gyri

12. The thinner, more delicate middle layer of the meninges.
   - ◯ septum
   - ◯ sulci
   - ◯ arachnoid
   - ◯ cortex

13. A site of union of common parts.
   - ◯ corpus callosum
   - ◯ connection
   - ◯ genu
   - ◯ commissure

14. The second major structure of the brain.
   - ◯ cerebellum
   - ◯ medulla
   - ◯ pituitary
   - ◯ cortex

15. The outermost layer of the meninges, which contacts the cranium.
   - ◯ pia mater
   - ◯ dura mater
   - ◯ mammillary body
   - ◯ diencephalon

16. An arched mass of white matter found in the depths of the longitudinal fissure.
   - ◯ splenium callosum
   - ◯ corpus callosum
   - ◯ septum callosum
   - ◯ medulla callosum

17. Part of the hypothalamus formed by the crossing of the optic nerves.
   - ◯ optic chism
   - ◯ optic crosswalk
   - ◯ optic connection
   - ◯ optic chiasm

18. Contains some of the most vital centers of body activity.
    - ◯ pia mater
    - ◯ diencephalon
    - ◯ adrenal
    - ◯ corpus oblongata

19. The midbrain.
    - ◯ midcephalon
    - ◯ sulci
    - ◯ mesencephalon
    - ◯ commissure

20. The innermost layer of the meninges.
    - ◯ pia mater
    - ◯ genu mater
    - ◯ dura mater
    - ◯ corpus matter

21. Part of the mesencephalon.
    - ◯ corporal quadrigemina
    - ◯ corpus quadrigemina
    - ◯ corpora quadrigemina
    - ◯ cortex quadrigemina

22. The "master gland."
    - ◯ pituitary
    - ◯ adrenal
    - ◯ neural
    - ◯ thyroid

CRANIAL NERVES

There are twelve pairs of cranial nerves that emerge from the undersurface of the brain to innervate structures of the head, neck, and trunk of the body. These nerves are primarily named for function and position. However, they are commonly tested as part of the physical exam and should be learned. In fact, cranial nerve testing is part of any routine neurological examination.

There are, as stated, twelve pairs of cranial nerves which are represented by Arabic numerals, as in cranial nerves 1 through 12. The numerals indicate the order that the nerves emerge from the brain from anterior to posterior. The individual name and function of each cranial nerve is listed below. You can refer to this chart for quick reference to cranial nerve functions.

You do not need to memorize all the information on this page; however, a good mnemonic device to help you remember the names of the cranial names in order is — On Old Olympus' Towering Top, A Fine Victorian Gentleman Viewed A Hawk. The first letter of each word corresponds to the first letter in each of the cranial nerves in order, 1-12.

Cranial Nerve	Function
1	Smell
2	Visual acuity/visual fields
3, 4	Pupillary reactions
3, 4, 6	Extraocular movements, including eye opening
5	Facial sensation, jaw movements, and corneal reflexes
7	Facial movements and gustation (taste)
8	Hearing, balance
9, 10	Swallowing, elevation of the palate, gag reflex and gustation
5, 7, 10, 12	Voice and speech
11	Shrugging the shoulders and turning the head

olfactory nerve: Cranial nerve 1. The sense of smell. There are numerous olfactory nerves that relay sensory impulses of smell from the membranes of the nasal cavity. Damage to these nerves results in a loss of smell.

optic nerve: Cranial nerve 2. Vision. This is a sensory-only nerve that conducts impulses from the retina of the eye. It originates in the back of the eyeball, and damage to these nerves results in blindness.

oculomotor nerve: Cranial nerve 3. This nerve controls all movement of the eyeballs. It is primarily a motor nerve. It comes out of the midbrain and serves four of the six eye muscles, as well as the muscle of the eyelid, the iris (which causes pupil dilation), and the ciliary body. Damage to these nerves can cause a droopy eyelid, constant dilated pupil, or the inability to rotate the eyeball.

trochlear nerve: Cranial nerve 4. This is a very small nerve, both sensory and motor, that innervates the superior oblique muscle of the eye.

trigeminal nerve: Cranial nerve 5. This is the largest of the cranial nerves. It is primarily sensory, but does send motor impulses to the muscles of mastication (chewing).

abducens nerve: Cranial nerve 6. This is a small nerve that provides both motor and sensory innervation to the lateral rectus eye muscle. Damage to this nerve causes the eyeball to be pulled medially, and makes it unable to move laterally at all.

facial nerve: Cranial nerve 7. This is a mixed nerve. The motor fibers innervate facial, scalp, and superficial neck muscles. The salivary glands are also innervated by this. The sensory fibers arise from the taste buds on the tongue. Damage to these nerves distorts taste perception, particularly with sweets, and causes the face to sag.

vestibulocochlear nerve: Cranial nerve 8. Hearing and equilibrium. This is also called the acoustic nerve. It is a sensory nerve that arises within the inner ear. The vestibular branch controls equilibrium and balance, while the cochlear portion controls hearing. Damage to these nerves can cause deafness or dizziness and inability to maintain balance.

glossopharyngeal nerve: Cranial nerve 9. This is a mixed nerve that innervates the tongue and pharynx. The sensory portion transmits impulses from the tonsils, salivary gland, and back third of the tongue. The motor fibers innervate the muscles of the pharynx that help with swallowing. Damage to these nerves would result in a loss of bitter and sour taste, or could cause difficulty swallowing.

vagus nerve: Cranial nerve 10. This arises from the medulla and has both motor and sensory fibers that serve autonomic organs of the thoracic and abdominal cavities. It is associated with such functions as breathing, heartbeat, hunger pangs, and peristalsis. One of its branches supplies the larynx and controls speech. Damage to both of these nerves would result in death; damage to only one would affect speech and swallowing.

accessory nerve: Cranial nerve 11. This is a motor nerve only. It innervates the muscles of the pharyngeal region as well as the sternocleidomastoid and trapezius muscles. Damage to this nerve would make it difficult to rotate the head or shrug the shoulders.

hypoglossal nerve: Cranial nerve 12. This supplies motor fibers to the muscles of the tongue. Damage would cause difficulty speaking, swallowing, or sticking out the tongue.

BRAIN ANATOMY

The following diagram depicts the cranial nerves, as well as the structures of the brain.

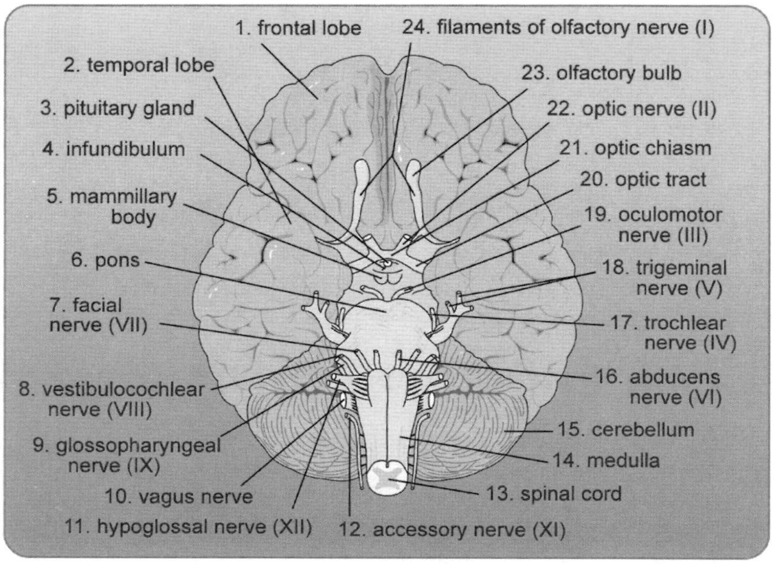

I. FILL IN THE BLANK.

In the blanks provided below, enter the terms corresponding to the numbers marked on the diagram. Use the word(s) in the box to fill in the blanks.

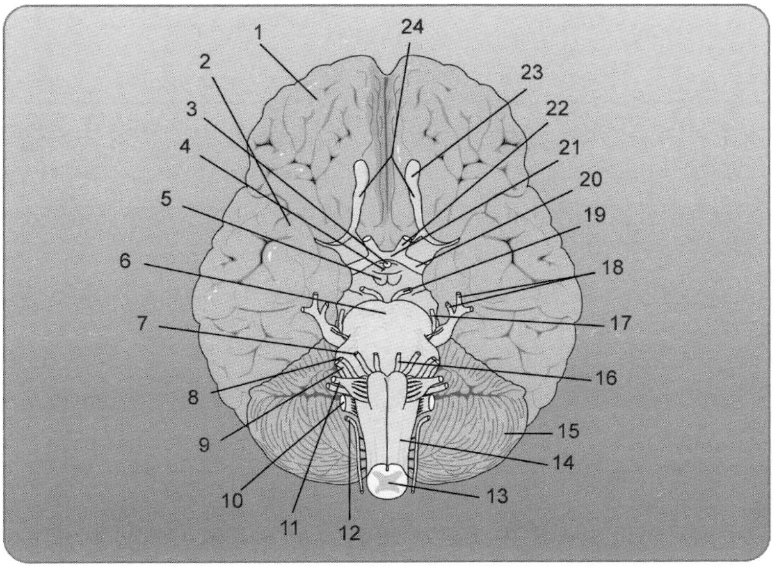

glossopharyngeal nerve
optic nerve
frontal lobe
vestibulocochlear nerve
cerebellum
pituitary gland
filaments of olfactory nerve
facial nerve
optic tract
mammillary body
abducens nerve
infundibulum
trigeminal nerve
accessory nerve
spinal cord
temporal lobe
vagus nerve
oculomotor nerve
optic chiasm
pons
trochlear nerve
hypoglossal nerve
medulla
olfactory bulb

1. ____________
2. ____________
3. ____________
4. ____________
5. ____________
6. ____________
7. ____________
8. ____________
9. ____________
10. ____________
11. ____________
12. ____________
13. ____________
14. ____________
15. ____________
16. ____________

17. ________________

18. ________________

19. ________________

20. ________________

21. ________________

22. ________________

23. ________________

24. ________________

II. MULTIPLE CHOICE.
Choose the best answer.

1. Nerves that resemble a horse's tail.
   - ◯ filum terminale
   - ◯ cauda equina
   - ◯ facial
   - ◯ cauda clonus

2. Nerve controlling the sense of smell.
   - ◯ vagus
   - ◯ accessory
   - ◯ trigeminal
   - ◯ olfactory

3. Innervates the thoracic and abdominal cavities.
   - ◯ vagal nerve
   - ◯ vagus nerve
   - ◯ efferent nerve
   - ◯ cauda nerve

4. The largest of the cranial nerves.
   - ◯ bigeminal
   - ◯ acoustical
   - ◯ conus medullaris
   - ◯ trigeminal

5. Controls hearing and balance.
   - ◯ cochlear
   - ◯ vestibular
   - ◯ vestibulocochlear
   - ◯ bigeminal

6. The nerve that controls vision.
   - ◯ trochlear nerve
   - ◯ olfactory nerve
   - ◯ oculomotor nerve
   - ◯ optic nerve

7. Point at the second lumbar vertebra, where the spinal cord tapers. It is cone shaped.
   - ◯ conus medullaris
   - ◯ bigeminal
   - ◯ lumbosacral
   - ◯ abducens

8. A small nerve to the lateral rectus eye muscle.
   - ◯ ocularis
   - ◯ clonus
   - ◯ filum terminale
   - ◯ abducens

9. Supplies motor fibers to the muscles of the tongue.
   - ◯ hypoglossal nerve
   - ◯ hyperglossal nerve
   - ◯ lingular fossa
   - ◯ hyperlingular nerve

10. A band of connective tissue that extends to the coccyx.
   - ◯ myconium terminale
   - ◯ filum terminale
   - ◯ sacrococcyx terminali
   - ◯ trigeminali

11. Controls all the movements of the eyeball.
   - ◯ occulomotor nerve
   - ◯ oculosensory nerve
   - ◯ oculomotor nerve
   - ◯ oculometer nerve

12. A mixed nerve of the tongue and pharynx.
   - ◯ hypoglossopharyngeal
   - ◯ glossopharyngeal
   - ◯ hyperglossopharyngeal
   - ◯ glossopharyngial

III. MATCHING.
Match the correct term to the definition.

1. ____ Cranial nerve 1: olfactory nerve
2. ____ Cranial nerve 2: optic nerve
3. ____ Cranial nerve 3: oculomotor nerve
4. ____ Cranial nerve 4: trochlear nerve
5. ____ Cranial nerve 5: trigeminal nerve
6. ____ Cranial nerve 6: abducens nerve
7. ____ Cranial nerve 7: facial nerve
8. ____ Cranial nerve 8: vestibulocochlear nerve
9. ____ Cranial nerve 9: glossopharyngeal nerve
10. ____ Cranial nerve 10: vagus nerve
11. ____ Cranial nerve 11: accessory nerve
12. ____ Cranial nerve 12: hypoglossal nerve

A. The sense of smell.
B. Hearing and equilibrium.
C. This nerve controls all movement of the eyeballs.
D. This is a small nerve that provides both motor and sensory innervation to the lateral rectus eye muscle.
E. This arises from the medulla and has both motor and sensory fibers which serve autonomic organs of the thoracic and abdominal cavities.
F. This supplies motor fibers to the muscles of the tongue.
G. This is mixed nerve that innervates the tongue and pharynx.
H. This is a mixed nerve. The motor fibers innervate facial, scalp, and superficial neck muscles. The salivary glands are also innervated by this. The sensory fibers arise from the taste buds on the tongue.
I. This is the largest of the cranial nerves. It is primarily sensory, but does send motor impulses to the muscles of mastication (chewing).
J. This is a motor nerve only. It innervates the muscles of the pharyngeal region as well as the sternocleidomastoid and trapezius muscles.
K. This is a very small nerve, both sensory and motor, which innervates the superior oblique muscle of the eye.
L. Vision.

SPINAL NERVES

The spinal nerves, as discussed briefly in the Central Nervous System unit, arise from the spinal cord between the vertebrae. There are 31 pairs and they are numbered according to the level of the vertebral column where they originate. After leaving the spinal cord, the spinal nerve forms large branches, called **rami**. The anterior rami form complex networks by subdividing into plexuses. **Plexuses** allow adjacent spinal nerves to provide neural pathways to regional body parts. In this manner, if one nerve is damaged or otherwise malfunctioning, other nerves arising from the plexus may compensate.

The phrenic nerves originate from the cervical plexus. The phrenic nerves innervate the diaphragm. Spinal cord injuries between C3–C5 can lead to death due to loss of diaphragmatic function.

There are four major plexuses: **cervical**, **brachial**, **lumbar**, **sacral** (sometimes combined into the lumbosacral) and a fifth smaller one, the **coccygeal**. The cervical plexus provides motor neurons to the muscles of part of the head, skin of the neck and upper shoulders. The brachial plexus innervates the shoulder and arm. The lumbar plexus provides sensory nerves to the abdominal wall, external genitalia, and outer thigh. The sacral plexus provides motor nerves to most of the lower extremity muscles. The coccygeal plexus provides sensory neurons to the skin of the coccyx.

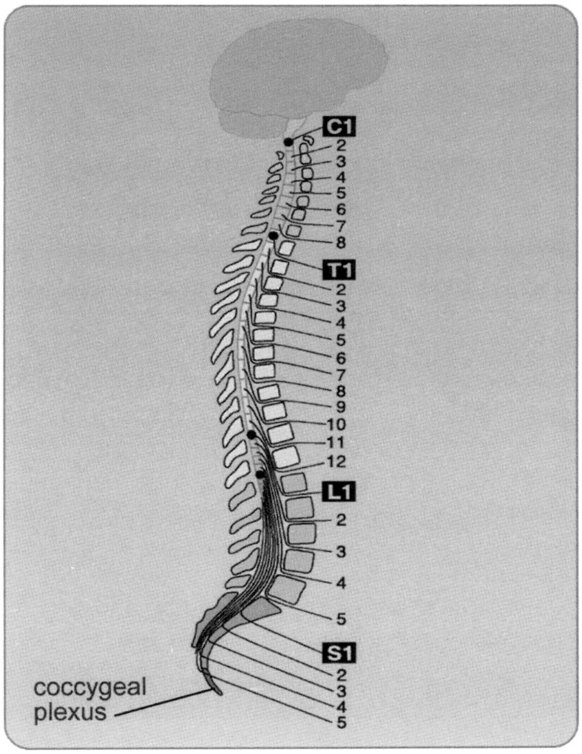

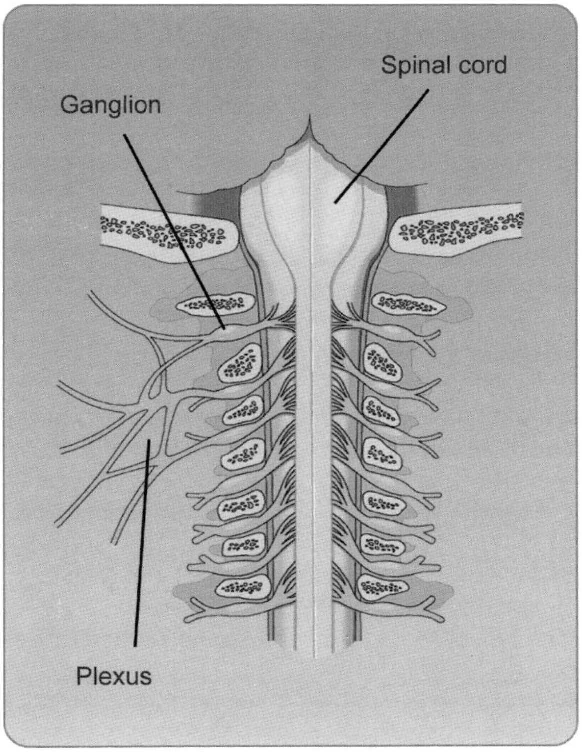

REFERENCES FOR CODERS

For more information about the neural plexuses, visit: www.ama-assn.org/atlas-of-human-body/nervous-system-groups

THE PERIPHERAL NERVOUS SYSTEM

After a nerve impulse goes from the brain to the spinal cord, it has to travel through the peripheral nerves to reach its destination. The peripheral nervous system, or PNS, is divided into **somatic** (voluntary) and **autonomic** (involuntary) systems. The somatic nerves serve the skeletal muscles—basically anything you can control consciously is served by the somatic nerves, and most everything else is controlled by the autonomic nerves. The **cranial nerves** and **spinal nerves** are the major structures of the Peripheral Nervous System. In the remainder of this unit we will investigate these two major categories of nerves.

To identify many of the nerves we cover in this unit you will need to locate them on the Elsevier's Anatomy Plates provided in your 3M Reference. You will not be required to memorize all the nerves and their precise locations; however, it is important that you be able to recognize their names and have an idea of the region of the body in which they occur.

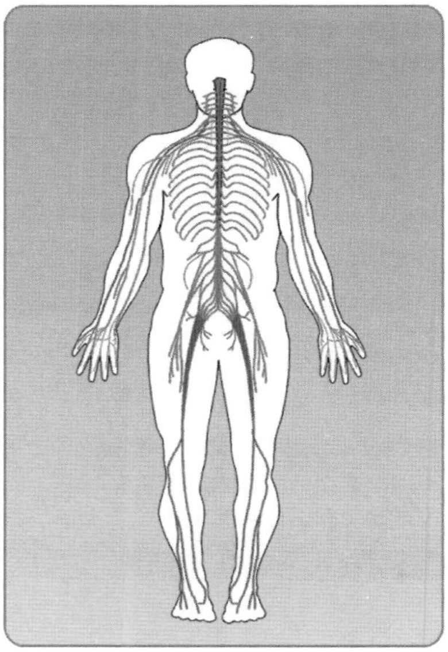

The peripheral nervous system

SENSORY AND MOTOR COMMUNICATION

The nervous system receives sensory inputs and sends motor outputs. Sensory or afferent signals are picked up by sensory receptors throughout the body and are sent via nerve fibers of the peripheral nervous system to the central nervous system. Motor or efferent signals are sent away from the central nervous system via nerve fibers, towards the peripheral nervous system and give energy or stimulation to the designated body organ or part.

Sensory input and motor output is further subdivided according to the regions of the body they serve, either somatic or visceral.

Highlights

Somatic: The somatic body region consists of the structures that lie outside the ventral body cavity (the skin, bones, and skeletal muscles).

Visceral: The visceral body region consists of the structures that lie within the ventral body cavity (the body cavity that contains the heart, lungs, intestines, kidneys, etc).

Somatic Sensory

General senses: These are the senses whose receptors are widespread throughout the outer parts of the body and include the senses felt on the skin (such as temperature, vibration, pain, pressure, touch) and proprioception (which informs us of the position and movement of our bodies).

Special senses: These are the senses whose receptors are located within a small or confined area of the body, such as sight, sound, smell, and equilibrium.

Somatic Motor

General motor: The supply of nervous energy to all of the muscles of the skeleton minus the pharyngeal arch muscles.

Branchial motor: This is the supply of nervous energy to the pharyngeal arch muscles.

Visceral Sensory

General senses: Include temperature, pain, and stretching of the visceral organs or parts of the body such as the stomach, lungs, heart, and digestive tract. Taste is also included in this category because the taste receptors are confined to the tongue and a portion of the surrounding area.

Visceral Motor

General motor: This is the supply of nervous energy to the glands, cardiac muscle, and smooth muscle that is basically the autonomic nervous system in that they are involuntarily stimulated to function.

I. **MATCHING.**
Match the correct term to the definition.

1. ___ Senses felt on the skin (temperature, vibration, touch, etc.) and proprioception (position and movement of the body).
2. ___ Supply of nervous energy to all muscles of the skeleton.
3. ___ Senses including taste, temperature, pain, and parts of the body such as the stomach, lungs, heart, and digestive tract.
4. ___ Supply of nervous energy to the glands, cardiac muscle, and smooth muscle.

A. Somatic Sensory
B. Visceral Sensory
C. Somatic Motor
D. Visceral Motor

NERVES OF THE HEAD AND NECK

After a nerve impuse goes from the brain to the spinal cord, it has to travel through the peripheral nerves to reach its destination. The **peripheral nervous system**, or PNS, is divided into **somatic** (voluntary) and **autonomic** (involuntary) systems. The somatic nerves serve the skeletal muscles—basically anything you can control consciously is served by the somatic nerves, and most everything else is controlled by the autonomic nerves.

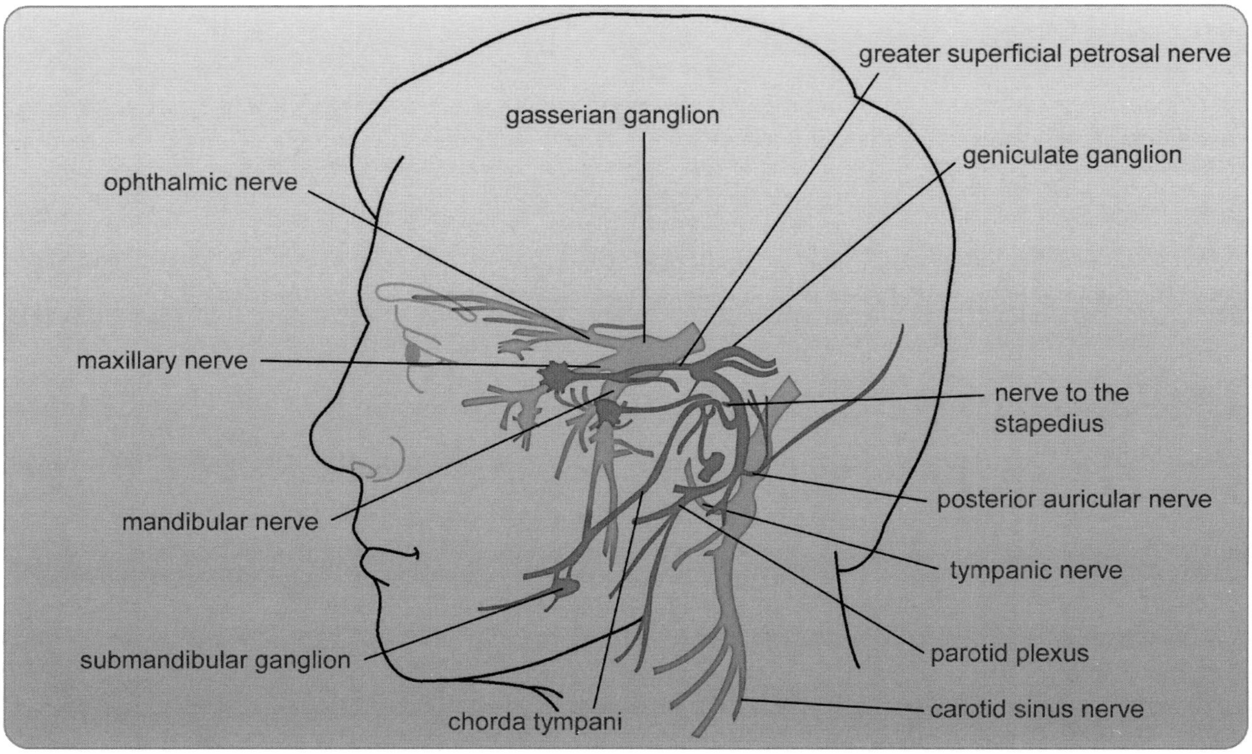

All of the nerves in the human body are named. We will not attempt to go into that much detail here. On the following pages use the images provided and the Elsevier's Anatomy Plates in your 3M reference to locate the bolded terms listed. To begin, locate these nerves in the Head and Neck:

- Carotid sinus nerve
- Mandibular nerve
- Maxillary nerve
- Lingual nerve
- Cochlear nerve
- Cervical nerve
- Greater occipital nerve
- Suboccipital nerve
- Great auricular nerve
- Facial nerve

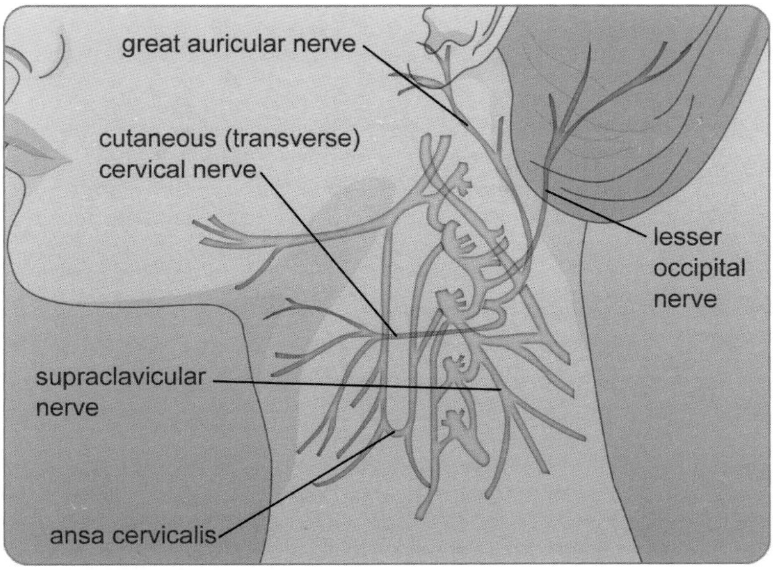

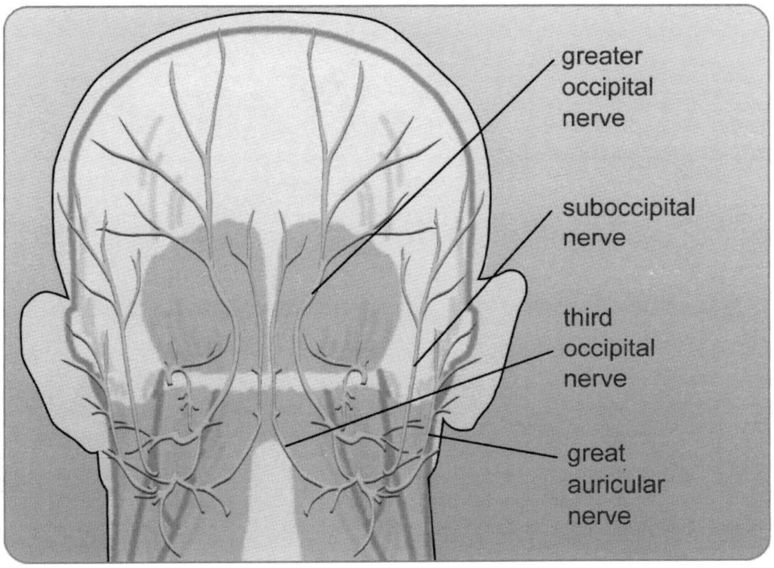

NERVES OF THE UPPER AND LOWER EXTREMITIES

Next we will look at the nerves of the upper and lower extremities. Remember that when the term "upper extremities" is used, the arms are being referred to. By the same token, "lower extremities" refers to the legs. Locate the structures below on the images provided or on the Elsevier's Anatomy Plates in the 3M Reference.

Upper Extremity:

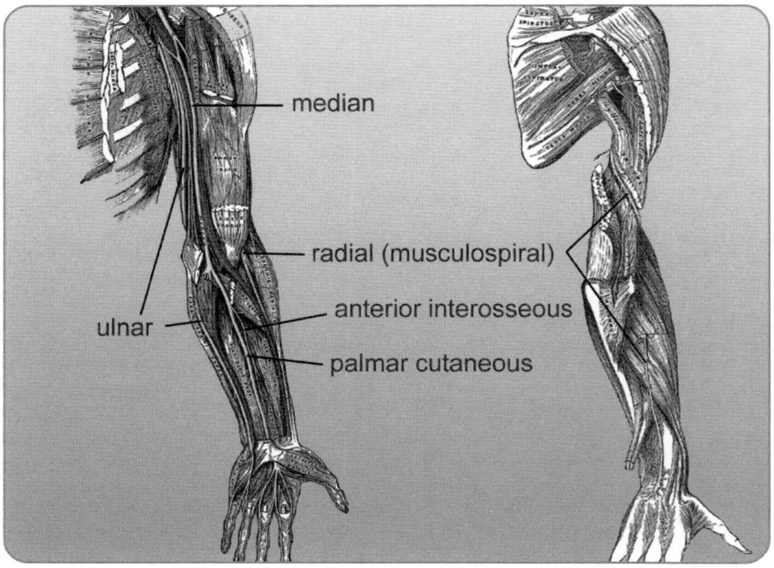

- Brachial Plexus
- Axillary nerve
- Median nerve
- Ulnar nerve
- Radial nerve

Lower Extremity:

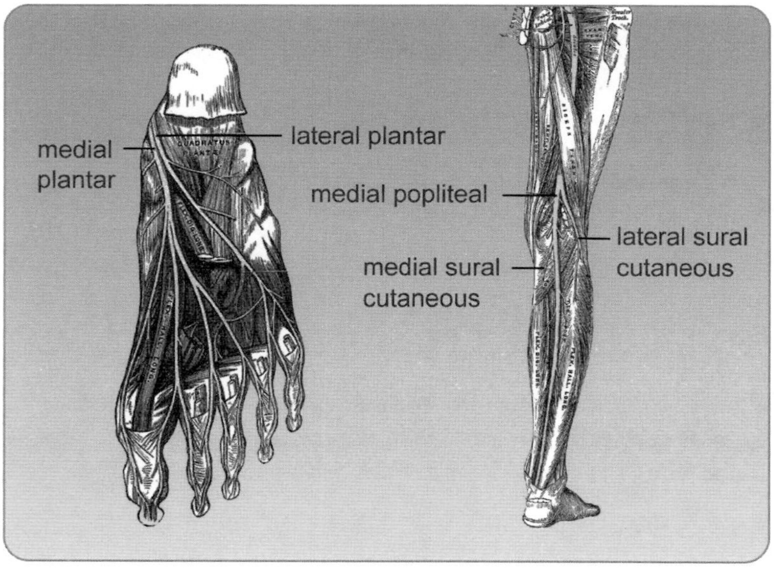

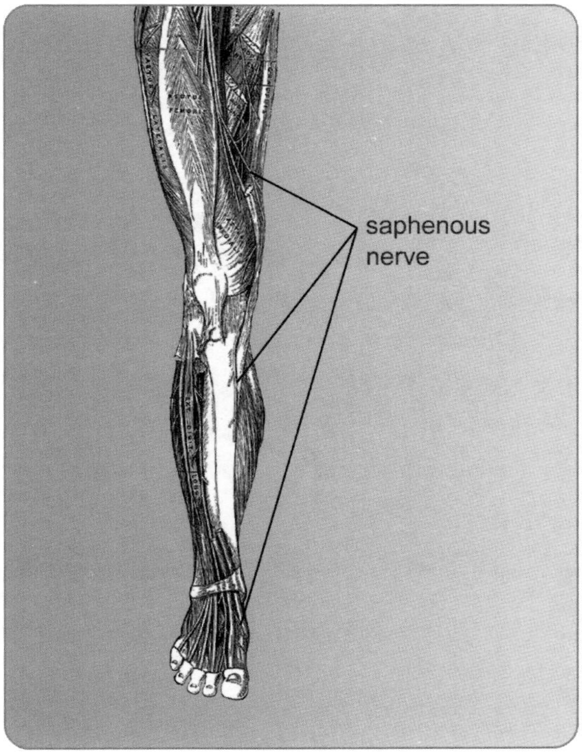

- Femoral nerve
- Saphenous nerve
- External popliteal nerve
- Sciatic nerve
- Ischiatic nerve
- Popliteal nerve
- Medial popliteal nerve
- Peroneal nerve (common fibular)
- Dorsal digital nerves
- Obturator nerve

NERVES OF THE TORSO

Let's move now to the nerves of the torso. You can probably guess by the names of some of these nerves, such as the pulmonary plexus and intercostal nerve, where they are located. Once again, locate the structures below on the images provided or on the Elsevier's Anatomy Plates in the 3M Reference.

- Cardiac plexus
- Phrenic Nerves (right and left)
- Celiac plexus
- Ilioinguinal nerve
- Superior gluteal nerve
- Subcostal nerve
- Pulmonary plexus
- Anterior and posterior vegal trunk
- Sacral plexus
- Iliohypogastric nerve
- Pudendal nerve
- Inferior gluteal nerve
- Intercostal nerves
- Dorsal scapular nerve
- Suprascapular nerve

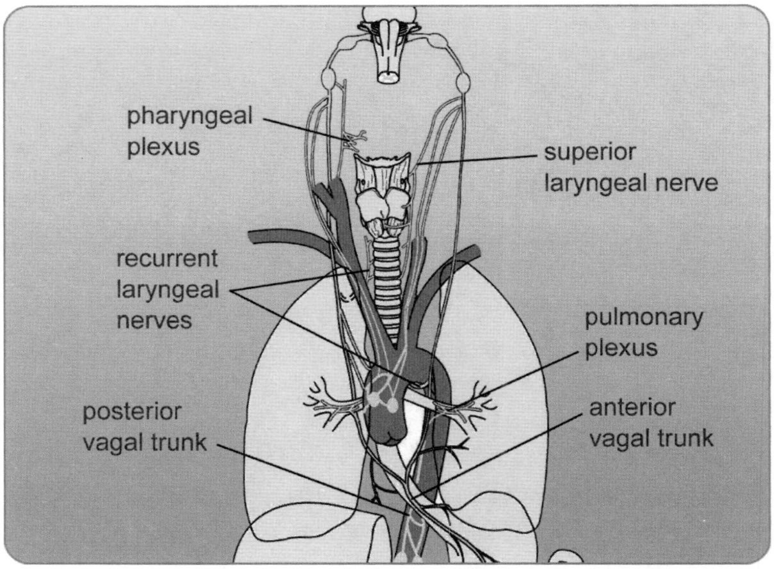

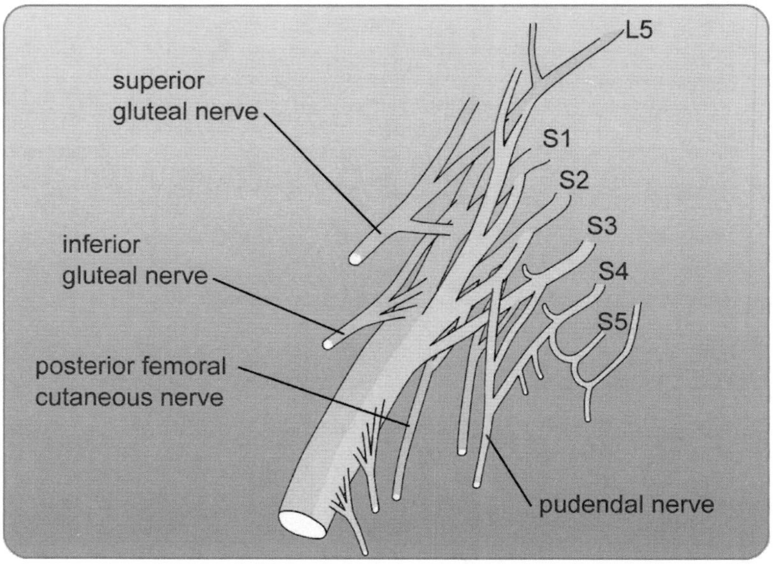

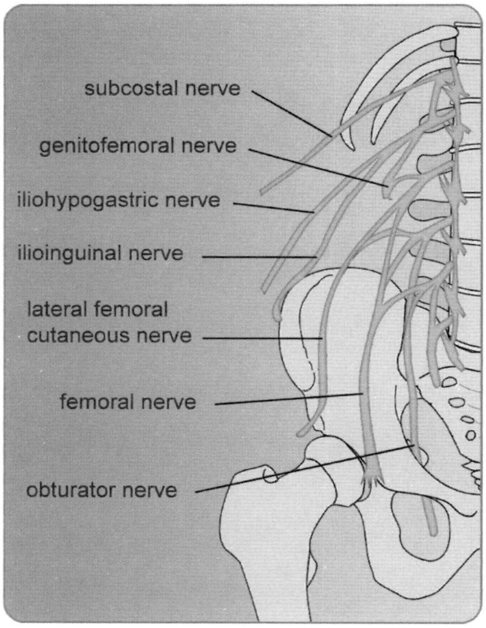

AUTONOMIC NERVES

The **autonomic** portion of the nervous system is a special sub-portion of the peripheral nervous system. The autonomic nerves either belong to the **parasympathetic** branch (digestion, breathing, slow heart rate, cellular metabolism) or the **sympathetic** branch (faster heart rate, "fight or flight" response). You will encounter the term *ganglion* among the names of the autonomic nerves. A **ganglion** is a cluster of neuronal cell bodies. Many of the ganglia of the autonomic nervous system lie along the **sympathetic trunk** (sympathetic chain) which is composed of bilateral bundles of nerve fibers, one on each side of the vertebral column. The sympathetic trunk extends from the base of the skull to the coccyx. For ICD-10 coding, you will need to know some of the different nerves of the autonomic nervous system. Find the list of autonomic nerves in the image provided.

- Sympathetic trunk (sympathetic chain)
- Greater, lesser, lumbar, sacral splanchnic nerves
- Celiac ganglion
- Superior and inferior mesenteric ganglion
- Hypogastric ganglion

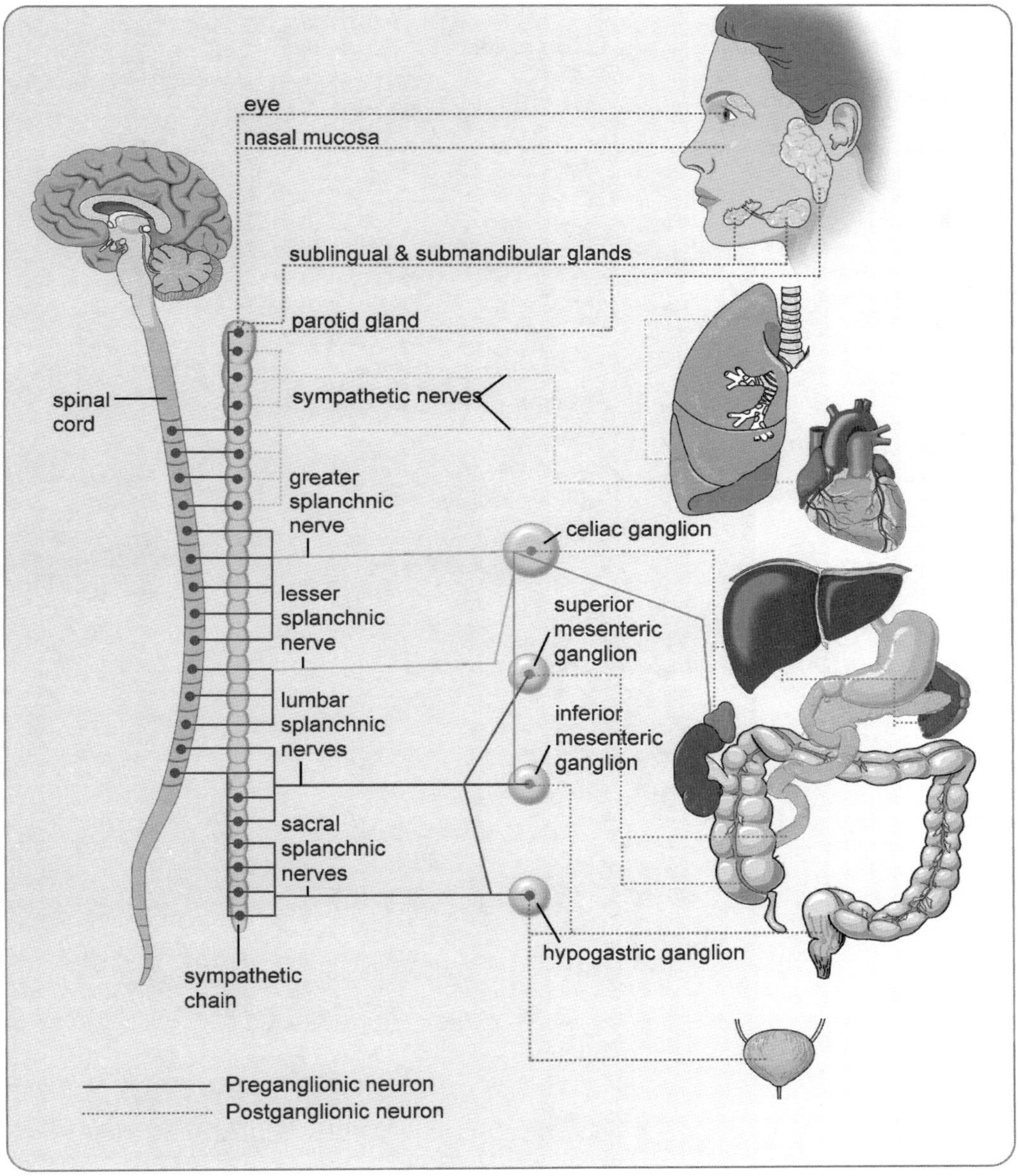

REVIEW: THE PERIPHERAL NERVOUS SYSTEM

I. FILL IN THE BLANK.

Using the word/word parts in the box, fill in the blanks.

filum terminale
conus medullaris
second lumbar
cauda equina
brain

1. The ________________ is the center of the nervous system.
2. The cone-shaped ending of the spinal cord is called the ________________.
3. The ________________ is a band of connective tissue arising from the conus medullaris.
4. Nerves branching out from the conus medullaris are called ________________.
5. The spinal cord ends at about the level of the ________________ vertebra.

II. MULTIPLE CHOICE.

Choose the best answer.

1. How many pairs of spinal nerves rise laterally from the spinal cord and externally through the foramina of the vertebral column?
   - ◯ 30
   - ◯ 31
   - ◯ 32
   - ◯ 33

2. The peripheral nervous system is made up of spinal nerves and _____ nerves.
   - ◯ autonomic
   - ◯ brain
   - ◯ cranial
   - ◯ motor innervation

3. The _____ System functions continuously and involuntarily, without conscious control.
   - ◯ autonomic nervous
   - ◯ peripheral nervous
   - ◯ central nervous
   - ◯ spinal nervous

4. The ANS function within which system?
   - ◯ Ancillary Nervous System
   - ◯ Central Nervous System
   - ◯ Peripheral Nervous System
   - ◯ both Central Nervous and Peripheral Nervous Systems

III. MATCHING.

Match the correct term to the definition. Answers may be used more than once.

1. ___ knee
2. ___ hand
3. ___ hip and upper leg
4. ___ foot
5. ___ thigh

A. femoral
B. tibial nerve
C. median nerve
D. sciatic nerve

UNIT 8

The Digestive System

THE DIGESTIVE SYSTEM - INTRODUCTION

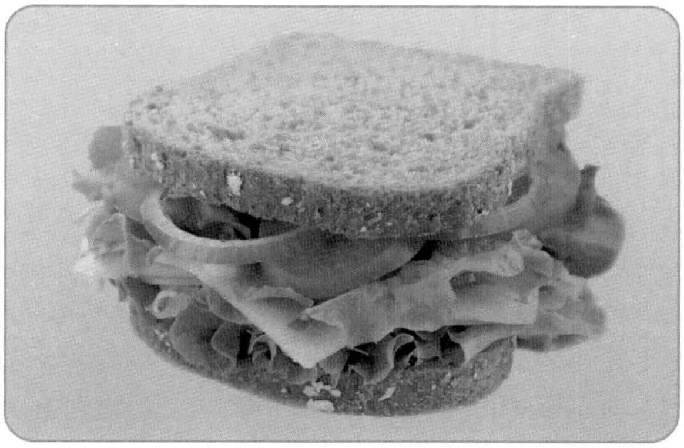

Just as bones and muscles are vital in supporting the human body, nutritious food and fluids are also vital to growth, repair, and production of body energy. The digestive system is the body system through which all consumed liquid and solid materials pass, enabling body organs to absorb and metabolize important nutrients.

Abdomen refers to the central part of the body from below the chest to the hips. The generic term *gut* is sometimes used as well; however, in medicine this generally refers to the developing GI (gastrointestinal) tract of an embryo. The term *viscera* (singular is *viscus*) is often used to designate the individual organs of digestion; however, the term is actually a general term for any organ of the abdominal or thoracic cavity. This would include digestive organs such as the liver and pancreas, but also respiratory organs such as the lungs. These are not specific medical anatomic terms, but rather a method of designating the external area specific to organs of digestion.

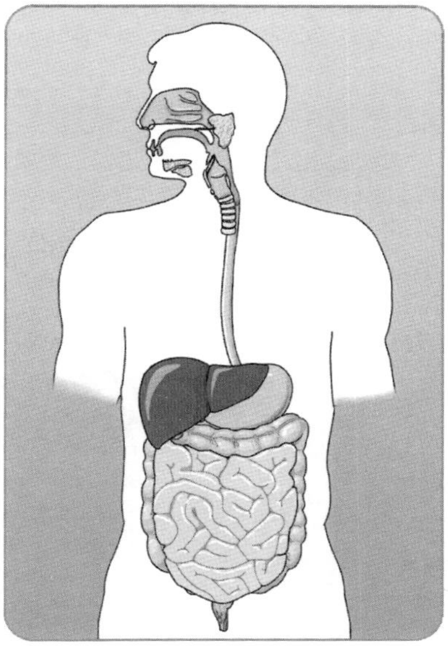

The digestive tract is a tube (lumen) that extends from the mouth to the anus. There are several organ systems connected along this path, such as the gallbladder, liver, pancreas, and salivary glands. Each organ has a specific function vital to the health of the human body, and the nutrients taken in through the digestive process are crucial to their ability to function. In other words, the digestive system consists of all of the parts of the body associated with solids and liquids from entrance by way of the mouth on down until every nutrient has been absorbed and the waste eliminated. Liquid waste is mostly eliminated through the urinary tract system; however, due to its close association with structures of the reproductive system, the urinary system will be introduced in a later unit.

MOUTH AND ASSOCIATED ORGANS

The structure and function of the digestive system begins with the **mouth (oral cavity)** and its associated organs. Food enters the mouth, is moistened by saliva, is masticated by the **teeth**, all while being manipulated and tasted by the **tongue**. The **lips (labia)** and cheeks hold food in the mouth (which is probably why your parents taught you to chew with your mouth closed).

Highlights

The oral cavity is divided into two sections: The vestibule and oral cavity proper.

Vestibule: Space between teeth and lips/cheeks.

Oral Cavity Proper: Space internal to the teeth (where tongue lies).

The oral cavity is divided into two sections: the **vestibule** and **oral cavity proper**. With your teeth and mouth shut tight, the vestibule is the space between the teeth and the lips or cheeks, and the oral cavity proper is the space internal to the teeth, where the tongue lies. The lining of the inside of the mouth is made of a stratified squamous epithelium, which protects it from abrasion due to hard or sharp foods during chewing. As you learned in the muscles unit of anatomy, the cheeks are formed by the buccinator muscles and the lips by the orbicularis oris muscle.

The part of the lips that we lick the most, where lipstick is applied and kisses are received or given, is called the **red margin**, with the line between the red of the lips and the skin above is the **vermilion border**. This is very thin and translucent tissue so the red color is actually derived from blood flow in the underlying capillaries. There are no sweat glands or salivary glands in the red margin of the lips so periodic moistening of the lips by the tongue is needed to prevent drying and cracking. The lips are connected to the inner mucosa of the gums by way of the superior and inferior **labial frenula** (singular, frenulum - which means "little bridle of the lip").

I. FILL IN THE BLANK.

Enter the correct word in the blank provided.

1. Another word for lips, the ______________ works with the cheeks to hold food in your mouth.
2. The space between the teeth and the lips or cheeks is called the ______________.
3. The ______________ is the space internal to the teeth that contains the tongue.
4. The______________ is the lining that protects the inside of the mouth from hard or sharp foods.
5. The area of the lips where lipstick is applied is called the ______________.
6. The line between the red of the lips and the skin is called the ______________.
7. The lips are connected to the gums with the______________.

PALATE

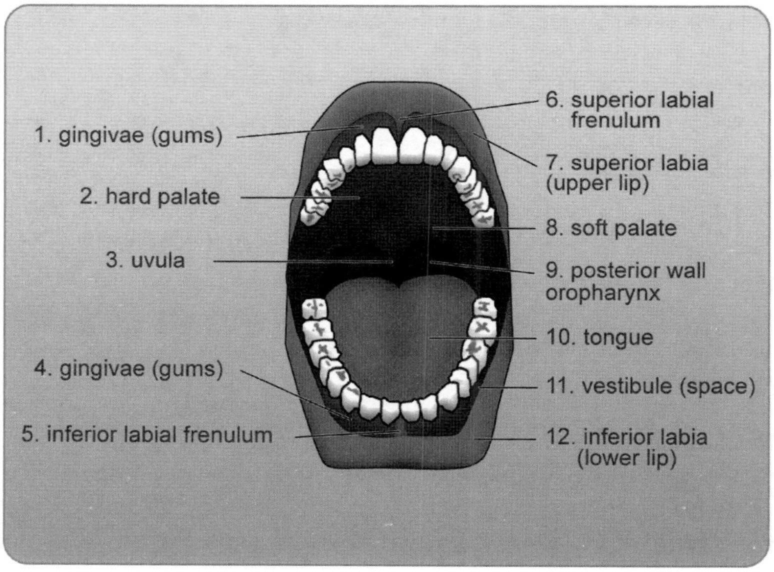

The palate forms the roof of the mouth and is made of two distinct sections, the hard palate and the soft palate. The **hard palate** is located anteriorly and the soft palate posteriorly. If you take a moment and place the tip of your tongue on the roof of your mouth just behind the teeth and gums and press, you will find the hard palate. The hard palate forms a rigid surface against which the tongue forces food during mastication. This hard surface is provided skeletal support by the maxilla and palatine bones. Now move your tongue to the back of the roof of your mouth just in front of your uvula and press again; this is the soft palate. The **soft palate** rises during swallowing to close off the **nasopharynx**. To see how this functions, try to breathe and swallow at the same time. The **uvula** is a finger-like piece of soft tissue that hangs down at the opening of the throat. It is anchored to the free edge of the soft palate.

It is helpful to note that many of the structures in the extreme upper digestive system are shared with the respiratory system, performing multiple important functions.

I. FILL IN THE BLANK.

Enter the bolded terms in the space provided.

1. **gingivae** ________________
2. **hard palate** ________________
3. **inferior labia** ________________
4. **inferior labial frenulum** ________________
5. **posterior wall oropharynx** ________________
6. **soft palate** ________________
7. **superior labia** ________________
8. **superior labial frenulum** ________________
9. **tongue** ________________
10. **uvula** ________________
11. **vestibule** ________________

II. FILL IN THE BLANK.

Refer to the image and enter the term corresponding to the following numbers. Use the words in the box to fill in the blanks.

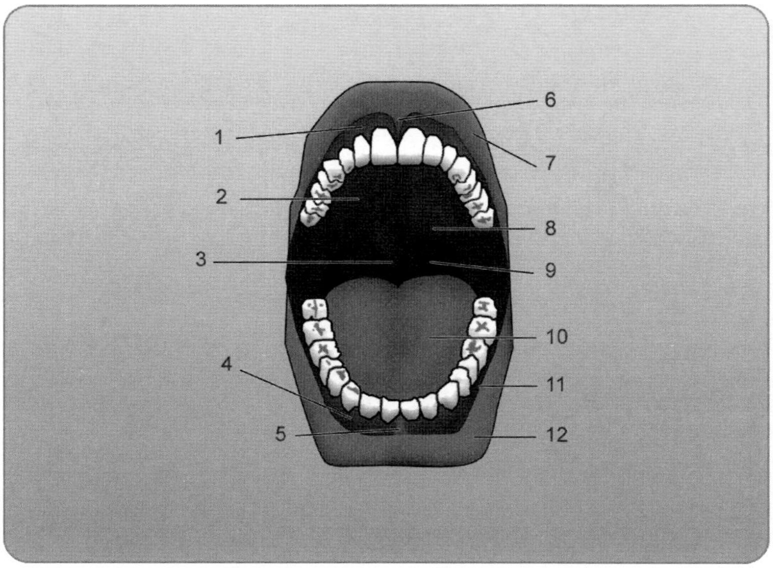

1. ____________
2. ____________
3. ____________
4. ____________
5. ____________
6. ____________
7. ____________
8. ____________
9. ____________
10. ____________
11. ____________
12. ____________

superior labia (upper lip)
gingivae (gums)
soft palate
posterior wall oropharynx
inferior labial frenulum
vestibule
inferior labia (lower lip)
superior labial frenulum
tongue
hard palate
gingivae (gums)
uvula

III. MULTIPLE CHOICE.
Choose the best answer.

1. Another name for an organ.
   - ◯ viscera
   - ◯ lumen
   - ◯ serosa
   - ◯ peristalsis

2. The hollow part of a tube.
   - ◯ lingual
   - ◯ perineum
   - ◯ mesentery
   - ◯ lumen

3. Another name for the mouth.
   - ◯ lingual
   - ◯ oral cavity
   - ◯ pharynx
   - ◯ mucosa

4. Term that means literally "pertaining to the cheek."
   - ◯ facial
   - ◯ alimentary canal
   - ◯ buccal
   - ◯ lingual frenulum

5. Refers to the GI tract of an embryo.
   - ◯ gut
   - ◯ abdomen
   - ◯ tummy
   - ◯ adventitia

6. Describes the body from the chest to the hips.
   - ◯ abdomen
   - ◯ dorsal mesentery
   - ◯ retroperitoneal
   - ◯ viscera

TONGUE

The tongue is a muscle that occupies most of the space on the floor of the mouth. The tongue serves several purposes:

- Contains **taste buds** for the ability to taste food and differentiate between sour, sweet, bitter, and spicy.
- Manipulates food that is being chewed by gripping it and repositioning it between the teeth for **mastication**.
- Helps mix saliva with food in order to form a compact mass or **bolus** of food.
- During swallowing, the tongue helps to push the food bolus or liquids into the pharynx for further digestion.
- In speech, the tongue aids in the formation of various consonants, such as d, k, l, n, t, and w.

> **Highlights**
>
> Extrinsic muscles allow the tongue to alter position.
>
> Intrinsic muscles allow the tongue to change shape.

The tongue is made up of two different types of muscles: extrinsic and intrinsic. Extrinsic muscles allow the tongue to change position, protrude, retract, move laterally, or wiggle. Intrinsic muscles allow the tongue to change shape to flat, round, firm, and relaxed.

We will look closer at the anatomy of the tongue on the following page, but first, locate the following structures in the image:

- Hard palate
- soft palate
- uvula
- palatine tonsil
- lingual tonsil
- tongue
- epiglottis

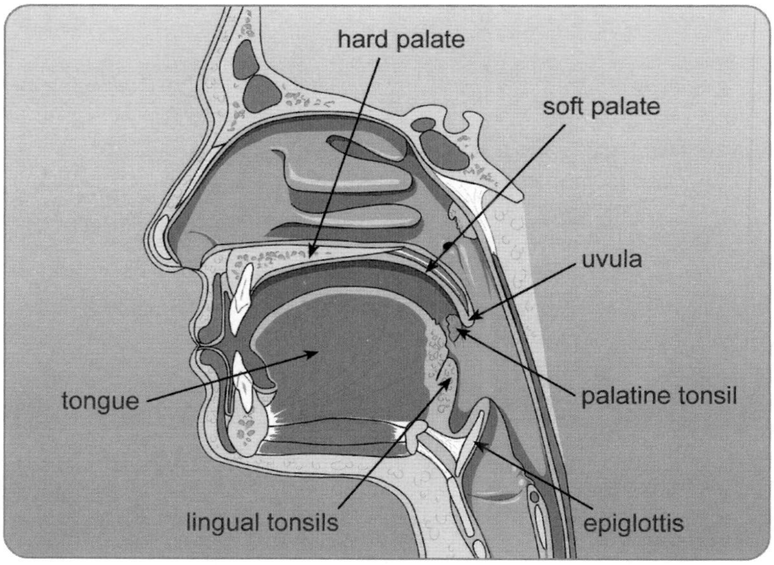

ANATOMY OF THE TONGUE

The tongue is secured to the floor of the mouth by the lingual frenulum. This secures the tongue into its position and limits its posterior movements so the tongue cannot be easily swallowed. When the lingual frenulum is abnormally short or long, a person is said to be "tongue-tied" (ankyloglossia), which distorts their speech and overly restricts tongue movement. This abnormality is corrected by snipping the **lingual frenulum**, once again allowing movement of the tongue and improving speech.

The superior surface of the tongue consists of three major types of projections:

- filiform papillae
- fungiform papillae
- circumvallate papillae

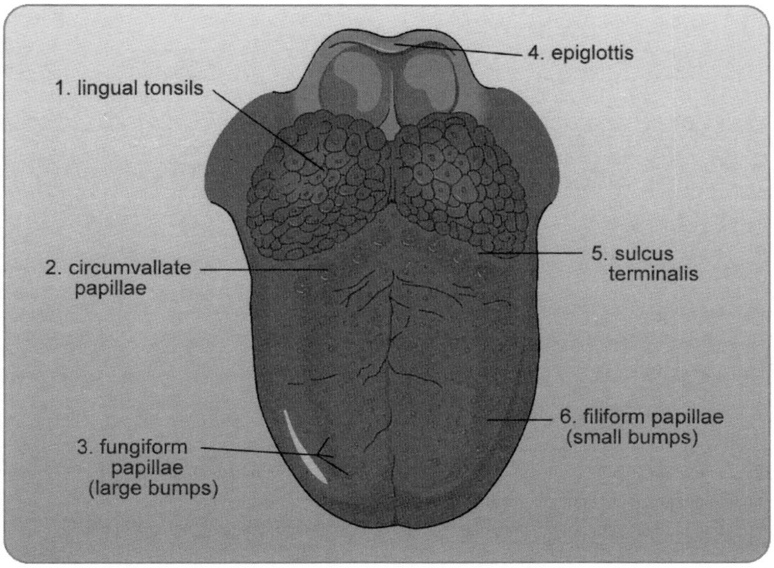

The **filiform papillae** lend a rough surface to the tongue, allowing it to grasp food and manipulate it during mastication. The filiform papillae are very numerous and give the tongue its whitish appearance, lining up in parallel rows.

The **fungiform papillae** have a vascular core that gives them a reddish appearance. Fungiform papillae, like their name "fungi," actually have a mushroom-like appearance.

Taste buds are located in the epithelium on the tops of fungiform papillae. Take a moment and look into a mirror at your tongue (in a very well lit room), and see if you can see these scattered fungiform papillae on the surface of your tongue. They are not as abundant as the filiform papillae but are more visible. As you may know, a swollen taste bud is a very painful and very visible malady that most individuals suffer on occasion.

Two-thirds of the way back on the tongue surface and anterior to the **sulcus terminalis** (a groove that marks the border between the mouth and the pharynx) lies the **circumvallate papillae**. There are 10–12 circumvallate papillae that lie in the shape of a V. These are individually surrounded by a circular ridge and the epithelium on the sides of these papillae contain more taste buds.

The posterior third of the tongue, or the root of the tongue, is considered part of the **oropharynx** and contains lingual tonsils. Many individuals who have had their palantine tonsils surgically removed can continue to get tonsillitis; however, this type of tonsillitis is called **lingual tonsillitis** and is treated with antibiotics.

I. FILL IN THE BLANK.

Enter the bolded terms in the space provided.

1. **circumvallate papillae** ________________
2. **epiglottis** ________________
3. **filiform papillae** ________________
4. **fungiform papillae** ________________
5. **lingual tonsils** ________________
6. **sulcus terminalis** ________________

II. FILL IN THE BLANK.

Refer to the image and enter the term corresponding to the following numbers. Use the words in the box to fill in the blanks.

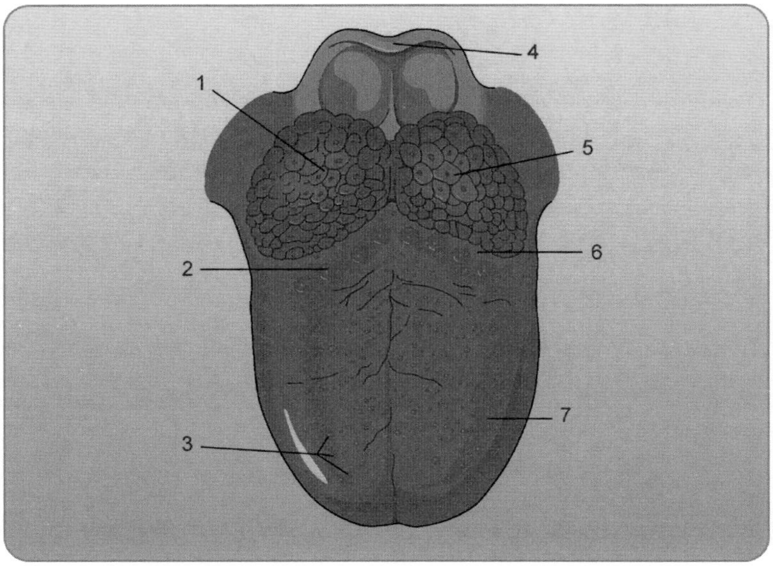

1. ____________
2. ____________
3. ____________
4. ____________
5. ____________
6. ____________
7. ____________

sulcus terminalis
lingual tonsils
filiform papillae
circumvallate papillae
lingual tonsils
epiglottis
fungiform papillae

III. MULTIPLE CHOICE.
Choose the best answer.

1. Elevations on the tongue.
   - ◯ papillae
   - ◯ serosa
   - ◯ omentum
   - ◯ buccal

2. Means pertaining to the tongue.
   - ◯ inguinal
   - ◯ oral
   - ◯ buccal
   - ◯ lingual

3. The tongue is connected to the floor of the mouth via the _____.
   - ◯ lingual frenulum
   - ◯ buccal
   - ◯ oral cavity
   - ◯ muscularis

TEETH

Our teeth allow us to masticate (chew) our food by tearing, grinding, and breaking it into tiny pieces that can then be digested. There are two sets of teeth (dentitions) present at birth. The first set to erupt are the **deciduous teeth (baby teeth)**, followed by the **permanent teeth**.

Underneath the deciduous teeth lie the permanent teeth. Between the ages of 5–12, the deciduous teeth are reabsorbed until they loosen and fall out.

Teeth fall into four classifications:

1. incisors
2. canines
3. premolars
4. molars

Teeth have different classifications. These classifications are made according to shape and function of the teeth. Teeth fall into four classifications: **incisors**, **canines**, **premolars**, and **molars**.

Shaped like a chisel, the main function of the incisor is to bite off pieces of food, the canines (eyeteeth/ cuspids) pierce and tear food, and premolars (bicuspids) and molars grind and mash food with a tremendous crushing power.

Teeth are surrounded by a pink, fleshy tissue called **gingiva (gums)**. Teeth consist of three main parts: **crown**, **neck**, and **root**.

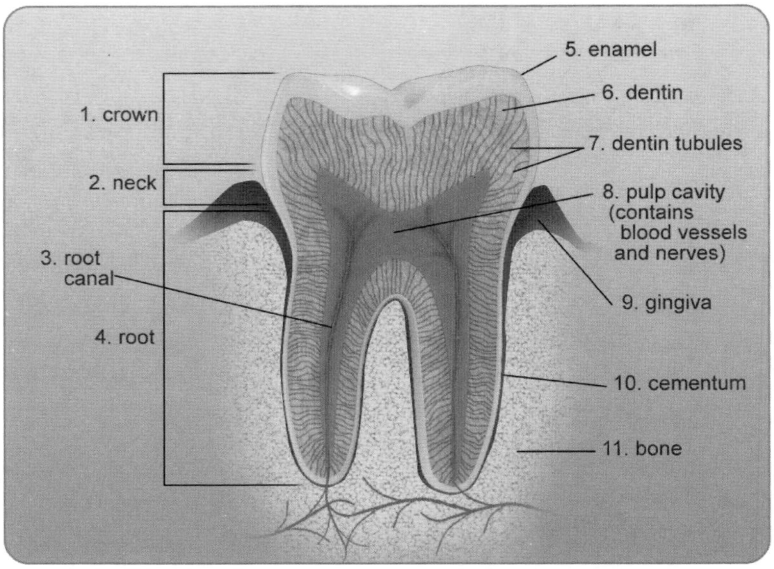

The crown is covered in **enamel**, which is the hardest substance in the body. It gives the teeth a white appearance and protects them from friction. Beneath the enamel is the **dentin**. This is considerably softer than enamel and is a yellowish, bony tissue. The innermost part of the tooth is the **pulp cavity**, which is filled with dental pulp, a loose connective tissue containing the nerve endings and blood vessels. This pulp supplies the tooth with nutrients and sensation. When a tooth is damaged by a blow or by a deep cavity, the pulp may become infected or even die. When this occurs, a **root canal** procedure must be performed. In this procedure the pulp is drilled out and the pulp cavity is sterilized and filled with a substance before the tooth can be capped.

The protective layer that covers the root is the **cementum** and the periodontal membrane actually holds the tooth in place. The crown and root meet near the gum line and form what is called the **neck** of the tooth.

Dental cavities or caries are a result of a gradual deterioration or demineralization of the tooth enamel and dentin due to bacteria. Dental plaque is a buildup of sugar, bacteria, and other debris that adheres to the surface of the teeth. These trapped sugars then metabolize and produce an acid that dissolves the calcium salts within the teeth. When the calcium salts have been leached out of the teeth, protein-digesting enzymes then destroy the remaining tooth matrix. Brushing teeth frequently helps to prevent dental cavities and tooth decay.

I. FILL IN THE BLANK.

Refer to the image and enter the term corresponding to the following numbers. Use the words in the box to fill in the blanks.

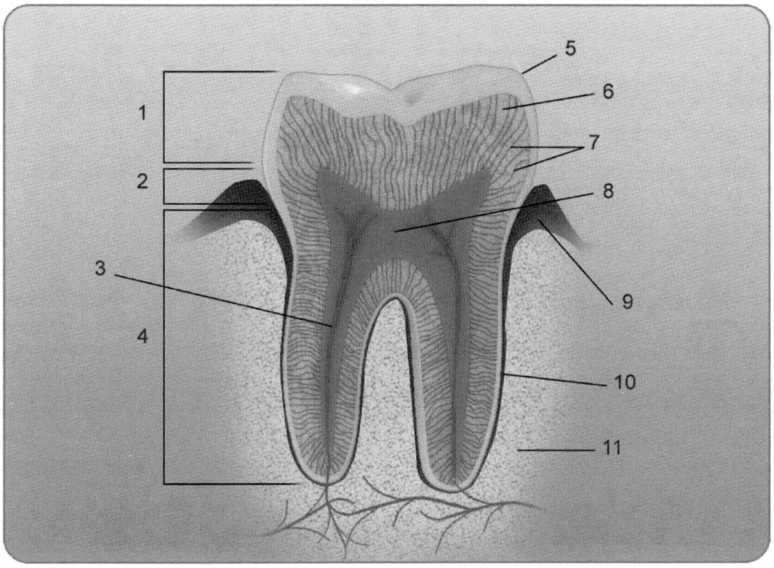

1. ________________
2. ________________
3. ________________
4. ________________
5. ________________
6. ________________
7. ________________
8. ________________
9. ________________
10. ________________
11. ________________

root canal
gingiva
crown
dentin
cementum
pulp cavity
enamel
bone
dentin tubules
root
neck

SALIVARY GLANDS

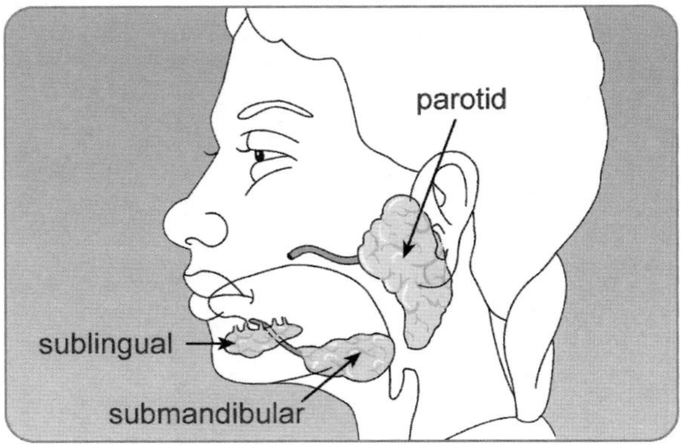

Salivary glands produce saliva, a complex mixture of water, ions, mucus, and enzymes. Saliva contains: a bicarbonate buffer that neutralizes bacteria-producing acids to help prevent tooth decay, proteins to stimulate the growth of good bacteria, and antiviral substances, antibodies, as well as a cyanide compound, which kills harmful microorganisms.

Saliva moistens the mouth, wets and dissolves food, and binds it into a bolus, allowing the enzymes in the saliva to start the digestive process before food is propelled towards the alimentary canal.

There are two distinct types of salivary glands: minor salivary glands and large extrinsic salivary glands.

The **minor salivary glands** are located throughout the mouth: in the mucosa of the tongue, palate, lips, and cheeks. They are responsible for maintaining a moist mouth.

Large extrinsic salivary glands lie external to the mouth, but their ducts connect to it. They secrete saliva only when we eat or when we anticipate eating. There are three pairs of extrinsic salivary glands:

1. parotid
2. submandibular
3. sublingual

Of these, the **parotids** are the largest. They are found in front of and below the external ear. The parotid ducts are called Stensen ducts. The **submandibular glands** are located just below the mandibular angle. Their ducts are the Wharton ducts. The smallest extrinsic salivary glands are the **sublingual glands**. They lie in front of the submandibular glands and are drained by the ducts of Rivinus.

PHARYNX

The **pharynx** has a role in both respiration and digestion. It is commonly referred to as the throat. There are three areas that make up the pharynx, including:

nasopharynx – the upper-most portion that starts at the back of the nasal cavity

oropharynx – the area from the soft palate to the hyoid bone

laryngopharynx – from the hyoid bone to the esophagus

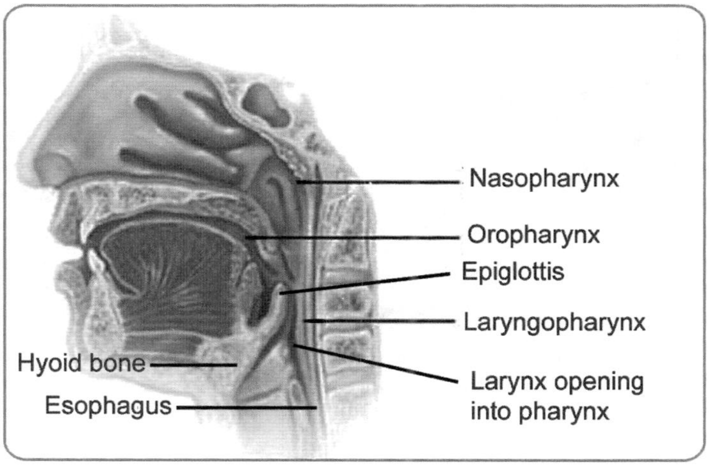

For digestion, the oropharynx is the most important part of the pharynx as it channels food to the esophagus during digestion and air to the trachea during respiration. The **epiglottis** covers the trachea during swallowing to prevent food or liquids from entering the trachea. The oropharynx is where the **palatine tonsils** are located. These are more commonly referred to as the tonsils and removed during a tonsillectomy.

The nasopharynx and laryngopharynx will be discussed with the anatomy unit for the respiratory system.

I. **MULTIPLE CHOICE.**
Choose the best answer.

1. The part of the pharynx most concerned with digestion is the (◯ laryngopharynx, ◯ oropharynx, ◯ nasopharynx, ◯ epiglottal pharynx).

2. The (◯ oropharynx, ◯ hyoid bone, ◯ epiglottis, ◯ uvula) prevents food or liquid from entering the trachea during swallowing.

ALIMENTARY CANAL

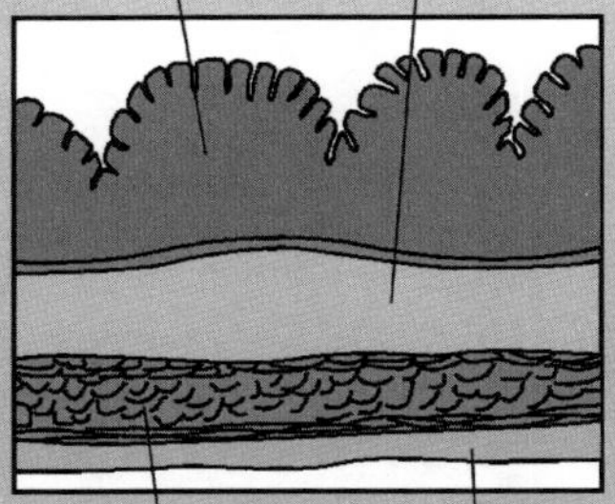

The main part of the digestive system is the alimentary canal. It is also called the GI tract (gastrointestinal tract). This is a generic term given for the tube that extends from the lips to the anus. It is coiled, varies in diameter, and the parts are identified individually. However, it never branches and is, in fact, a single continuous tube. The alimentary canal is approximately nine meters (or 30 feet) long and is made up of four layers of tunica (coat or covering).

- Serosa
- Muscularis, consisting of the inner and outer muscularis
- Submucosa
- Mucosa

Tunica Serosa

This is the outermost covering of the alimentary canal within the abdominal cavity. In most of the digestive tract (stomach and intestines), it consists of a thin layer of loose connective tissue covered by **mesothelium** (a type of squamous epithelium [single layer of skin cells] that lines body cavities within the peritoneal cavity). This structure is also referred to as **visceral peritoneum**, as it covers all of the vital organs.

In the abdominal cavity, the serosa surrounding the tube of the alimentary canal fuses together to form a suspensory structure called **mesentery**. This structure houses blood vessels and nerves that supply the digestive tract and is continuous for the length of the cavity lining. Outside of the abdominal cavity, the digestive tube connects to such structures as the esophagus and rectum by way of a layer of connective tissue called the **tunica adventitia**.

Tunica Muscularis (inner and outer)

This gives the alimentary canal the ability to be motile (having the ability of spontaneous movement). In most of the alimentary canal, muscularis consists of two thick layers (inner and outer muscularis) of smooth muscle (involuntary muscles with a single nuclei, spindle-like in appearance). The muscle fibers of the inner layer are aligned circularly, whereas those in the outer layer are aligned longitudinally. This combination of circular and longitudinal smooth muscle gives the tube an ability to perform complex movements that squeeze and propel solid or liquid nutrients in the lumen (a process called **peristalsis**). Additionally, the muscularis contains valves or **sphincters**. These are especially thickened circular muscles that occur in strategic places within the canal to regulate food passage. Between the inner circular and outer longitudinal layers of smooth muscle is another critical component of the digestive tract's nervous system—the myenteric (muscle + intestine) plexus.

Tunica Submucosa

This layer lies between the mucosal and inner muscularis layers. This layer is highly vascular (containing many blood vessels). It is composed of elastic and collagen fibers, and its function is to serve the mucosal layer. The submucosa also contains the submucous plexus, a critical component of the digestive tract's nervous system that provides nervous control to the mucosa.

Tunica Mucosa

This is the innermost layer of the alimentary canal that lines the lumen (the hollow part of a tube or organ) of the digestive tract. Of the four tunic layers, the mucosa is the most widely varied. It allows the lumen the ability to perform digestive tasks along its length. Included within the tunica mucosa are epithelial cells vital to the functions of nutrient absorption. Beneath the epithelium, but still within the tunica mucosa, is a layer called the lamina propria, which is loose connective tissue. Blood vessels and lymphatics course through the lamina propria to supply the epithelium. Beneath the lamina propria is the lamina muscularis mucosae, a thin layer of smooth muscle that allows the mucosa to move and fold.

Three primary functions of this layer are:

Distention: the state of being enlarged or allowing for an increased capacity. This occurs most notably in the stomach.

Absorption: the process of absorbing or assimilating nutrients, such as in the small intestine, or the absorption of water in the colon.

Secretion: where the glandular parts secrete digestive enzymes into the cavity to break down food, such as in the stomach.

I. **FILL IN THE BLANK.**

Refer to the image and enter the term corresponding to the following numbers. Use the words in the box to fill in the blanks.

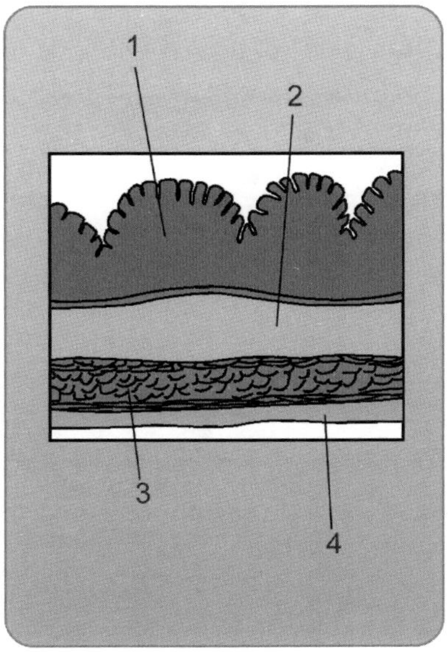

1. ________________
2. ________________
3. ________________
4. ________________

tunica muscularis
tunica mucosa
tunica serosa
tunica submucosa

STRUCTURES OF THE ALIMENTARY CANAL

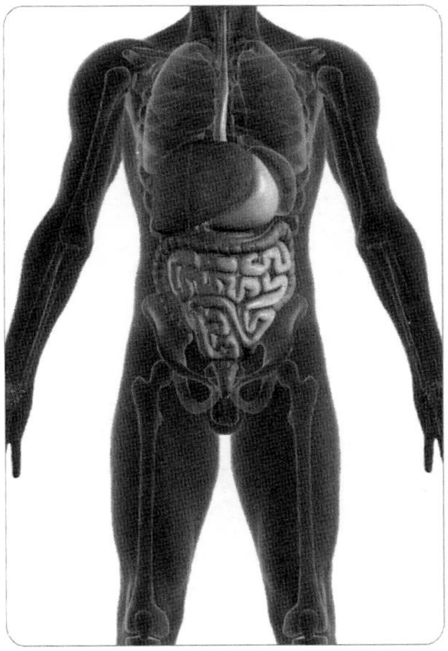

As you are exposed to the examination, diagnosis, and treatment of gastrointestinal disorders in individual reports, the term "alimentary canal" or even "gastrointestinal tract" are far too general to be practical from a medical perspective, and thus you will rarely see them in transcribed reports. The same is true of larger components of the GI tract. The large intestine is a familiar term to many people from basic biology in high school or college; however, in a medical context this term is too general to be useful. It is necessary for medical practitioners to determine a specific component of the large intestine, such as the sigmoid colon or hepatic flexure, where a problem may exist. It is these individual parts of the tract that are identified on x-rays, CT scans, or in operative procedures.

In addition to the individual organs that make up the digestive system, there are many microscopic glandular structures that are found in the walls of the GI tract.

There are also larger secretory organs (such as the liver and pancreas) whose products are transmitted through ducts within the GI tract. These secretions break fats into fatty acids, proteins into amino acids, and carbohydrates into simple sugars. Only after food is broken down is it able to be used by the body for nutrition.

Essentially, the greater part of the gastrointestinal tract itself is contained within the abdominal cavity. The abdominal cavity is lined by the **parietal peritoneum**. On the back (or the dorsal side) the peritoneum itself forms long, thin sheets of tissue that support the GI tract. This is called the **dorsal mesentery**. Each organ or structure within the abdominal cavity also has its own protective lining called **visceral peritoneum** or **serosa**.

Where two organs are next to each other, double folds of peritoneum called **omentum** pass between them to support and transmit vessels and nerves to and from the organs. This omentum also protects the organs from excessive rubbing that would break down outer organ walls.

The omentum is divided into two sections:

1. The **lesser omentum** extends from the lesser curvature of the stomach to the underside of the liver.
2. The **greater omentum** extends from the greater curvature of the stomach to the transverse colon.

There are some abdominal organs positioned outside the peritoneal cavity, meaning they are not covered by peritoneum. These are referred to as **retroperitoneal** and include the pancreas, kidneys, most of the duodenum, and the abdominal aorta.

If you think about it, you already know a great deal about the process of digestion. For example, you take food into your mouth (also called the oral or buccal cavity). You taste it, chew it, and swallow it. The mouth and its components (e.g., lips, teeth, tongue) are vital to the process of digestion. The terms for these particular structures are part of our everyday vernacular, so they will not be further discussed in this chapter. However, there are, of course, medical designations for the same terms.

A lip is a labium (plural: labia), and lingual means "pertaining to the tongue." The tongue is connected to the floor of the mouth by the lingual frenulum. You know that lingua refers to the tongue, and a frenulum is a general term for a membrane that curbs or limits the movement of an organ or part. Finally, the tongue has many small elevations on it that are called papillae. These are also important in the process of digestion.

That specialty of medicine that deals specifically with digestion and problems associated with it is **gastroenterology**. In a hospital setting, gastroenterology is part of the medical record and will be integrated together with many other specialties. Consider 30 feet of digestive tract, and you can imagine the numerous problems that can occur.

Additionally, factor in how important the intake of food or nutrition is to sustaining life. Illnesses related to digestion and nutrition and the treatment of such illnesses is a major part of medicine. It will be necessary for you to be familiar with the anatomical structures found in this unit.

I. MULTIPLE CHOICE.
Choose the best answer.

1. The lining of the abdominal cavity.
   - ◯ parietal perineum
   - ◯ omentum
   - ◯ viscera
   - ◯ parietal peritoneum

2. The branch of medicine dealing with digestion.
   - ◯ genitourinary
   - ◯ gastroenterology
   - ◯ gastrologist
   - ◯ gerentologist

3. The outer and final layer of the GI tract.
   - ◯ omentum
   - ◯ serosa
   - ◯ adventitia
   - ◯ retroperitoneal

4. The process of assimilating nutrients.
   - ◯ gastroenterology
   - ◯ absorption
   - ◯ distention
   - ◯ secretion

5. Double folds of peritoneum.
   - ◯ serosa
   - ◯ omentum
   - ◯ peritoneum
   - ◯ adventitia

6. A term for releasing enzymes to break down food.
   - ◯ secretion
   - ◯ secretive
   - ◯ distending
   - ◯ peristalsis

7. Another term for visceral peritoneum.
   - ◯ submucosa
   - ◯ serosa
   - ◯ mucosa
   - ◯ adventitia

8. The canal which makes up most of the digestive system.
   - ◯ digestive canal
   - ◯ alimentary canal
   - ◯ gastroenterology canal
   - ◯ absorptive canal

9. The layer responsible for contraction.
   - ◯ muscularis
   - ◯ collagen
   - ◯ lumen
   - ◯ serosa

10. Organs not covered by the peritoneum.
    - ◯ peritoneal
    - ◯ viscera
    - ◯ retroperitoneal
    - ◯ submucosa

11. Long, thin sheets of tissue that support the GI tract.
    - ◯ serosa
    - ◯ lumen
    - ◯ dorsal mesentery
    - ◯ peritoneum

12. The approximate length of the GI tract.
    - ◯ 40 feet
    - ◯ 25 feet
    - ◯ 30 feet
    - ◯ 13 feet

13. The second layer surrounding the lumen.
    - ◯ serosa
    - ◯ submucosa
    - ◯ viscera
    - ◯ omentum

14. The state of being enlarged.
    - ◯ distention
    - ◯ retention
    - ◯ absorption
    - ◯ intention

15. Along with elastic fibers, this comprises the submucosal layer.
   - ◯ papillae
   - ◯ serosa
   - ◯ muscularis
   - ◯ collagen

16. The process by which the body moves food throuth the alimentary canal.
   - ◯ swallowing
   - ◯ peristalsis
   - ◯ secretion
   - ◯ absorption

17. The liver and pancreas are ______ organs.
   - ◯ inguinal
   - ◯ absorptive
   - ◯ secretory
   - ◯ mucosal

18. Extending from the larger curvature of the stomach to the transverse colon.
   - ◯ adventitia
   - ◯ greater omentum
   - ◯ parietal peritoneum
   - ◯ lesser omentum

19. Not a function of digestion.
   - ◯ absorption
   - ◯ secretion
   - ◯ distention
   - ◯ support

REVIEW: UPPER DIGESTIVE STRUCTURES

I. SPELLING.

Determine if the following words are spelled correctly. If the spelling is correct, leave the word as it has already been entered. If the spelling is incorrect, provide the correct spelling.

1. papilae ____________________
2. gastrointerology ____________________
3. distension ____________________
4. lingual ____________________
5. peritoneum ____________________
6. mucosa ____________________
7. mesentary ____________________
8. omentum ____________________
9. lumen ____________________
10. paristalsis ____________________

II. MATCHING.

Match the correct term to the definition. Enter only the letter in the space provided (no punctuation).

1. ____ The outer layer of the of the portion of the alimentary canal within the abdominal cavity.
2. ____ Double folds of peritoneum.
3. ____ The hollow part of a tube or tubular organ.
4. ____ Organs not covered by the peritoneum.
5. ____ Another name for the mouth.
6. ____ Describes the body from the chest to the hips.
7. ____ Extends from the larger curvature of the stomach to the transverse colon.
8. ____ Refers to the GI tract of an embryo.
9. ____ Means pertaining to the tongue.
10. ____ Term which means literally "pertaining to the cheek."

A. oral cavity
B. omentum
C. gut
D. lumen
E. greater omentum
F. abdomen
G. tunica serosa
H. buccal
I. lingual
J. retroperitoneal

III. MULTIPLE CHOICE.
Choose the best answer.

1. The branch of medicine dealing with digestion.
   - ◯ gastrenterology
   - ◯ gastroenterology
   - ◯ gastronterology
   - ◯ gastric enterology

2. The lining of the abdominal cavity.
   - ◯ parietal perineum
   - ◯ parietal peroneum
   - ◯ parental peritoneum
   - ◯ parietal peritoneum

3. Elevations on the tongue.
   - ◯ papillae
   - ◯ papilla
   - ◯ papilae
   - ◯ parpellae

4. Another name for organs.
   - ◯ viscera
   - ◯ visera
   - ◯ vicera
   - ◯ vissera

5. The process of assimilating nutrients.
   - ◯ absarption
   - ◯ absorption
   - ◯ absorpsion
   - ◯ absorptive

6. The tongue is connected to the floor of the mouth via the __________.
   - ◯ lingual frenulum
   - ◯ lingual phrenulum
   - ◯ lingual frenulem
   - ◯ lingual phrenulem

7. Along with elastic fibers, this comprises the submucosal layer.
   - ◯ colagen
   - ◯ collajen
   - ◯ colagin
   - ◯ collagen

8. The process by which the body moves food throuth the alimentary canal.
   - ◯ parastalsis
   - ◯ peristalsis
   - ◯ paristalsis
   - ◯ peristolsis

9. The approximate length of the GI tract.
   - ◯ 30 meters
   - ◯ 30 inches
   - ◯ 30 feet
   - ◯ 3 feet

10. Not a function of digestion.
   - ◯ absorption
   - ◯ secretion
   - ◯ distention
   - ◯ support

MAJOR STRUCTURES OF THE DIGESTIVE SYSTEM

The following are figures of the major structures of the digestive system. Note the placement of the individual components of the alimentary canal.

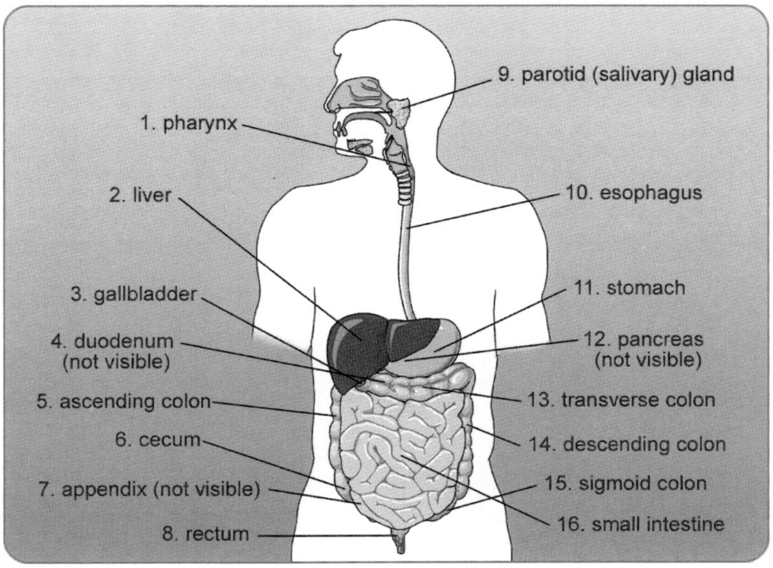

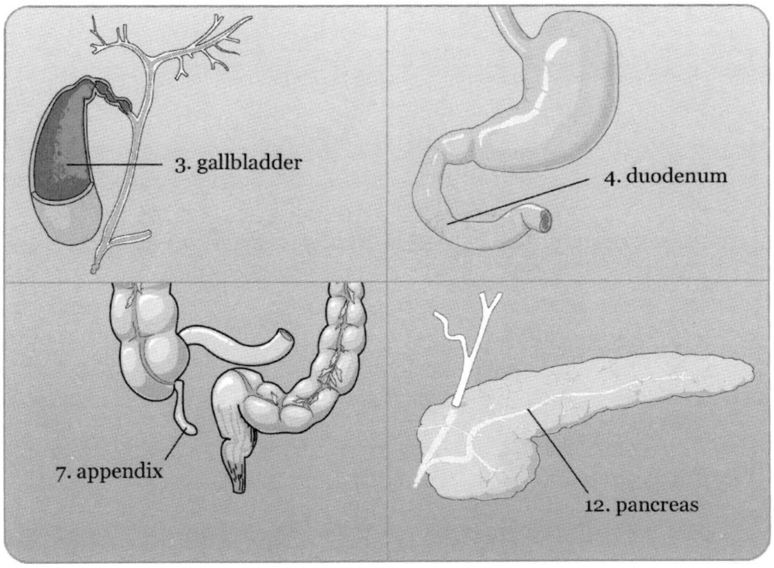

I. **FILL IN THE BLANK.**

Please enter the numbered terms in the blanks provided. Use the word(s) in the box to fill in the blanks.

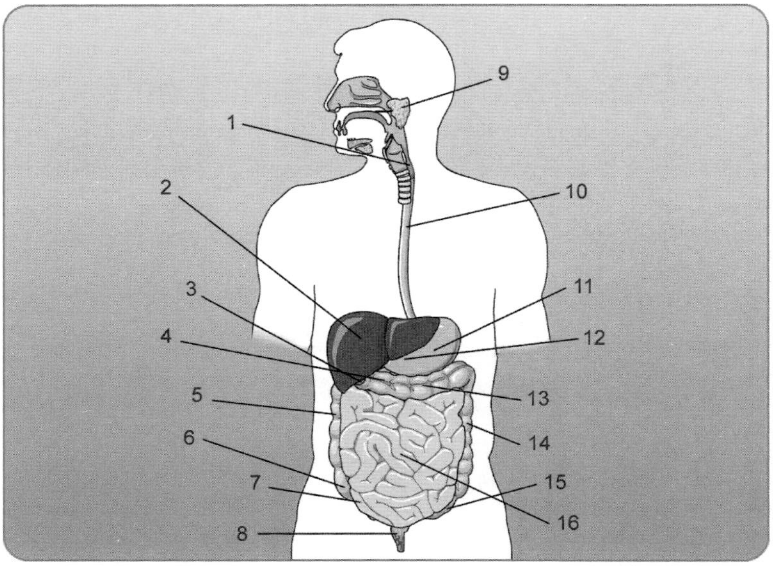

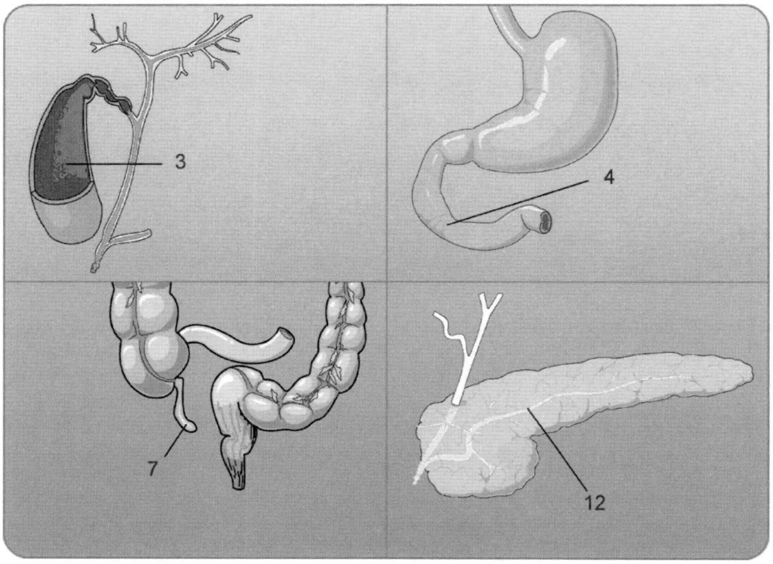

1. ________________
2. ________________
3. ________________
4. ________________
5. ________________
6. ________________
7. ________________
8. ________________
9. ________________
10. ________________
11. ________________
12. ________________
13. ________________
14. ________________
15. ________________
16. ________________

parotid (salivary) gland
small intestine
duodenum
transverse colon
gallbladder
sigmoid colon
ascending colon
descending colon
appendix
esophagus
pharynx
pancreas
rectum
liver
stomach
cecum

MOUTH AND ESOPHAGUS

Before continuing, it may be easier for you to learn additional terms if you are better acquainted with their nature and function.

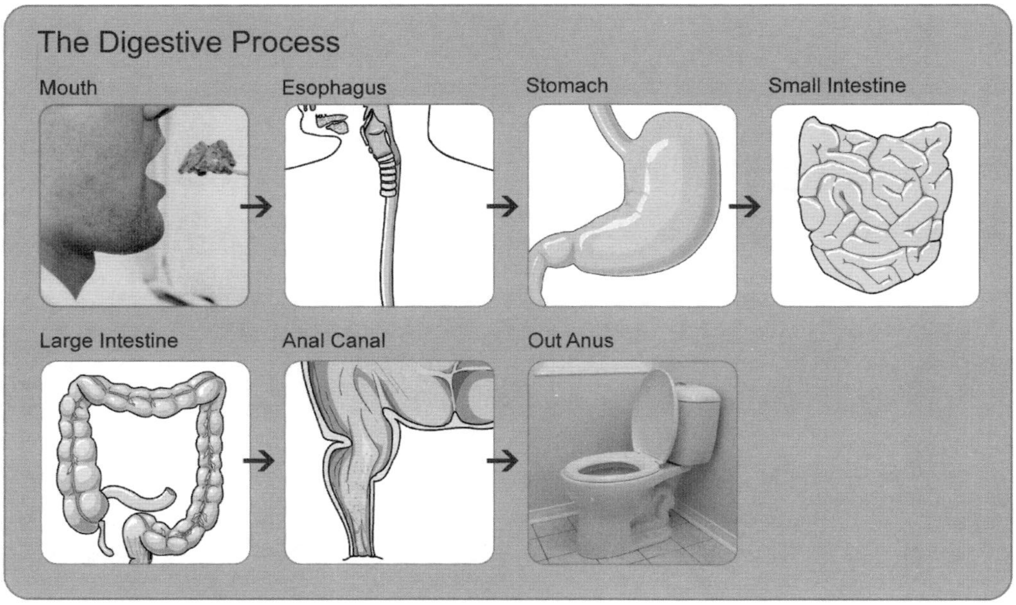

Mouth, Esophagus, Stomach

Common sense dictates that your mouth is where you put your food. This is the very beginning of the digestive process.

Next, you use your teeth to chew food or break it down into smaller particles that are easier for your body to process. To move on to the next phase, you swallow. At this point food enters the pharynx, which serves as a common passageway for both the respiratory system (which will be discussed in greater detail soon) and the digestive system.

There are separate components of the pharynx. The nasopharynx is a posterior continuation of the nasal cavity and is not actually part of the digestive system. The uvula is a small, fleshy mass that hangs from the soft palate, just above the base of the tongue. The oropharynx is a combination of the roots *oro-* (meaning relationship to the mouth) and *pharynx*, and extends from the soft palate within the mouth to the level of the hyoid bone. Also in this region is the epiglottis, which is a lid-like structure composed of cartilage that hangs over the entrance to the larynx to prevent food from entering the larynx or trachea upon swallowing.

The esophagus is the part of the alimentary canal that connects the pharynx to the stomach. It is a muscular tube that is about 25 cm long. The muscular function of the esophagus is not voluntary, but carries food quickly from one place to another.

There are eight steps that occur to get food from the mouth to the stomach:

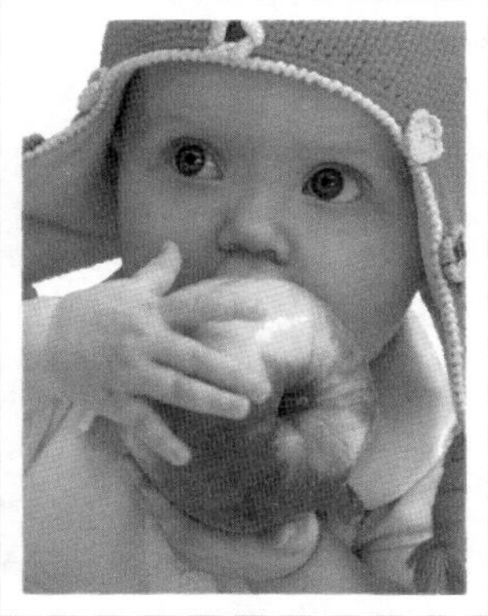

1. The food is chewed up and moistened with saliva to become a bolus, or a rounded mass of food.
2. The bolus is pushed to the back of the mouth by the tongue and the cheeks.
3. The soft palate and pendant uvula seal off the nasal cavity.
4. The tip of the tongue pushes up against the top of the mouth while the base of the tongue pushes the food down, and the sides of the pharynx contract.
5. The hyoid bone and the larynx are elevated.
6. The bolus pushes down on the epiglottis, which blocks the trachea.
7. A contraction of the pharynx pushes the bolus into the esophagus, past the larynx.
8. Another wave of contractions pushes the bolus through the esophagus to the stomach. The muscles of the neck and throat then relax and return to their normal breathing position.

I. **MATCHING.**
Match the correct term to the definition.

1. ____ pharynx
2. ____ uvula
3. ____ oropharynx
4. ____ epiglottis
5. ____ esophagus

A. small, fleshy mass hanging from the soft palate
B. lid-like structure that hangs over the entrance to the larynx
C. extends from the soft palate in the mouth to the level of the hyoid bone
D. part of the alimentary canal that connects the pharynx to the stomach
E. passageway for the respiratory and digestive system

STOMACH

The stomach is the most distended portion of the alimentary canal. It serves primarily as storage for food before it passes into the intestines. Although some digestion occurs at this point, food is primarily converted into a pasty material called **chyme**.

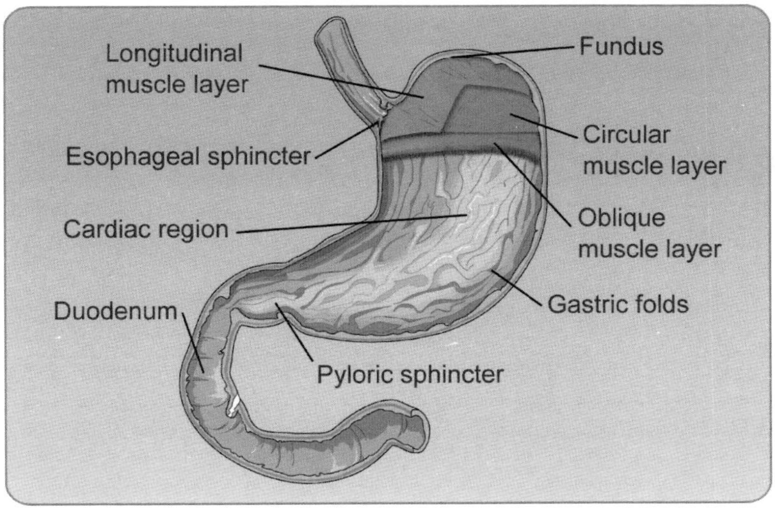

The stomach has three mechanical tasks. First, it stores the swallowed food and liquid. To do this, the muscle of the upper part of the stomach relaxes to accept large volumes of swallowed material via the lower esophageal sphincter. The second job is to mix up the food, liquid, and digestive juice produced by the stomach. The stomach muscle tissue is made up of several muscle types, thereby allowing the "mixer" effect that is necessary to change the bolus into material that can be metabolized. The third task of the stomach is to empty its contents slowly into the small intestine through the pyloric sphincter.

The stomach consists of four major parts and two curvatures:

1. The **cardiac orifice** is the junction between the esophagus and the stomach. This is also frequently referred to as the gastroesophageal junction (GE junction). The muscles here are in a constant state of contraction in order to prevent the stomach contents from flowing backward.
2. The **fundus** is the dome-shaped portion of the stomach that extends slightly above the cardiac orifice.
3. The **body** of the stomach is the widest portion and is located between the lesser and greater curvatures.
4. The **pylorus** of the stomach is the last area of the stomach, just before the duodenum.
5. The **lesser curvature** is the smaller curve at the more superior aspect of the stomach.
6. The **greater curvature** is the large curve that makes up the inferior border of the stomach.

I. MATCHING.
Match the correct term to the definition.

1. ____ fundus
2. ____ pyloric sphincter
3. ____ lower esophageal sphincter

A. dome-shaped portion of stomach
B. controls opening into the stomach
C. controls opening into the small intestine

SMALL INTESTINE

The small intestine is where most absorption of nutritional elements occurs in the gastrointestinal tract. The small intestine has three major parts: the duodenum, jejunum, and ileum. The **duodenum** is curve-shaped, resembling an imperfect circle. The **jejunum** is the next portion of the small intestine, followed by the **ileum**. While these parts are not distinct to the naked eye, their functions and internal anatomy differ. For instance the jejunum has more mucosal folds than the ileum and is slightly wider.

The small intestine is approximately 20 feet long!

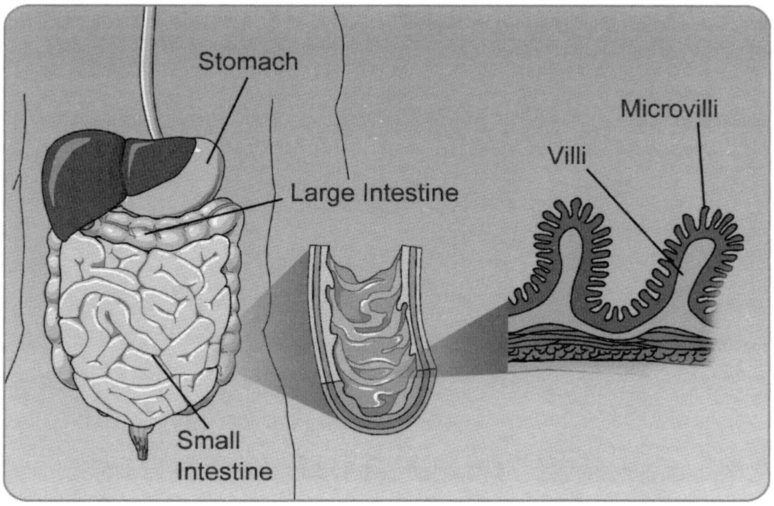

The lining (mucosa) of the small intestine contains many folds that are covered with tiny finger-like projections called **villi**. The villi are covered with microscopic projections called **microvilli**. The villi and microvilli create a very large surface area, enhancing absorption. Specialized cells in the small intestine allow materials to pass through the lining into the blood.

LARGE INTESTINE

The most distal portion of the alimentary canal is the **large intestine**. It is so named because at 6 cm in diameter, it is the widest portion of the canal. It is here that most water is absorbed and feces are formed. The large intestine is about 5 feet long. There are other differences from the small intestine. There are no villi in the large intestine. There are three distinct longitudinal muscles, teniae coli, that run the length of the large intestine. There is also a series of bulges in the wall of the large intestine called **sacculations** or **haustra**.

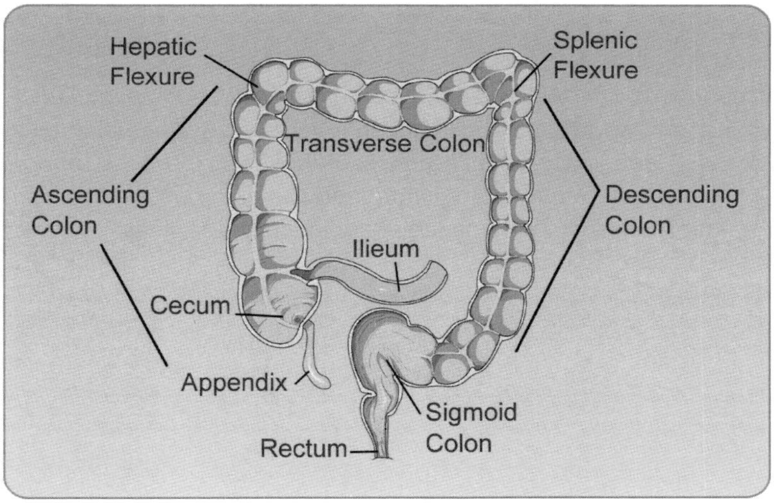

It is divided into four major regions:

Cecum – The first portion of the large intestine, the cecum, opens into the colon and is where the **appendix**, a small finger-like projection, is attached to its medial portion.

Colon – The second portion of the large intestine is the colon. Different areas of the colon have specific terms assigned to them. Continuing from the cecum in an upward direction is the **ascending colon**. At the liver, the colon bends sharply, an area referred to as the **hepatic flexure**. The colon then extends in a horizontal direction, called the **transverse colon**. At the left abdominal wall, there is another sharp bend in the colon called the **splenic flexure**. At this point, the colon continues in a downward direction and is called **descending colon**. Finally, the colon terminates in an S-shaped bend that is referred to as the **sigmoid colon**.

Rectum – The third portion of the large intestine is the rectum, located between the sigmoid colon and the anal canal.

Anus/Anal Canal – The anal canal forms a muscular opening in the muscles of the pelvic floor that is called the **anus**. This is surrounded by both involuntary and voluntary muscular sphincters.

REFERENCES AND ADDITIONAL ACTIVITIES FOR CODERS

http://anatomyarcade.com/ (Please note that there are some advertisements on this site. We do not endorse any products advertised.)

http://msjensen.cehd.umn.edu/WEBANATOMY/

LARGE GLANDULAR ORGANS OF THE DIGESTIVE SYSTEM

Although the alimentary canal comprises most of the digestive system, there are a few glandular accessory organs that secrete directly into the alimentary canal via ducts, and these are important to digestion. They include the liver, the gallbladder, and the pancreas.

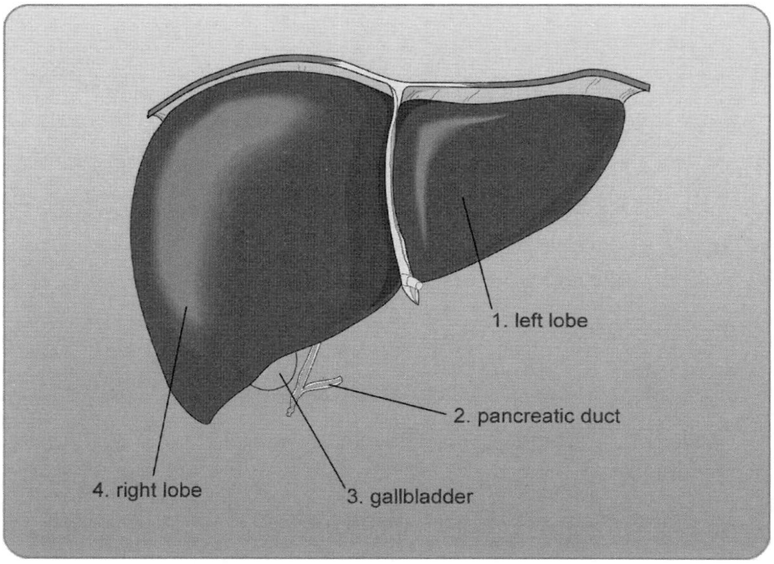

The Liver

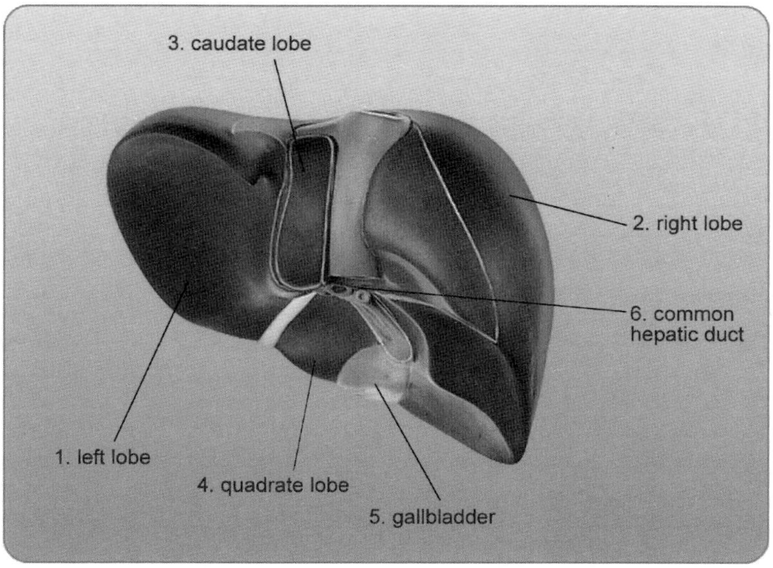

The Anterior of the Liver

The **liver** is the largest gland in the body. It is composed of four lobes:

- the left lobe (largest portion)
- the right lobe
- the caudate lobe
- the quadrate lobe

The two main lobes are on the front while the two smaller lobes are on the back of the liver. Within the lobes are many liver lobules that produce bile. Bile is continuously secreted into the intestines through two hepatic ducts that merge to form the **common hepatic duct**. Between meals, **bile** is stored in the gallbladder. At mealtime it is squeezed out of the gallbladder through the common bile duct and into the duodenum to mix with the fat in food. The bile acids dissolve fat into the watery contents of the intestine, much like detergents dissolve grease from a frying pan. The liver also aids the body in detoxifying certain substances, drugs, for example.

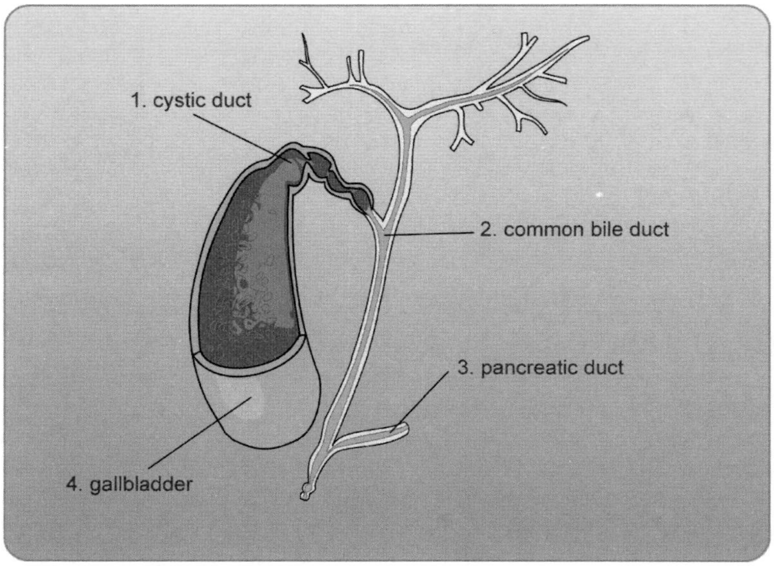

The Gallbladder

The **gallbladder** is a sac-like organ that is attached to the undersurface of the liver. It stores and concentrates bile. The **cystic duct** drains the gallbladder. It unites with the **hepatic duct** to form the **common bile duct** that conveys bile into the duodenum.

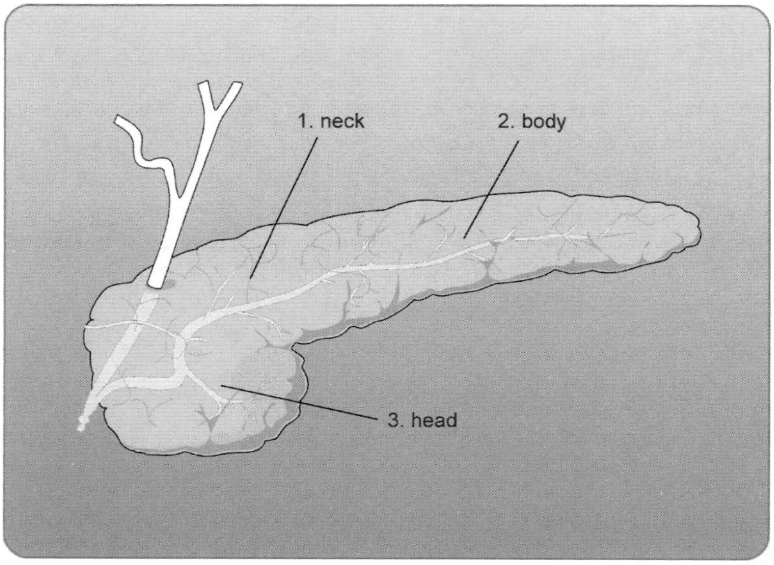

The Pancreas

Finally, the **pancreas** is involved in both the digestive and the endocrine systems. For its role in digestion, it creates juices and secretes them into the **pancreatic duct**, which empties into the common bile duct to enter the duodenum for the breakdown of foods.

I. FILL IN THE BLANK.

Using the word/word parts in the box, fill in the blanks.

liver
gallbladder
pancreas

1. The organ that creates and secretes juices into the duodenum for breakdown of foods is the ________________.
2. The largest gland in the body, that also produces bile, is the ________________.
3. The organ that stores and concentrates bile is the ________________.

REVIEW: DIGESTIVE STRUCTURES

I. MULTIPLE CHOICE.
Choose the best answer.

1. Which of the following is not an accessory organ?
   - ◯ splenic flexure
   - ◯ liver
   - ◯ pancreas
   - ◯ gallbladder
2. Part of the small intestine that receives secretions from the liver and pancreas.
   - ◯ splenic flexure
   - ◯ duodenum
   - ◯ spleen
   - ◯ fundus
3. Where small and large intestines meet.
   - ◯ iliocecal valve
   - ◯ splenic flexure
   - ◯ cecum
   - ◯ ileocecal valve
4. Bend in the colon, left of the abdomen.
   - ◯ duodenum
   - ◯ splenic flexure
   - ◯ ileocecal valve
   - ◯ stomach

5. 15-cm portion of the large intestine.
   - ◯ rectum
   - ◯ cecum
   - ◯ small intestine
   - ◯ esophagus

6. Finger-like structure off the cecum.
   - ◯ spleen
   - ◯ uvula
   - ◯ rectum
   - ◯ appendix

7. Cartilage that hangs over the larynx.
   - ◯ epiglottis
   - ◯ uvula
   - ◯ tonsil
   - ◯ frenulum

8. The most distended portion of the alimentary canal.
   - ◯ abdomen
   - ◯ stomach
   - ◯ bolus
   - ◯ duodenum

9. Between the pharynx and the stomach.
   - ◯ uvula
   - ◯ cecum
   - ◯ esophagus
   - ◯ appendix

II. FILL IN THE BLANK.

Use the word(s) in the box to fill in the blanks.

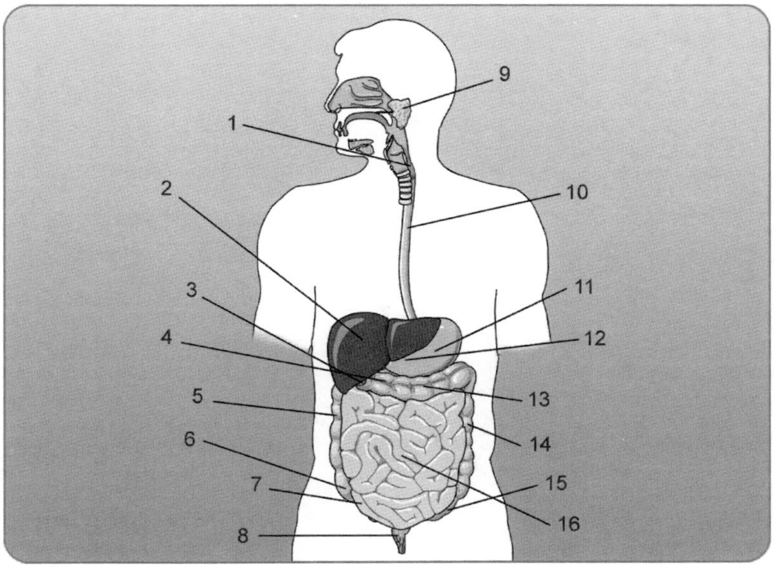

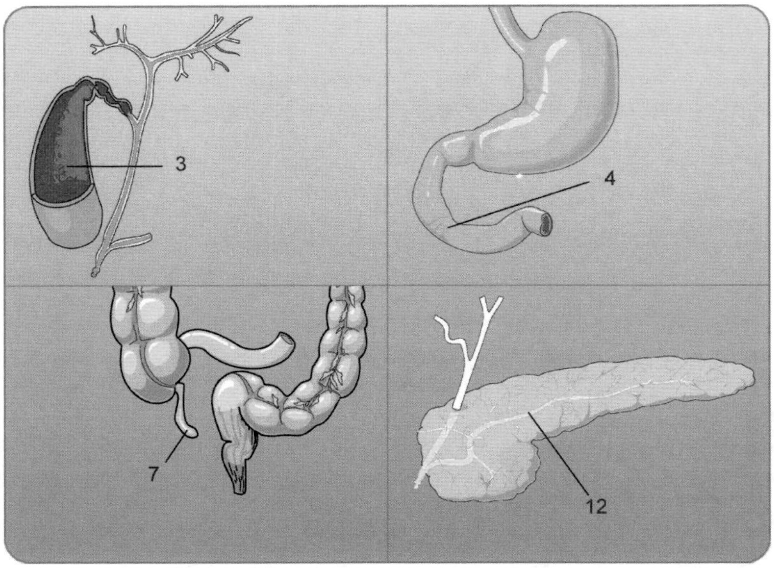

1. ____________________
2. ____________________
3. ____________________
4. ____________________
5. ____________________
6. ____________________
7. ____________________
8. ____________________
9. ____________________
10. ____________________
11. ____________________
12. ____________________
13. ____________________
14. ____________________
15. ____________________
16. ____________________

transverse colon
gallbladder
small intestine
duodenum
pancreas
ascending colon
parotid (salivary) gland
descending colon
pharynx
appendix
esophagus
sigmoid colon
liver
stomach
cecum
rectum

UNIT 9

The Respiratory System

THE RESPIRATORY SYSTEM - INTRODUCTION

The respiratory system works in close combination with the circulatory system to provide a constant supply of oxygen (O_2) to every cell in the body and to remove all gaseous waste (carbon dioxide or CO_2) from the body. Its structures allow life-giving gas exchange between the blood and the atmosphere. This is the primary function of respiration.

The respiratory system is responsible for important secondary functions as well. These include vocalization (speech), or the production of sound as air passes over the vocal cords; assistance with abdominal compression that occurs during micturition (urination), defecation, and parturition (childbirth); and the natural reflexes of coughing and sneezing, which assure that the respiratory system is kept clean.

Highlights

The respiratory system performs the following important functions:

- Gas exchange between blood and atmosphere
- Speech
- Assistance with abdominal compression
- Natural reflexes (sneezing/coughing)

There are many mechanisms that facilitate the functions of the respiratory system, with a variety of body parts working in concert to keep the body oxygenated. **Pulmonology** is the name for the science that is concerned with the anatomy, physiology, and pathology of the lungs.

RESPIRATION

The respiratory tract begins at the lips and nostrils and ends at the lungs. The respiratory system also consists of structures that are important in digestion, such as the mouth and the pharynx.

The respiratory system is broken down into the upper respiratory system and the lower respiratory system. The upper respiratory system is "all in your head" (and upper throat) and is comprised of the **nasal cavity**, **nares**, **larynx**, hard palate, soft palate, and **pharynx**. The lower respiratory system begins with the **trachea** and encompasses the **lungs** and **bronchi**.

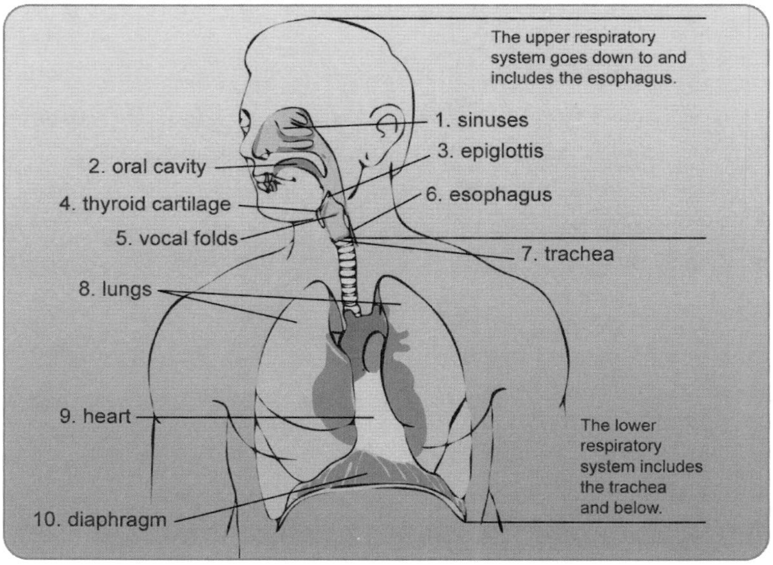

The Respiratory System

Although respiration (or the lack thereof!) can be voluntary, like holding your breath for example, respiration is a largely involuntary process controlled by the brain, and it consists of two basic functions:

1. **Ventilation**: This is the process of moving air in and out of the lungs. It can be done naturally by the body, or artificially by machines in cases of inadequate or absent breathing.

   a. **Inspiration**: Inspiration occurs when the **diaphragm** (the musculomembranous partition separating the abdominal and thoracic cavities and the major inspiratory muscle) contracts to create a slight vacuum in the chest cavity, allowing the lungs to expand and draw air from the airway inward to the lungs.
   b. **Expiration**: At the end of this cycle expiration occurs. This is when the chest wall and diaphragm relax. This, combined with the natural elasticity of the lungs, expels the air. During a very deep inspiration, the capacity of the chest cavity is maximized. All of the muscles—the scalenus anterior, pectoralis major, and sternocleidomastoid—contract to elevate the ribs. You can feel this process yourself by placing your hands on your ribcage and taking a deep breath. Then, with your nose plugged and your mouth tightly shut, attempt to suck in air. You should not be able to feel your ribs elevate as in the previous exercise.

2. **Diffusion**: This term means "the process of becoming widely spread." Specifically, oxygen is carried to every cell of the body by passing first through the pulmonary alveoli to the blood. Finally, carbon dioxide is released from the cells back into the blood, carried through the pulmonary alveoli, and released back out of the respiratory tract and into the atmosphere.

I. FILL IN THE BLANK.

Refer to the image and enter the terms corresponding to the following numbers. Use the words in the box to fill in the blanks.

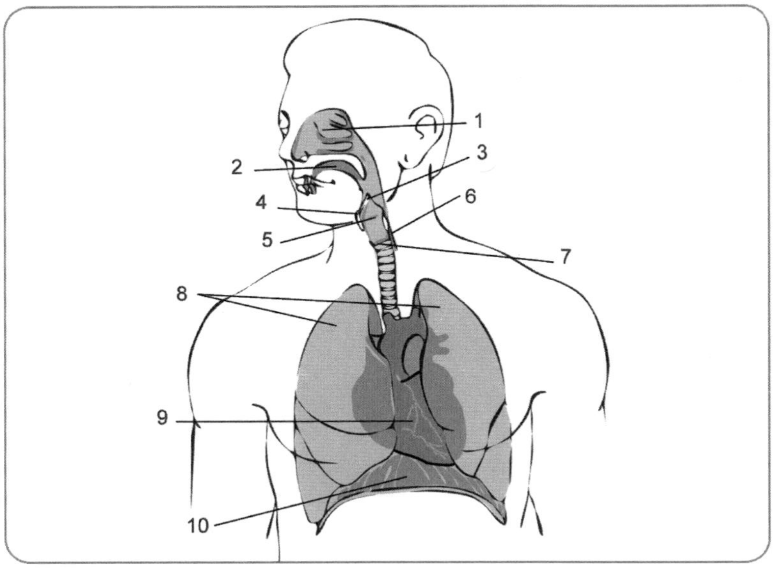

1. ________________
2. ________________
3. ________________
4. ________________
5. ________________
6. ________________
7. ________________
8. ________________
9. ________________
10. ________________

thyroid cartilage
heart
epiglottis
trachea
diaphragm
sinuses
esophagus
vocal folds
oral cavity
lungs

GROSS RESPIRATORY

Several physical requirements must be met in order for ventilation and diffusion to be effective. First, the actual structures in which the gaseous exchange takes place must have thin, permeable walls (or membranes) so that diffusion can easily occur- i.e., the **alveoli**, which are located at the ends of the bronchioles. In addition, these membranes must be kept moist to permit optimal gas exchange. A rich blood supply is also a necessary factor - there are very dense capillary beds that surround each alveolus. (There are 300-400 million alveoli per lung.) Furthermore, the gaseous exchange must take place deeply enough within the body so that the incoming air can be made sufficiently warm. Lastly, a pump must operate to effectively replenish the supply of air.

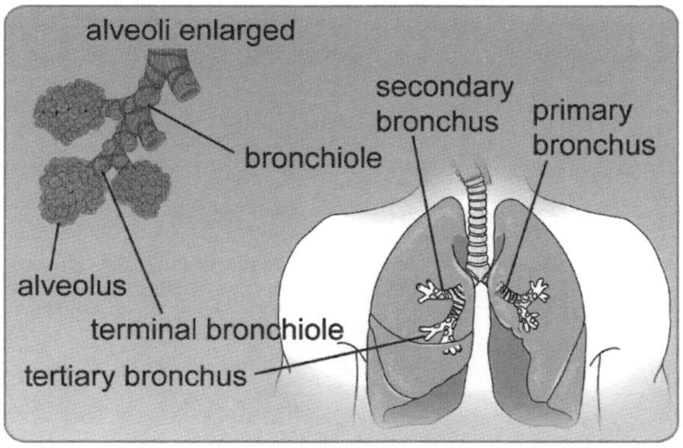

Some structures are part of more than one system. For example, the oral cavity (mouth) is the beginning point of the digestive system AND an important point for air entry into the respiratory system.

Some structures are part of both the respiratory and digestive systems. For the most part, the basic structures of the respiratory system should not be difficult for you to learn, but a couple of items should be noted. First, the external **naris** refers to one nostril. The plural form is **nares** and it is more commonly used. **Bronchus** is also singular, with the plural form being **bronchi**. Here, too, the plural is the more commonly used form.

Here is a slightly different diagram of the respiratory system. Note the nasal cavity (which houses some of the sinuses), the external naris, the hard and soft palates (within the oral cavity), and the right and left pulmonary bronchi.

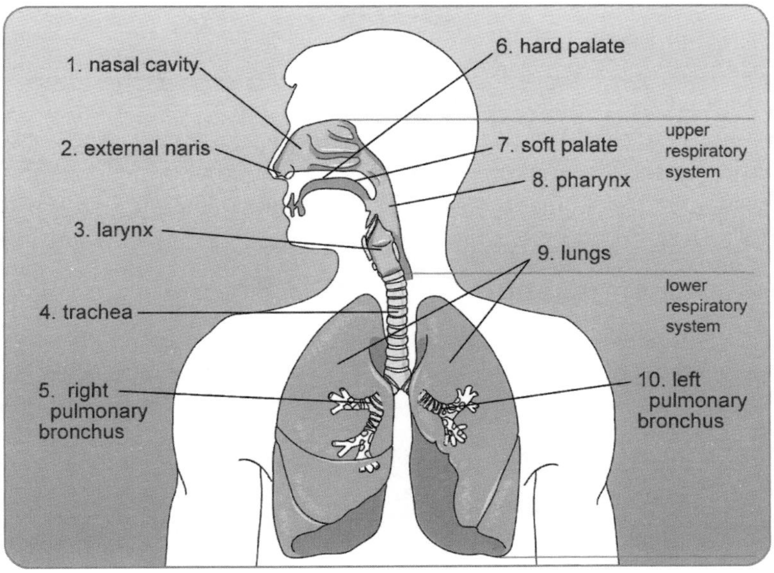

I. **FILL IN THE BLANK.**

In the blanks below, refer to the image and enter the term corresponding to the following numbers. Use the word(s) in the box to fill in the blanks.

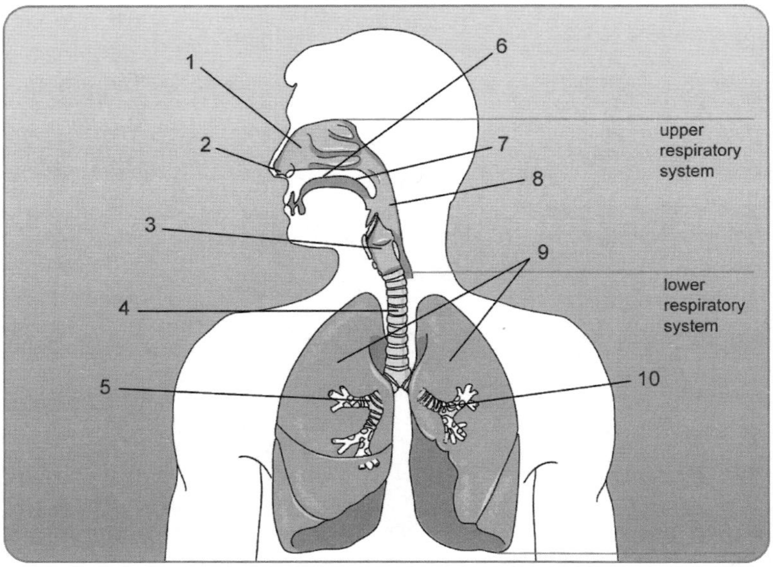

1. ________________
2. ________________
3. ________________
4. ________________
5. ________________
6. ________________
7. ________________
8. ________________
9. ________________
10. ________________

external naris
left pulmonary bronchus
pharynx
nasal cavity
hard palate
trachea
right pulmonary bronchus
lungs
larynx
soft palate

II. FILL IN THE BLANK.

Determine if the anatomical part belongs to the upper or lower respiratory system. Fill in the blank with either "upper" or "lower."

1. lungs ________________
2. soft palate ________________
3. pharynx ________________
4. right pulmonary bronchus ________________
5. nasal cavity ________________
6. larynx ________________
7. left pulmonary bronchus ________________
8. trachea ________________
9. hard palate ________________
10. external naris ________________

NASAL CAVITY

Air can be taken in simultaneously through the oral and nasal cavities. It can also be taken in through only the oral cavity or only the nasal cavity just as effectively. Unless there is some obstruction, people take in most of their oxygen through the nasal cavity. This is divided into two equal cavities by the **nasal septum** that serves as the partition. The perpendicular **ethmoid** and **vomer** bones, along with septal cartilage, make up the nasal septum. Each side opens into the **external nares** (nostrils). There are also internal (posterior) nares or **choanae** (singular choana) that link the external nares to the nasopharynx.

Highlights

Functions of the nasal cavity:

1. Warm, moisten, and clean air
2. Sense of smell
3. Sound resonation (singing/speech)

The bones that make up the nose are the frontal, nasal, palatine, maxillae, and conchae (also called turbinates). The **conchae**, or **turbinate**, bones create a passageway for air; this passage is called the meatus. Air enters through the external naris, travels up the **meatus** (which is often designated in sections—anterior, middle, posterior), passes through the choana, and into the nasopharynx.

The nasal cavity itself serves three major functions:

1. It warms, moistens, and cleans the inhaled air. Epithelium refers to the covering of various surfaces of the body, both internal and external, including the linings of small cavities and vessels. The nasal epithelia cover the conchae (turbinate bones) and serve to warm, moisten, and clean the air that is taken in. The epithelial lining contains many blood vessels that enable it to warm the air. These vessels are the source of nosebleeds (medical term—epistaxis). Nasal hairs are also present in this lining and sometimes extend outside the nostrils. These are actually filters for microscopic particles that might otherwise be inhaled.
2. It is the olfactory center. One of the senses is also an integral function of the nasal cavity—the sense of smell. The medical term for this is **olfaction**. The olfactory epithelia are located in the upper posterior part of the nasal cavity and are associated with the reception of odors. The olfactory system protects the body by alerting it to harmful contaminants in the air, as well as to potential dangers in foods. Of course, it is responsible for certain pleasant associations: the smell of baking cookies or sizzling hamburgers, the perfume of flowers, or the scent of aftershave.
3. The third function of the nasal cavity is related to sound production. The nasal cavity serves as a resonating chamber for the voice. As such, it prolongs and intensifies the sound vibrations created by the voice box (larynx), thus aiding in speech production and enhancing vocal music.

nasal septum: The partition that divides the two equal cavities of the nose.

perpendicular ethmoid: One bone that makes up the nasal septum.

vomer: One bone that makes up the nasal septum.

external nares: The nostrils.

choanae: Internal nares that link the external nares to the nasopharynx.

conchae bones: Also called turbinate bones, they create a passageway for the air.

meatus: The passage created by the conchae where air flows.

nasopharynx: The nasal portion of the pharynx.

I. TRUE/FALSE.
Mark the following true or false.

1. The medical term for the sense of smell is olfaction.
   - ◯ true
   - ◯ false

2. The nasal cavity has nothing to do with sound production in the human body.
   - ◯ true
   - ◯ false

3. Epithelia cover the conchae to warm, moisten, and clean air taken in through the nose.
   - ◯ true
   - ◯ false

SINUS CAVITIES

Certain bones of the face are configured to create air spaces. These interosseous spaces are called the **paranasal sinuses**. They are named after the bones that create them—**maxillary**, **frontal**, **sphenoid**, and **ethmoidal** (or ethmoid). They communicate with the nasal cavity and assist in respiration by warming and moistening inspired air. They also allow for lessening the weight of the skull without compromising its strength. Unfortunately, these warm, moist sinuses are susceptible to infection. Sinus infections are quite common, so familiarize yourself with the location and names of the various sinus cavities.

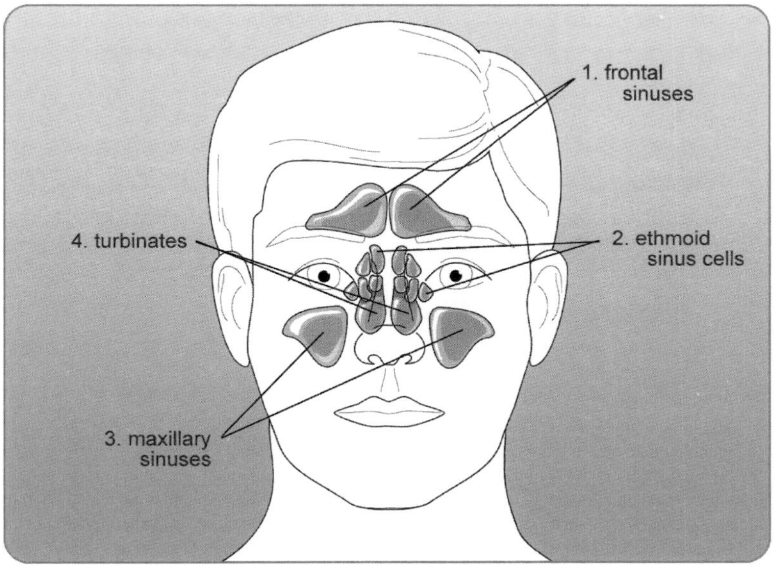

I. FILL IN THE BLANK.

Use the word(s) in the box to fill in the blanks.

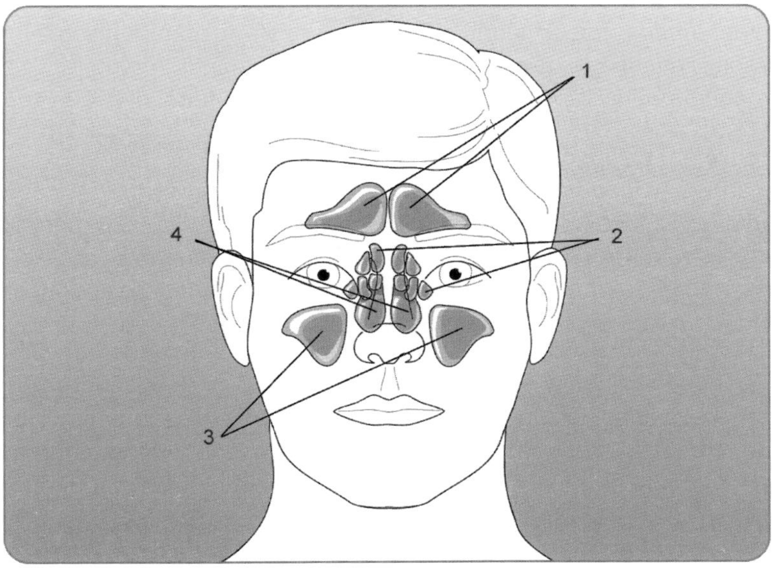

1. ________________
2. ________________
3. ________________
4. ________________

maxillary sinuses
turbinates
ethmoid sinus cells
frontal sinuses

PHARYNX

The pharynx is the passageway that connects the nasal and oral cavities to the larynx. It is divided into three distinct regions based upon function:

> The pharynx is the passageway that connects the nasal and oral cavities to the larynx.

1. First is the **nasopharynx**. This is only respiratory in function. It is the uppermost portion of the pharynx. The paired auditory, or eustachian, tubes connect the nasopharynx to the cavities of the middle ear. The **pharyngeal tonsils**, more commonly called adenoids, are found in the posterior wall of this cavity.
2. Second is the **oropharynx**. This is the middle portion of the pharynx. **Palatine tonsils** are located at the back and side (posterolateral) wall of the oropharynx, and **lingual tonsils** are found at the base of the tongue. Tonsils are small, rounded masses of tissue. When used generically, (as in "he had his tonsils out") the reference is to the palatine tonsils. Tonsillitis, an infection of the palatine or lingual tonsils, can occur even after a tonsillectomy (excision or removal of the tonsils).
3. The third and final portion of the pharynx is the **laryngopharynx**. This is the lowermost portion. The respiratory and digestive tracts diverge here at the laryngopharynx. Food and fluids enter the esophagus, and air goes into the larynx.

I. FILL IN THE BLANK.

Using the word/word parts in the box, fill in the blanks.

pharynx
oropharynx
laryngopharynx
nasopharynx

1. The respiratory and digestive tracts diverge at the ________________.
2. The ________________ is only respiratory in function.
3. The passageway that connects the nasal and oral cavities to the larynx is the ________________.
4. The ________________ is where the palatine tonsils are found.

LARYNX AND TRACHEA

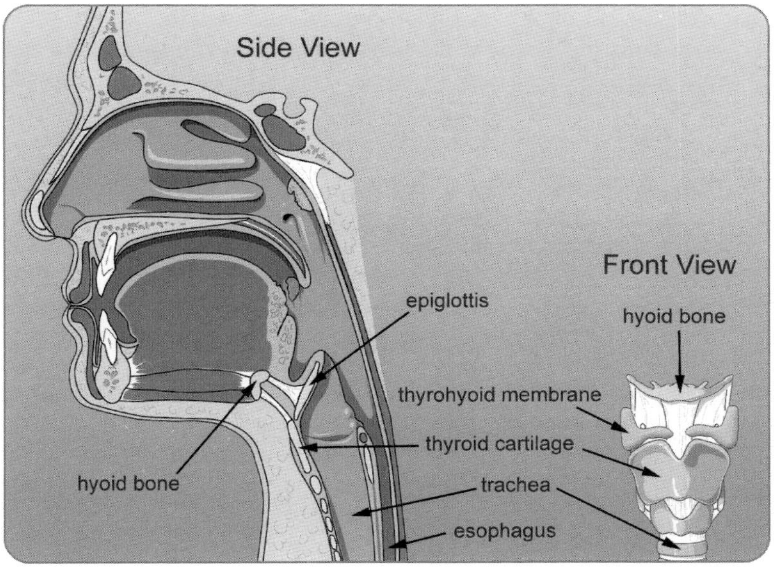

The **larynx** (voice box) begins at the oropharynx and extends down to the opening of the trachea. The larynx is the entrance to the lower respiratory tract. Its three main functions are:

1. Control of the airflow between the pharynx and the trachea.
2. Prevent food or fluid from getting into the trachea and thus into the lungs upon swallowing.
3. Produce the sound vibrations. This last function gives rise to the term **voice box**. Another term for the voice box is the **glottis**.

The larynx is composed of nine cartilages, the largest being called the **thyroid cartilage**. This is more prominent in males than in females and is also called the **Adam's apple**.

The lower end of the larynx is made up of ring-shaped **cricoid cartilage**. A pair of **arytenoid cartilages** are situated above the cricoid and are attached to the vocal cords. The **vocal cords** are actually a pair of strong connective tissue bands stretched across the upper opening of the larynx. They are sometimes referred to as the *true* vocal cords. The false vocal cords (also called ventricular folds) support the true vocal cords but are not actually used in sound production. The true vocal cords vibrate to cause sound as air moves across them.

The larynx opens at its lower end into the **trachea** (also called the windpipe), a rigid tube that is approximately 4.5 inches in length, which connects the larynx to the bronchi. A series of 16 to 20 C-shaped hyaline cartilage rings make up the wall of the trachea. The open part of the C is at the back of the trachea and is covered by connective tissue and smooth muscle. This allows for the trachea to be rigid but flexible, yet still allows for the lumen of the tube to be permanently open.

Two additional terms need to be introduced at this point that are also mentioned with the digestive system. The **epiglottis** is the flap of cartilage that covers the windpipe (trachea) when swallowing occurs, preventing food and liquids from entering the trachea. The small conical piece of flesh that hangs down from the posterior portion of the soft palate is called the **uvula**. It is a remnant left as the soft palate forms during fetal development. It is used in the production of sounds in some languages other than English.

When you inhale tiny dust particles, they stick to the mucous layer of the trachea, and the cilia (minute, hair-like processes) sweep those particles upwards to the pharynx where they are removed by coughing. Smoking and air pollution destroy the cilia, thus allowing contaminants to enter the lungs.

I. FILL IN THE BLANK.

In the blanks provided below, refer to the image and enter the term corresponding to the following numbers. Use the word(s) in the box to fill in the blanks.

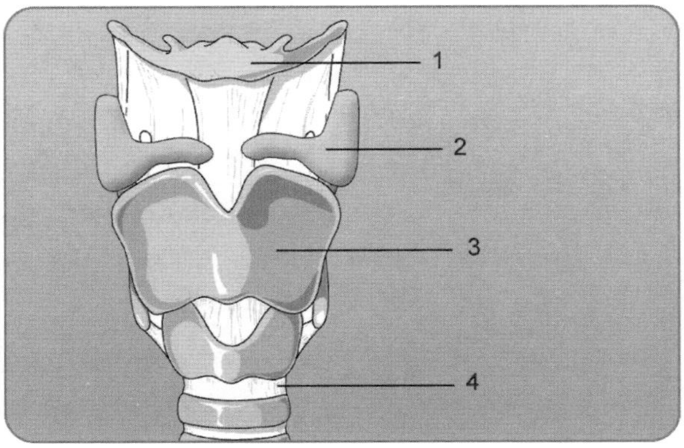

1. ____________________
2. ____________________
3. ____________________
4. ____________________

thyroid cartilage
trachea
thyrohyoid membrane
hyoid bone

II. FILL IN THE BLANK.

In the blanks provided below, refer to the image and enter the term corresponding to the following numbers. Use the word(s) in the box to fill in the blanks.

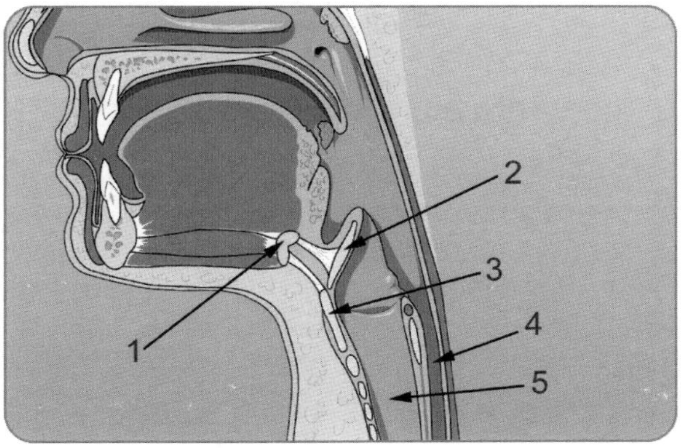

1. ______________
2. ______________
3. ______________
4. ______________
5. ______________

esophagus
hyoid bone
trachea
thyroid cartilage
epiglottis

BRONCHI

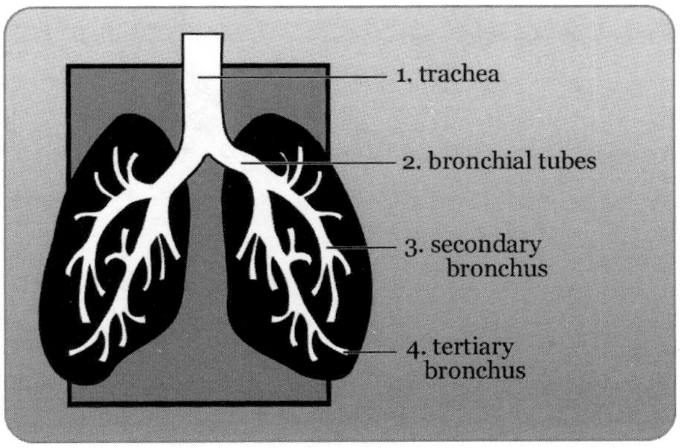

The trachea bifurcates, or divides, into two branches at its most distal portion and forms the **bronchi**. The bifurcation is reinforced by a cartilaginous plate called the **carina**.

At the bifurcation of the trachea, the respiratory tract divides into a right and left pulmonary bronchus. These structures are called bronchial trees because they are composed of respiratory tubes that branch off and get progressively smaller in diameter. Like the trachea, each bronchus is made up of cartilaginous rings to keep the lumen open as it goes into the lung. As the branches get smaller, they are called **secondary bronchi** and **segmental** (or **tertiary**) **bronchi**. (The term *tertiary* actually means third in order.) The bronchi then branch into even smaller tubules called **bronchioles**.

Many terminal bronchioles deep in the lungs mark the end of the respiratory tract proper. The terminal bronchioles do continue to branch into alveolar ducts that lead into alveolar sacs containing individual alveoli, the basic functional units of the respiratory system. Through them the exchange between alveolar gas and pulmonary capillary blood takes place. Each lung contains an estimated 350 million alveoli.

I. **FILL IN THE BLANK.**

In the blanks provided below, refer to the image and enter the term corresponding to the following numbers. Use the word(s) in the box to fill in the blanks.

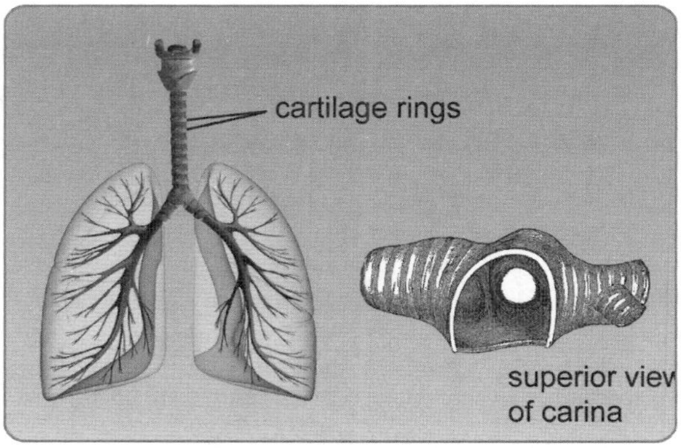

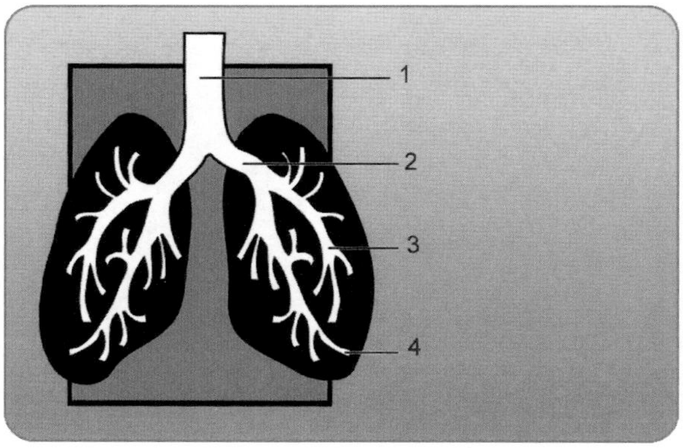

1. ______________
2. ______________
3. ______________
4. ______________

secondary bronchus
trachea
tertiary bronchus
bronchial tubes

THE LUNGS AND THORACIC CAVITY

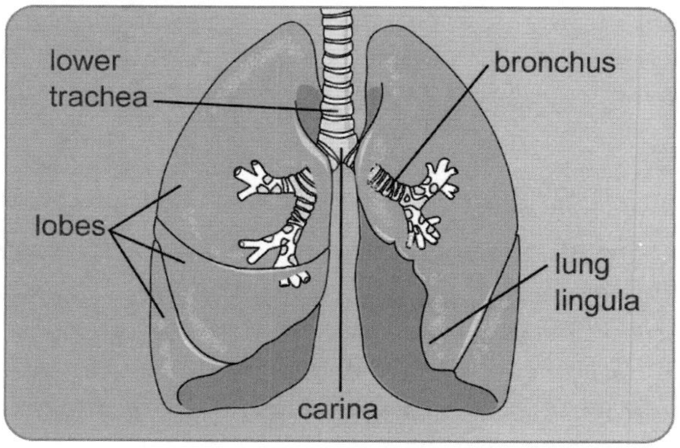

The **lungs** are cone-shaped organs in the thoracic cavity. The base of each lung is located at the diaphragm, and the apex, or top, of each lung is slightly above the clavicle, or collar bone. The **hilum** of the lung is where the primary bronchi and pulmonary blood vessels enter each lung.The lungs are separated from each other by the **mediastinal space** and its contents, which constitutes the **mediastinum**. It contains several organs and structures, including the heart, trachea, esophagus, lymph nodes, nerves, and major circulatory branches.

The left lung is slightly smaller than the right and is designated as having a **superior** (upper) and **inferior** (lower) lobe. However, there is a projection from the anterior aspect of the upper lobe of the left lung, called the **lingula**.

The right lung is divided into three lobes: the **superior** (upper), **medial** (middle), and **inferior** (lower). The lobes of both lungs are then further divided into smaller lobules that contain the alveoli.

The lungs are located in the pleural divisions of the thoracic cavity. The **parietal pleura** is a serous membrane that lines the entire thoracic cavity. A separate pleural sac (**visceral pleura**) encases each lung. The space between the visceral pleura and the parietal pleura provides lubrication to eliminate friction between the lungs and the parietal pleura, making respiration painless. Additionally, the shape of the thoracic cavity and the way the ribs are attached to the spine, allows the volume of the thoracic cavity to increase during inspiration.

REVIEW: THE LUNGS AND THORACIC CAVITY

I. MATCHING.
Match the correct term to the definition.

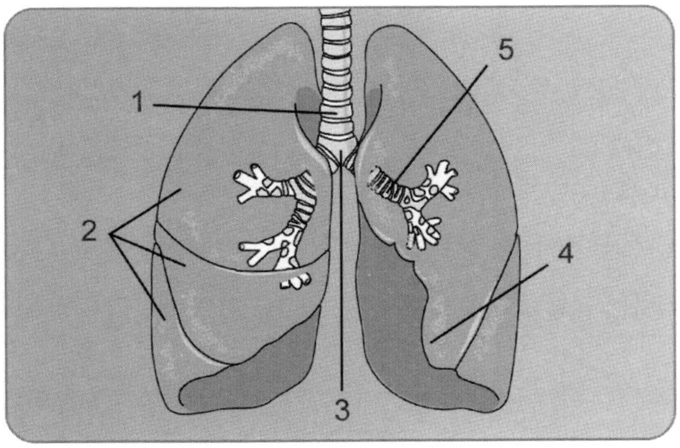

1. ___
2. ___
3. ___
4. ___
5. ___

A. lung lingula
B. carina
C. lower trachea
D. lobes
E. bronchus

RESPIRATORY TERMINOLOGY

Term	Definition
septum	Partition between the two sides of the nasal cavity.
ethmoid	Perforated like a sieve, such as the ethmoid bone.
vomer	Bone of the nasal septum.
choana(e)	Link from external nares to nasopharynx.
turbinates	Another name for conchae.
meatus	Passageway in the body, especially an opening on the surface.
epithelium	Lining of small cavities.
epistaxis	Nosebleed.
olfaction	Sense of smell.

olfactory epithelia	Lines the olfactory region of the nasal cavity.
paranasal sinuses	Air spaces contained by certain bones of the face.
maxillary sinus	One of the paired paranasal sinuses located in the body of the maxilla.
frontal sinus	One of the paired irregular shaped paranasal sinuses located in the frontal bone.
sphenoid sinus	One of the paired paranasal sinuses in the anterior part of the body of the sphenoid bone.
ethmoidal sinus	One of the paranasal sinuses located within the ethmoid bone.
auditory	Pertaining to the sense of hearing.
eustachian	Tube connecting the nasopharynx to the middle ear.
adenoids	Pharyngeal tonsils.
laryngopharynx	Where the respiratory and digestive systems diverge.
thyroid	Gland situated in the lower part of the front of the neck.
cricoid	Ring-shaped cartilage making up the lower larynx.
arytenoid	Vocal cord cartilage.
bifurcates	Divided into two branches.
bifurcation	Site where a single structure divides into two.
carina	Cartilaginous plate of the trachea.
bronchial tree	Another name for pulmonary bronchus.
tertiary	Third in order.
bronchioles	One of the subdivisions of the branched bronchial tree.
alveolar ducts	Small passages connecting the respiratory bronchioles and the alveolar sacs.
alveoli	Functional units of the respiratory system.
mediastinal space	Space separating the lungs.
mediastinum	Mass of tissues and organs separating the two pleural sacs.
lobules	Division of lung lobes.
pleura	Serous membrane of the thoracic cavity.
visceral	Pleura which is adherent to the outer surface of the lung.
parietal	Pleura that lines the thoracic wall and diaphragm.

UNIT 10

The Endocrine System

THE ENDOCRINE SYSTEM - INTRODUCTION

The human body uses various "biofeedback mechanisms" to monitor the conditions within cells, tissues and organs. For instance, in the genitourinary system, the presence or absence of certain male and female hormones have different effects on the body and play important roles in the reproductive cycle. In this unit, we will discuss the central structures of the endocrine system and how the hormones that they secrete help to maintain the body's normal state (homeostasis).

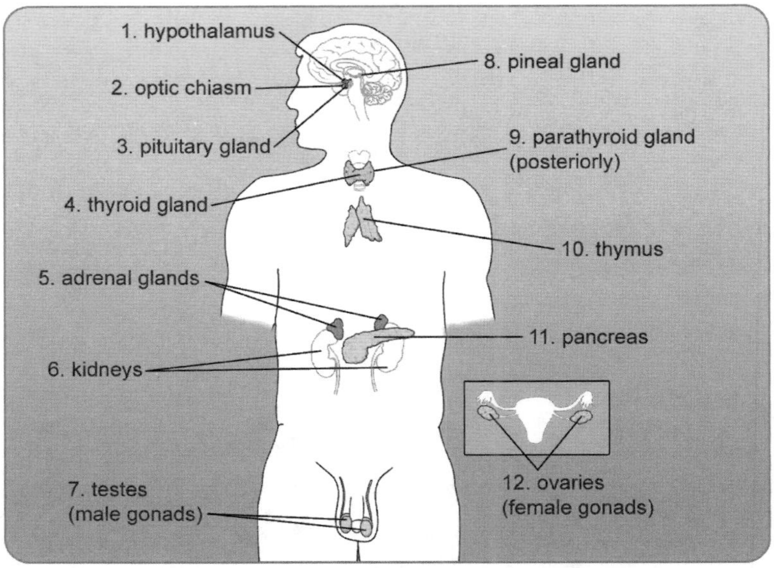

The many different glands in the human body are classified into two distinct groups:

- **Exocrine glands**, (exo = outside) such as sweat glands, salivary glands, and mucous glands, secrete fluids that are transported via ducts to their appropriate destinations and function within a particular body system.
- **Endocrine glands**, (endo = within) on the other hand, constitute their own body system. They are ductless and secrete chemicals, called **hormones**, directly into the blood. These hormones (chemical messengers) are then transported through the blood to specific organs in the body. When they arrive at the target organ, the hormone causes a stimulant or suppressive action on a specific type of cell or tissue.

The glands that comprise the **endocrine system** are the pituitary, thyroid, parathyroids, pancreas, adrenals, gonads, pineal, and thymus. Additionally, mucosal cells within the duodenum and placenta are considered part of the endocrine system. They are located in various anatomic locations:

- the pituitary gland attached to the undersurface of the brain
- the thyroid in the neck
- the thymus in the chest
- the adrenals on the superior portion of the kidneys
- the gonads of the male and female sex glands located in their respective reproductive systems
- the pancreas in the abdominal cavity
- the pineal gland located in the midbrain

HYPOTHALAMUS AND PITUITARY GLAND

The **pituitary gland**, also called the **hypophysis**, is about 1 cm in diameter and is located beneath the brain in a bony receptacle of the sphenoid bone called the sella turcica. It is attached to the underside of the brain by a stalk called the **infundibulum**.

The cerebral arterial circle (circle of Willis) surrounds the pituitary gland and provides it with blood exchange. The pituitary gland is actually composed of two distinct masses of tissue: **anterior lobe** and **posterior lobe**.

The anterior lobe is derived from the top of the pharynx and is the glandular portion. The posterior lobe is derived from the nervous system. They both fuse together to form a single organ.

The pituitary gland is often referred to as the master gland because it is responsible for the regulation of so many body activities. The release of hormones from the pituitary gland is controlled by the brain, specifically the hypothalamus.

Highlights

Hormones secreted by the pituitary:

- Growth hormone (GH)
- Thyroid stimulating hormone (TSH)
- Adrenocorticotropic hormone (ACTH)
- Follicle stimulating hormone (FSH)
- Luteinizing hormone (LH)
- Prolactin
- Oxytocin
- Vasopressin

Eight important hormones are secreted by the pituitary, six via the anterior lobe and two via the posterior lobe. These hormones are:

Growth hormone (GH): This regulates the growth of all body tissue and is very active during adolescence.

Thyroid stimulating hormone (TSH): This regulates the activity of the thyroid gland.

Adrenocorticotropic hormone (ACTH): This assures normal function of the adrenal cortex. It also works on all cells to help break down fats.

Follicle stimulating hormone (FSH): In the male this stimulates the testes to produce sperm; in the female it stimulates the production of estrogen.

Luteinizing hormone (LH): This works in conjunction with FSH to induce ovulation and produce progesterone. In the male, this is called interstitial cell stimulating hormone (ICSH) and stimulates the testes to produce testosterone.

Prolactin: This hormone works with other hormones to initiate the secretion of milk by the mammary glands.

Oxytocin: This causes the uterus to contract during labor, as well as stimulates the mammary glands to let down milk. This is generated by the hypothalamus through the posterior lobe.

Vasopressin: This has two separate functions: to constrict the blood vessels causing increased blood pressure, and to permit the kidneys to reabsorb water. This is also a posterior lobe hormone.

The **hypothalamus** receives input from the autonomic nervous system, visual cortex (determining the amount and quality of light for regulating circadian rhythms), blood-born molecules (insulin, etc.), and stress levels, among many other stimuli. The hypothalamus analyzes these inputs and releases either neural impulses to the appropriate secretory organ, or it releases endocrine hormones to affect the actions of the pituitary gland.

hypophysis: Another name for the pituitary gland.

infundibulum: The stalk that attaches the pituitary gland to the brain.

circle of Willis: This surrounds the pituitary gland and provides it with blood exchange.

growth hormone: Regulates the growth of body tissues.

thyroid stimulating hormone: Regulates the thyroid gland.

adrenocorticotropic hormone: Assures normal function of the adrenal cortex and breaks down fats.

follicle stiumulating hormone: Stimulates testes to produce sperm in males, stimulates production of estrogen in females.

luteinizing hormone: Works with FSH to induce ovulation and produce progesterone.

prolactin: Works with other hormones to initiate secretion of milk by the mammary glands.

oxytocin: Causes uterine contractions during labor and stimulates the mammary glands.

vasopressin: Constricts blood vessels causing increased blood pressure and permits kidneys to reabsorb water.

THYROID AND PARATHYROID GLANDS

The **thyroid gland** is positioned just below the larynx. It is a flat structure that is roughly the shape of a shield, consisting of two lobes that lie on either side of the trachea and are connected by a broad isthmus. This is the largest of the endocrine glands, weighing between 20 and 25 gm, and has both a rich blood and lymph supply. It is comprised of many round hollow sacs, called **follicles**, which synthesize the thyroid hormones and store them. In between the follicles are epithelial cells that also produce a hormone.

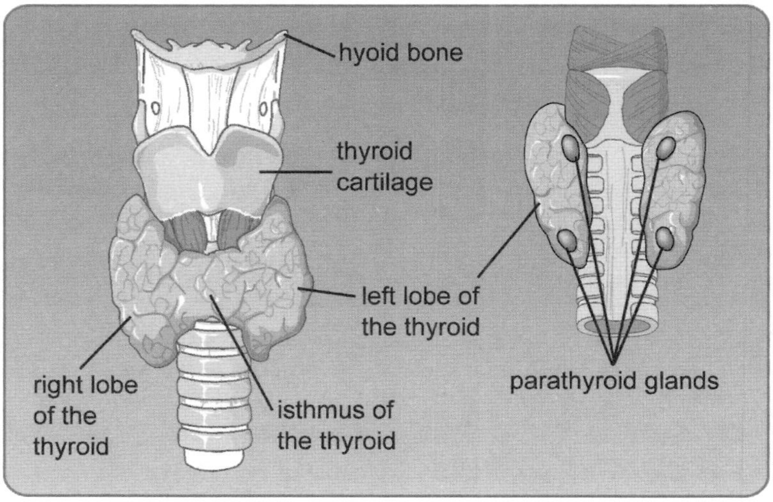

Two hormones are produced by the thyroid gland. The first is **thyroid hormone (TH)** which is a name that applies to two similar molecules **T3 (triiodothyronine)** and **T4 (thyroxine)**. These are stored in the follicles and are utilized to regulate basal metabolic rate (the rate at which the body uses oxygen to transform nutrients into energy). They regulate normal growth and development, including mental processes and sexual maturity. The second hormone, **thyrocalcitonin** or **calcitonin**, regulates the calcium balance of the blood. All three hormones are made up primarily of **iodine**, which is essential for normal thyroid function.

Embedded on the posterior surface of the lateral lobes of the thyroid gland, but structurally distinct from it, are four **parathyroid glands**, two superior and two inferior.

The hormone secreted by the parathyroids is called **parathormone (PTH)**. This hormone regulates the ratio of calcium and phosphorus in the blood and bone tissues.

I. **FILL IN THE BLANK.**

In the blanks provided below, refer to the image and enter the term corresponding to the following numbers. Use the word(s) in the box to fill in the blanks.

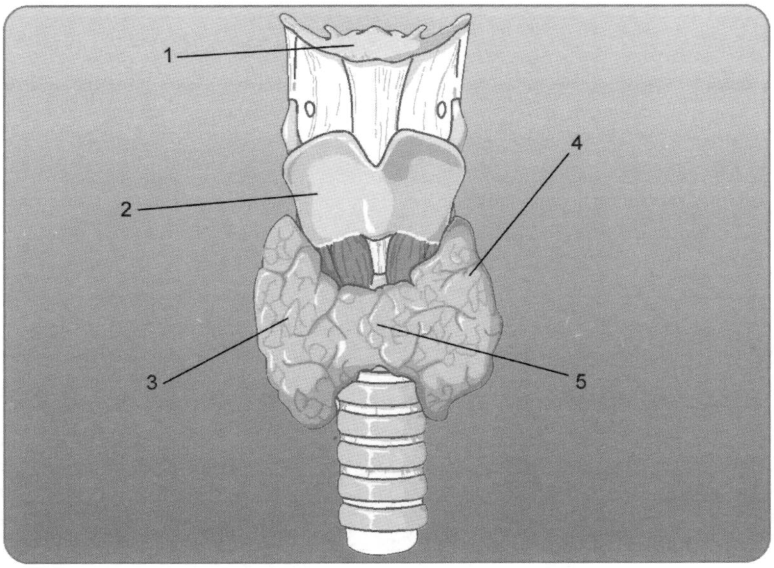

1. ________________
2. ________________
3. ________________
4. ________________
5. ________________

right lobe of thyroid gland
hyoid bone
isthmus of thyroid gland
left lobe of thyroid gland
thyroid cartilage

II. **FILL IN THE BLANK.**

Enter the correct word in the blank provided.

1. The hormone that regulates normal growth and development is the________________.
2. Hormones in the thyroid are primarily made up of ________________.
3. The thyroid gland is positioned just below the ________________.

larynx
thyrocalcitonin
iodine
thyroid hormone
parathyroid

4. The hormone ________________ regulates the calcium balance in the blood.
5. Four ________________ glands are embedded on the posterior surface of the lateral lobes.

ADRENAL GLANDS

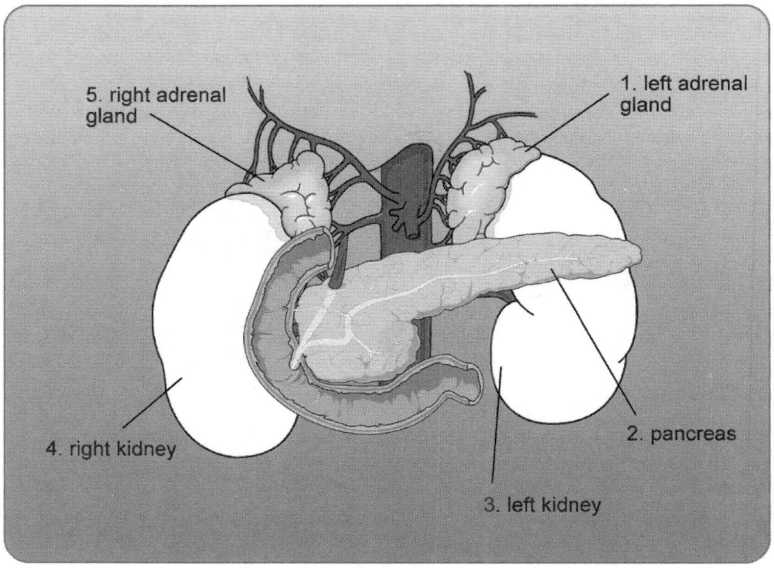

Triangular-shaped **adrenal glands** sit atop each kidney. Each one has an outer cortex and an inner medulla that individually function as separate glands. The inner medulla produces two hormones, **epinephrine** (also called adrenaline) and **norepinephrine**. These two hormones increase cardiac output and heart rate, dilate coronary vessels, increase mental alertness, increase respiratory rate, and elevate the overall metabolic rate. They are responsible for the "flight or fight" reaction under stressful conditions.

The outer cortex produces a variety of hormones, including **cortisol** to regulate carbohydrate and protein metabolism, **aldosterone** to control fluid and electrolyte balance, and **androgen** (male hormones) that affect the growth of body and facial hair.

In all, approximately 30 hormones are produced by the adrenal glands, and modern medicine does not fully understand the interplay and effects of all of them.

Highlights

The adrenal glands are also called the **suprarenal** glands.

I. MATCHING.
Using the above image, match the correct term to its number.

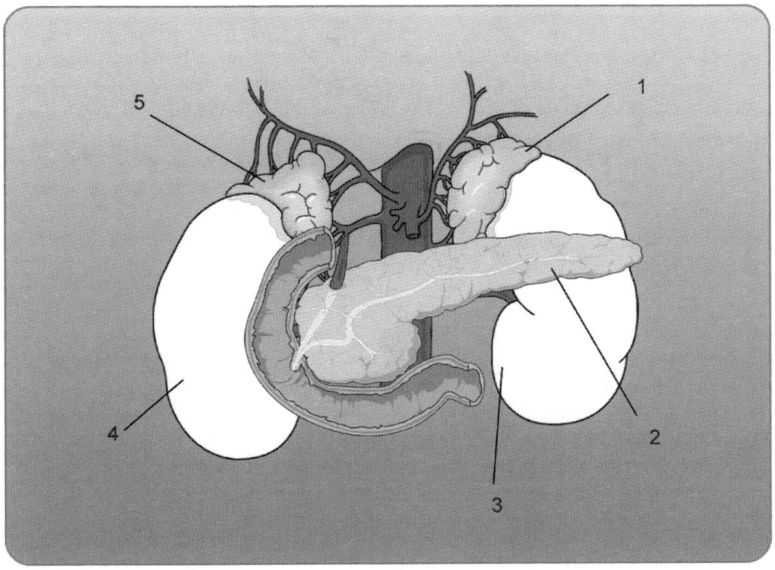

1. ___
2. ___
3. ___
4. ___
5. ___

A. pancreas
B. right adrenal gland
C. left adrenal gland
D. right kidney
E. left kidney

PANCREAS

As discussed in the Digestive System unit, the **pancreas** is involved in both the digestive and the endocrine systems. For its role in digestion, it creates juices and secretes them into the duodenum via a duct (exocrine gland) for the breakdown of foods.

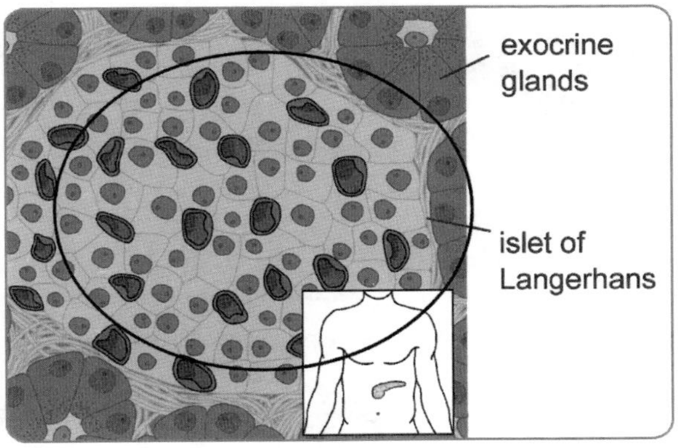

The endocrine portion of the pancreas consists of scattered clusters of cells called the **islets of Langerhans**. Two types of cells make up these clusters: alpha cells and beta cells. The hormones produced by them are taken up in the blood and do not enter the duct system of the pancreas.

Islet cell transplantation is an experimental procedure that has been used to treat Type I Diabetes.

The **alpha cells** produce a hormone called **glucagon**. This converts glycogen into glucose and increases the level of glucose in the blood. The **beta cells** produce a hormone called **insulin** that lowers the blood sugar and increases the cellular utilization of glucose. Together these hormones are essential for the metabolism of carbohydrates. There are two rare cell types as well:

- Delta cells that secrete somatostatin
- F (PP) cells that secrete pancreatic polypeptide (a hormone that may inhibit pancreatic exocrine activity)

I. **MATCHING.**
For each function or structure listed below, indicate whether it is part of the exocrine or endocrine function of the pancreas.

1. ____ production of glucagon
2. ____ secretion of enzymes to break down carbohydrates and proteins
3. ____ production of insulin
4. ____ islets of Langerhans

A. exocrine
B. endocrine

GONADS (MALE AND FEMALE)

Gonads are male and female sex glands. They produce both sex hormones and sex cells. In the male, the **interstitial cells** of the **testes** produce and secrete the male sex hormone **testosterone**. This controls the development and function of the male secondary sex organs, as well as the secondary sexual characteristics. It is also responsible for regulating the male sex drive.

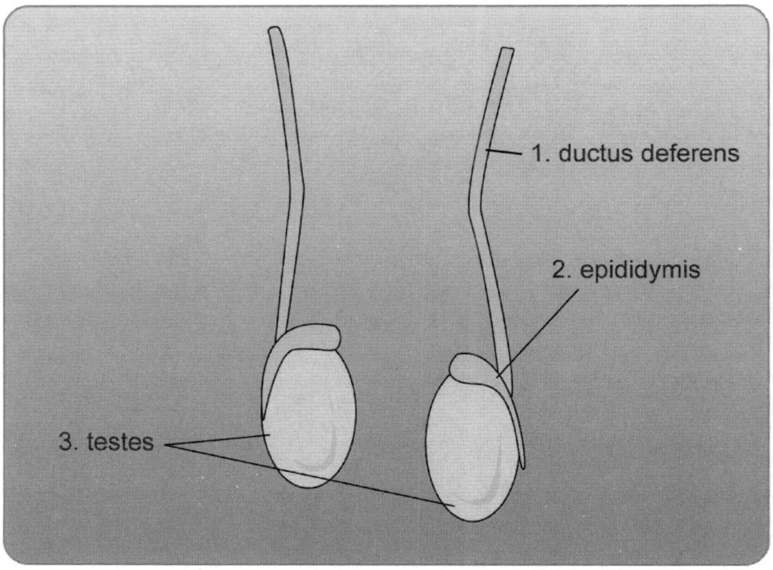

Generally, the hormones produced by the **ovaries** are responsible for the development and function of secondary sex organs, menstrual changes of the uterus, secondary sexual characteristics (including hair growth), the regulation of the female sex drive, and preparation of the uterus and female system for pregnancy.

I. **FILL IN THE BLANK.**

In the blanks provided below, refer to the image and enter the term corresponding to the following numbers. Use the word(s) in the box to fill in the blanks.

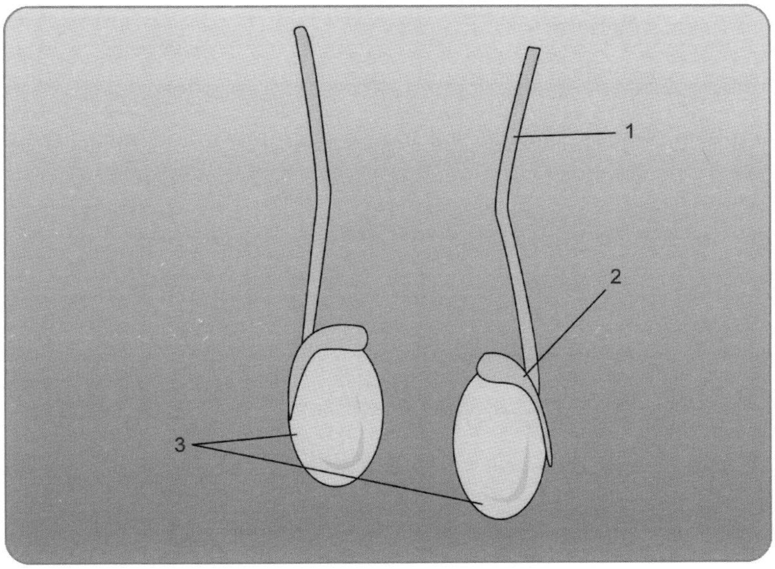

1. ________________
2. ________________
3. ________________

epididymis
testes
ductus deferens

PINEAL GLAND, DUODENUM, AND PLACENTA

The **pineal gland**, or **epiphysis**, is a cone-shaped body less than 1 cm at its widest dimension, which is attached to the third ventricle of the brain. The gland itself undergoes a regression after age seven and contains sand-like structures after age 15. It releases a hormone called **melatonin** that plays a role in sexual maturation and in maintaining daily body rhythms.

> There is a great deal that is not yet known about the endocrine system. Some hormones are still being isolated and identified, and their functions are not yet clear. These may become important in medicine as they continue to be studied.

The last components of the endocrine system are the **duodenum**, the **placenta**, and the **thymus**. There are cells present in the mucosal layer of the duodenum that secrete a hormone called secretin, which stimulates the pancreas to secrete digestive juices. The placenta, an organ that provides nutrient and waste exchanges between mother and fetus, also functions as an endocrine gland. It secretes at least three hormones that ensure a normal pregnancy. The thymus gland secretes a group of hormones which appear to play an important role in the mechanism of immunity.

As a medical employee, it is not necessary for you to understand the function and interrelationships of all hormones; however, many common diseases and problems arise from inadequate function or destruction of endocrine glands. For example, diabetes mellitus, the failure of the pancreas to produce insulin, is extremely common and several serious complications arise from it.

I. FILL IN THE BLANK.

Using the word/word parts in the box, fill in the blanks.

thymus
melatonin
epiphysis
placenta

1. Another name for the pineal gland is the ________________.
2. The ________________ gland secretes hormones that play an important role in immunity.
3. ________________ plays a role in sexual maturation and maintaining daily body rhythms.
4. The ________________ secretes at least three hormones that ensure a normal pregnancy.

ENDOCRINE TERMINOLOGY – LESSON 1

exocrine: Secretes fluids that are transported via "ducts" to their appropriate destinations and function within a particular body system.

endocrine: Secretes chemicals, called hormones, directly into the blood.

pituitary: Referred to as the master gland because it is responsible for the regulation of so many body activities.

thyroid: Secretes hormones that regulate normal growth and development, including mental processes and sexual maturity.

parathyroids: Hormone secreted by the parathyroids is called parathormone (PTH). This hormone regulates the ratio of calcium and phosphorus in the blood and bone tissues.

pancreas: Functions as both an exocrine and endocrine gland.

adrenals: Triangular-shaped glands that sit atop of each kidney. Each one has an outer cortex and an inner medulla that individually function as separate glands.

gonads: Male and female sex glands. They produce both sex hormones and sex cells.

pineal: Releases a hormone called melatonin that plays a role in sexual maturation and in maintaining daily body rhythms.

hypophysis: Another name for the pituitary gland.

sella turcica: Bony receptacle located beneath the brain which contains the pituitary gland.

infundibulum: A stalk which attaches the pituitary gland to the underside of the brain.

circle of Willis: Surrounds the pituitary gland and provides it with blood exchange.

hypothalamus: Controls the release of hormones from the pituitary gland.

adrenocorticotropic: Hormone that assures normal function of the adrenal cortex. It also works on all cells to help break down fats.

luteinizing: Works in conjunction with FSH to induce ovulation and produce progesterone.

ENDOCRINE TERMINOLOGY - LESSON 2

prolactin: Hormone that works with other hormones to initiate the secretion of milk by the mammary glands.

vasopressin: Constricts the blood vessels causing increased blood pressure, and permit the kidneys to reabsorb water.

isthmus: Connects the two lobes of the thyroid gland.

thyroxine: Regulates normal growth and development, including mental processes and sexual maturity.

calcitonin: Regulates the calcium balance of the blood.

islets of Langerhans: Endocrine portion of the pancreas that consists of scattered clusters of cells.

glucagon: Converts glycogen into glucose and regulates the level of glucose in the blood.

insulin: Increases the cellular utilization of glucose.

epinephrine: Increases cardiac output and heart rate, dilates coronary vessels, increase mental alertness, increases respiratory rate, and elevates the overall metabolic rate.

norepinephrine: Increases cardiac output and heart rate, dilates coronary vessels, increase mental alertness, increases respiratory rate, and elevates the overall metabolic rate.

adrenaline: Another name for epinephrine and norepinephrine.

aldosterone: Controls fluid and electrolyte balance.

androgen: Affects the growth of body and facial hair.

epiphysis: Another name for the pineal gland.

melatonin: Plays a role in sexual maturation and in maintaining daily body rhythms.

UNIT 11

The Urinary System

THE URINARY SYSTEM - INTRODUCTION

The urinary system, also called the excretory system and the genitourinary system, works closely with the circulatory system. The urinary system is responsible for eliminating metabolic wastes from the body in the form of urine. However, there are three additional important functions for which the urinary system is responsible:

- The regulation of the fluid content (water) in the body.
- Controlling the acid-base balance in the body.
- Maintaining electrolyte balance.

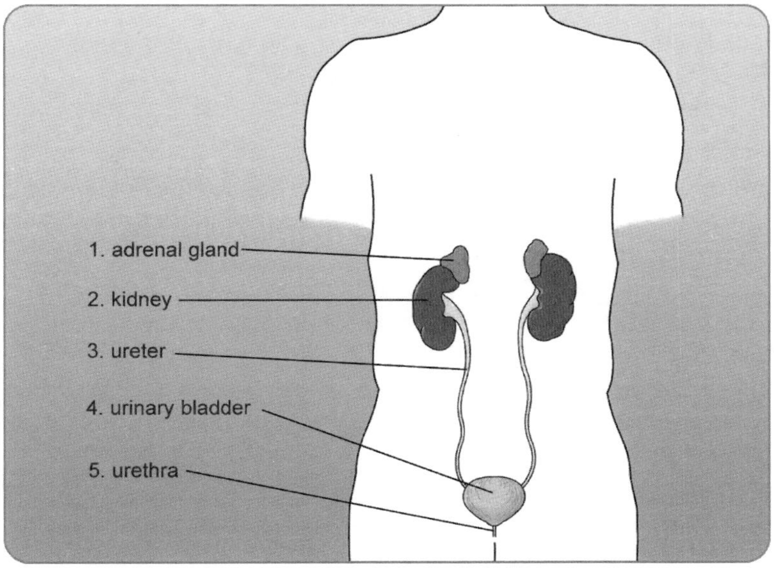

The urinary system is often studied in combination with the reproductive system. This is logical, especially since these two systems actually share structures in the male reproductive system. However, whereas reproduction is not essential to the sustenance of life, the urinary system is vital.

As mentioned above, this system is closely associated with the circulatory system. In fact, approximately 25% of the blood that is pumped from the left ventricle in every cardiac cycle is distributed into the kidneys for filtration.

The urinary system consists of the kidneys, ureters, bladder, and urethra.

The adrenal glands are located at the upper pole of each kidney and will be discussed in a separate lesson.

KIDNEYS

The term **renal** means pertaining to the kidneys. Additionally, the combining form *nephr/o–* also means pertaining to the kidneys.

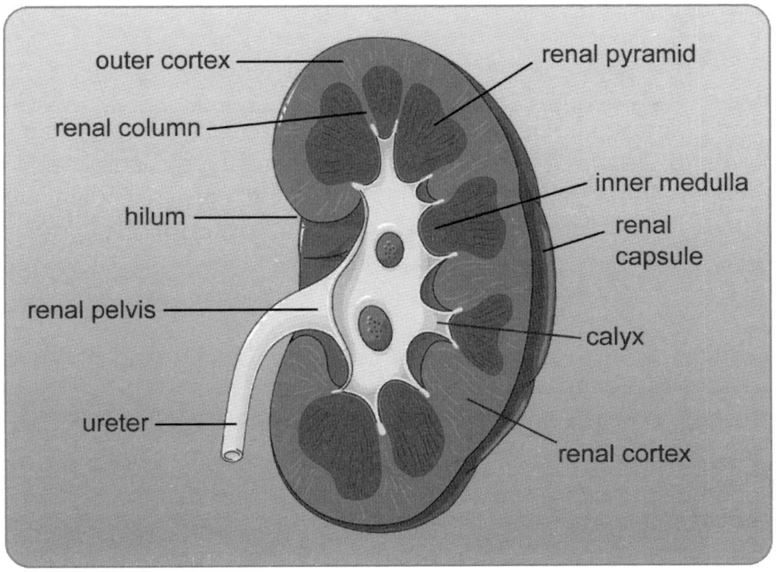

The kidneys lie on either side of the vertebral column and are located high up in the abdominal cavity, behind the peritoneal cavity. Thus, their position is **retroperitoneal**.

There are two kidneys, and they are designated left and right. The left kidney is usually slightly higher than the right. Both kidneys are embedded in fatty tissue for protection and measure approximately 10–12 cm in length. They are lima-bean shaped with the medial margin forming a concave depression called the renal **hilum**. Arteries, vessels, nerves and the ureter are transmitted through the hilum.

Each kidney is surrounded by a thin capsule and is made up of two distinct regions:

1. Outer **cortex**
2. Inner **medulla**

The cortex is not uniform in thickness, but has wedges of cortical tissue called **renal columns (columns of Bertin)**. Furthermore, the cortex contains many thousands of microscopic filtration units called nephrons. **Nephrons** are the functional units of the kidney. They filter waste products out of the blood to be evacuated in the urine and reabsorb usable products such as ions, glucose and amino acids to be utilized in the body. Nephrons are situated within the highly vascular tissue of the renal cortex and extend into the renal medulla. Within the medulla there are 8-15 **renal pyramids** that are separated by **renal columns**. The apex of each pyramid projects into a **minor calyx**, where urine is collected. Each minor calyx empties its contents into a **major calyx**. All major calices empty into the funnel shaped cavity called the **renal pelvis**, to be emptied into the **ureter**.

I. MULTIPLE CHOICE.
Choose the best answer.

1. The renal vessels exit the kidneys at the _____.
   - ◯ outer cortex
   - ◯ renal hilum
   - ◯ inner medulla
   - ◯ renal columns

2. The medical term used when referring to the kidneys is _____.
   - ◯ retroperitoneal
   - ◯ kidneys
   - ◯ renal
   - ◯ medulla

3. The kidney is made up of which two of the following distinct regions?
   - ◯ outer cortex and inner medulla
   - ◯ left and right
   - ◯ concave hilum and renal vessels
   - ◯ calyx and papilla

4. What is the name for the thousands of microscopic filtration units?
   - ◯ nephrons
   - ◯ renal columns
   - ◯ calices
   - ◯ papilla

5. The kidneys are located _____.
   - ◯ near the lungs
   - ◯ behind the peritoneal cavity
   - ◯ in the lower abdomen
   - ◯ on the same side of the vertebral column

KIDNEY - MICROSCOPIC ANATOMY

The filtration, re-absorption, and secretion functions that take place within the kidneys are very complex and dependent on the presence or absence of metabolic molecules, such as sodium and chloride. While we will not cover the physiologic processes performed in the kidneys, a brief description of the anatomic structures involved is included here.

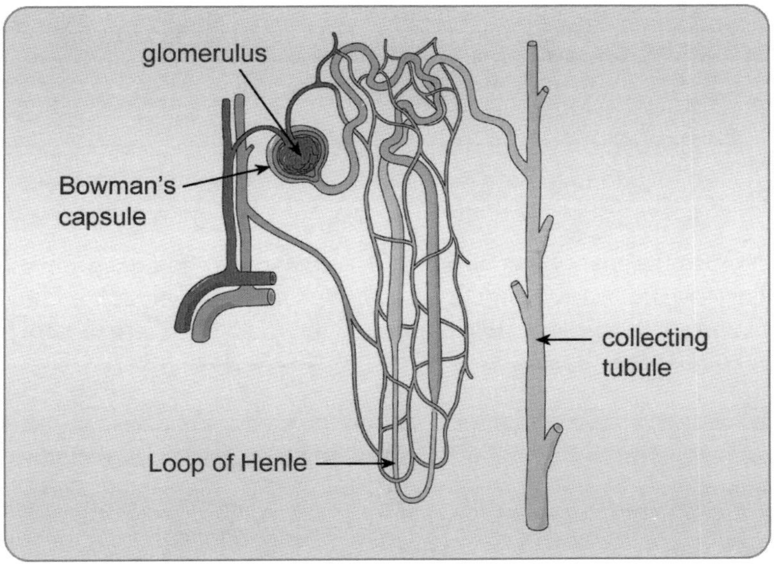

Nephrons are where the urine formation takes place. There are approximately 1 million nephrons in the cortex of each kidney.

There are two main parts to each nephron: the renal corpuscle and the renal tubule. The **renal corpuscle** is made up of the Bowman's capsule and glomerulus (the main filter of the nephron). The filtered fluid from the glomerulus flows into the Bowman's capsule. This filtrate is processed in the nephron to form urine. **Renal tubules** collect the byproducts to be secreted by the kidneys via the ureters. Glucose, sodium, water, and amino acids are then reabsorbed via blood vessels in the **loop of Henle**.

URETERS, BLADDER, AND URETHRA

The **ureters** transfer urine from the kidneys to the **urinary bladder** and are also located in the retroperitoneal area. Each ureter is approximately 25 cm in length and is comprised of three distinct portions:

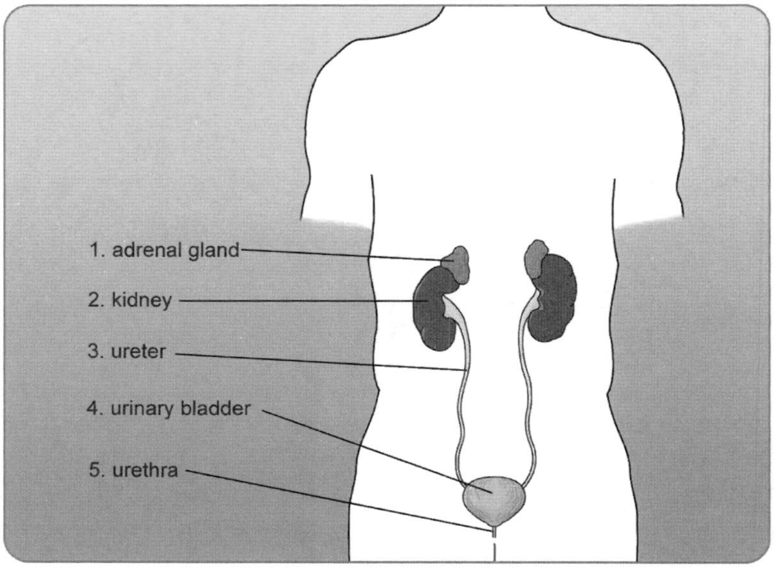

1. The upper (or proximal) ureter is formed by the calices, which funnel together and empty into the renal pelvis.
2. The lumen of the ureter and the bladder is lined with transitional epithelium that is unique to the urinary system because it appears to be squamous (meaning flat or scale-like) when distended with urine, but cuboidal (shaped like a cube) at other times.
3. The urinary bladder is a storage sac for urine. It abuts the uterus and vagina in females and is located above the prostate gland in males. Within the bladder there is a triangular area formed by two ureteral openings and a single urethral opening. This is called the **trigone**.

The **urethra** is a tubular structure that transports the urine from the bladder to outside the body. In the female body, the urethra is a simple tube about 4 cm in length that empties urine through a urethral orifice into the vestibule between the labia minora. In the male body, the urethra is approximately 20 cm long and S–shaped (because of the penis).

The process of eliminating urine from the bladder is called **micturition**. Two sphincter muscles control the passage of urine through the urethra. In medical reports, dictators often use the term **voiding**, which means casting out waste matter, when referring to the process of urination.

I. FILL IN THE BLANK.

Using the word/word parts in the box, fill in the blanks.

micturition
calices
trigone
voiding
bladder

1. The ________________ abuts the uterus and vagina in females and is located above the prostate gland in males.
2. The triangular area formed by two ureteral openings and a single urethral opening is called the ________________.
3. ________________ is the process of eliminating urine from the bladder.

4. The upper ureter is formed by the ________________ which funnel together and empty into the renal pelvis
5. A term in medical records often used in reference to the urination process is ________________.

URINARY TERMINOLOGY

kidney: One of a pair of organs located in the right and left side of the abdomen which help filter the blood and aid in urine excretion.

adrenal gland: One of a pair of small glands, each of which sits on top of one of the kidneys.

retroperitoneal: External to or posterior to the peritoneum.

hilum: Anatomic nomenclature for a depression or pit at the part of an organ where vessels and nerves enter.

renal cortex: The outer part or substance of the kidney.

renal medulla: The inner part or substance of the kidney.

ureter: Transfers urine from the kidneys to the urinary bladder. The human body has two and they are located in the retroperitoneal area.

urinary bladder: The urinary bladder is a storage sac for urine.

renal: Pertaining to the kidneys.

urethra: Tubular structure which transports urine from the bladder to outside the body.

column of Bertin: Inward extensions of the cortical structure of the kidney between the renal pyramids.

malpighian corpuscles: A body that forms the beginning of a nephron, consisting of a glomerulus surrounded by the glomerular capsule (an expanded portion of the renal tubule).

micturition: Process of eliminating urine from the bladder.

urethral orifice: The opening between the bladder and the urethra at one corner of the bladder trigone.

trigone: Triangular area within the bladder formed by two ureteral openings and a single urethral opening.

squamous: Flat or scale-like.

renal papilla: The blunted apex of a renal pyramid, found in the inner zone of the renal medulla and projecting into a renal sinus.

transitional epithelium: Lining of the lumen of the ureters and the bladder.

renal pyramids: The conical masses that make up the substance of the renal medulla; they contain the loops of Henle, the collecting ducts, and the straight arterioles of the kidney.

calyx: The recesses of the renal pelvis that enclose the renal pyramids.

URINARY ANATOMY

I. FILL IN THE BLANK.

In the blanks provided below, refer to the image and enter the term corresponding to the following numbers. Use the word(s) in the box to fill in the blanks.

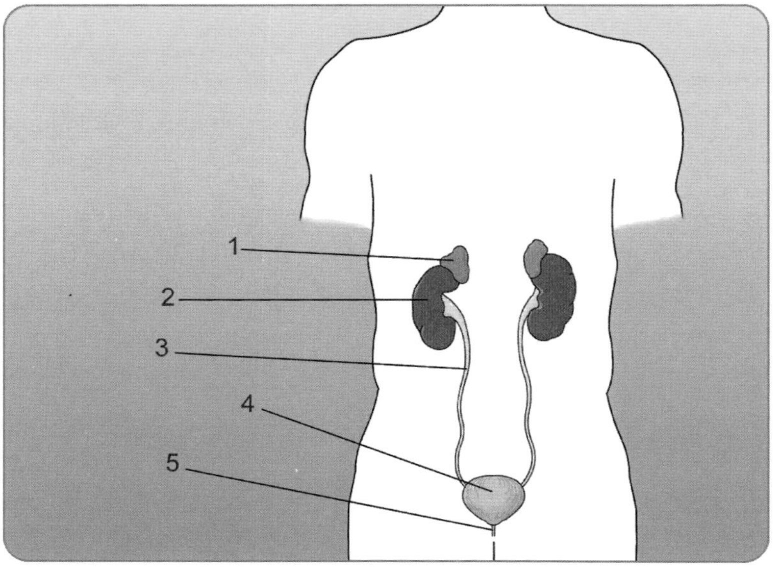

1. ______________
2. ______________
3. ______________
4. ______________
5. ______________

urinary bladder
kidney
urethra
adrenal gland
ureter

REVIEW: URINARY ANATOMY

I. MULTIPLE CHOICE.
Choose the best answer.

1. The storage sac for urine.
   - ◯ ureteral sac
   - ◯ urinary bladder
   - ◯ hillum
   - ◯ ureter

2. The process of eliminating urine from the bladder.
   - ◯ micturition
   - ◯ corte
   - ◯ menstruation
   - ◯ ureteral drainage

3. The outer portion of the kidney.
   - ◯ cortex
   - ◯ vortex
   - ◯ ureter
   - ◯ adrenal glands

4. Means literally behind the peritoneum.
   - ◯ anteperitoneal
   - ◯ biperitoneal
   - ◯ multiperitoneal
   - ◯ retroperitoneal

5. The depression or pit on the kidney where vessels and nerves enter.
   - ◯ medulla
   - ◯ adrenal glands
   - ◯ hilum
   - ◯ urethral orifice

6. The opening between the bladder and urethra.
   - ◯ prepuce
   - ◯ cortex
   - ◯ urethral orifice
   - ◯ ureter

7. A combining form from Medical Word Building that means pertaining to the kidneys.
   - ◯ nephr/i
   - ◯ nephr/o
   - ◯ naphri/o
   - ◯ nephri/o

8. Wedge of cortical tissue.
   - ◯ corpuscle of Bertin
   - ◯ column of Bertin
   - ◯ Column of Bertin
   - ◯ column of Bertan

9. Structure that transfers urine from the kidney to the bladder.
   - ◯ renal glands
   - ◯ adrenal glands
   - ◯ ureter
   - ◯ urethral orifice

10. The inner portion of the kidney.
   - ◯ medulla
   - ◯ medallion
   - ◯ medullary
   - ◯ medulian

11. Caps on the kidneys.
   - ◯ renal glands
   - ◯ electrolyte glands
   - ◯ ureter glands
   - ◯ adrenal glands

UNIT 12

The Reproductive System

THE REPRODUCTIVE SYSTEM - INTRODUCTION

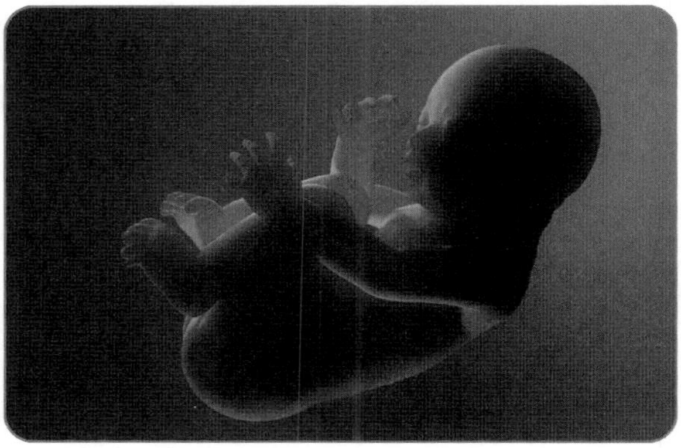

The reproductive system is not vital to the function and health of the human body, but it exists to perpetuate the species and pass genetic material from one generation to another. Most of the smallest details of human reproduction occur cyclically within the human male and female and are not, therefore, significant to the function of the body as a whole.

An incredible amount of information is currently available on the process of human reproduction. Because of this knowledge, laboratories in clinics and hospitals throughout the world are able to recreate many of the natural reproductive functions on behalf of couples who struggle with infertility.

The focus of this unit will be on understanding the basic structure of both sexes and the potentiality for disease and not on the overall process of reproduction. Additionally, this unit will contain information on the urinary or excretory system. The urinary system is closely related to the reproductive system in that they are anatomically close and even share certain organs, especially in the male.

It is necessary for male and female anatomy, as they relate to the reproductive system, to be studied separately. The first part of this unit will discuss the female reproductive system. This includes the parts necessary to both create and sustain life prior to and following birth, including the nourishment of a newborn child.

UTERUS AND VAGINA

The structures of the female reproductive system can be grouped based on their location in the body into either the **internal** or **external reproductive organs**. Collectively, these organs are responsible for menstruation, the production of sexual components to create fetuses and for providing nourishment to the fetus during pregnancy and after (breast feeding).

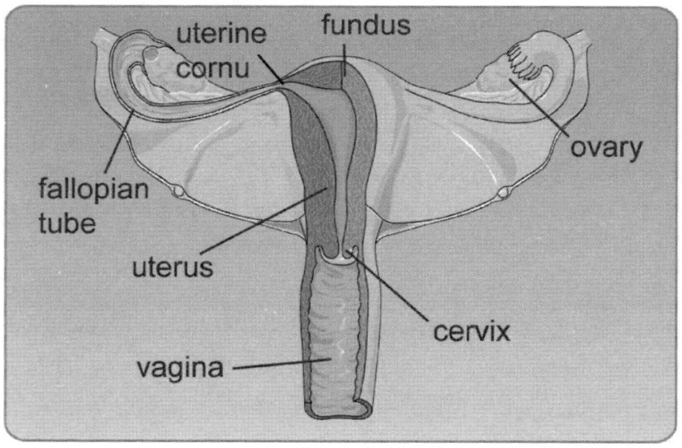

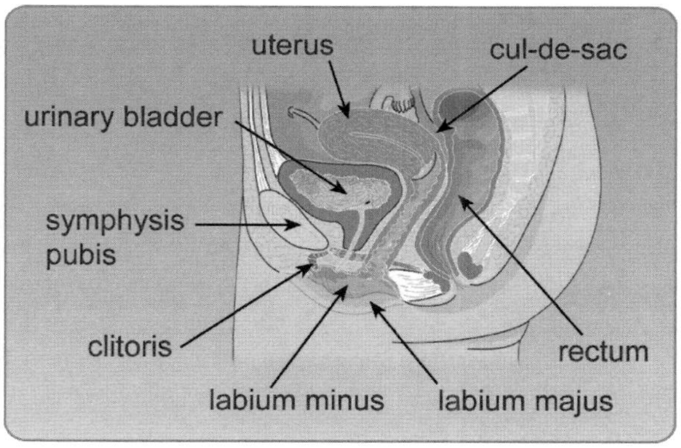

The female has four primary internal sex organs:

- vagina
- uterus
- fallopian tubes
- ovaries

The **vagina** is a muscular tube about 3 inches in length that passes from the cervical opening, or os, of the uterus to the vulva, outside of the body. A recessed area around the cervix is called the **fornix**. The vagina functions as a receptacle for the penis during sexual intercourse, a repository for sperm, a passageway for the discharge of menstrual flow, and as the birth canal for parturition (the birthing process).

The uterus is a hollow, thick-walled, muscular organ that is shaped somewhat like an inverted pear. Positioned between the urinary bladder and the rectum, the uterus is not firmly attached and can be tilted (for example, when the bladder is full). The main portion of the uterus is called the body. The tapered distal portion is the cervix. And the uppermost portion is referred to as the **fundus uteri**. The two areas at the upper corners of the uterus are called the **uterine cornu** (cornu refers to "horn-shaped").

The wall of the uterus is composed of three layers. The inner lining, or **endometrium**, undergoes changes based on the menstrual cycle. The middle layer of the uterus is called the **myometrium**. It has three layers of smooth muscle (hence the prefix **myo-**) that are thicker at the fundus and thinner at the cervix. The perimetrium is the external layer of tissue that partially surrounds the uterus. It does not cover the cervix and only a part of the uterine body.

Another important structure in the female anatomy is called the **cul de sac**, or **Pouch of Douglas**. It is an extension of the peritoneal cavity between the rectum and back wall of the uterus.

The term "cul-de-sac," aside from being any *blind pouch or cavity that is closed at one end*, is used specifically to refer to the rectouterine pouch. This area is prone to infection, and it is not uncommon to see procedures performed on this body part, such as a culdoscopy or culdocentesis.

OVARIES AND FALLOPIAN TUBES

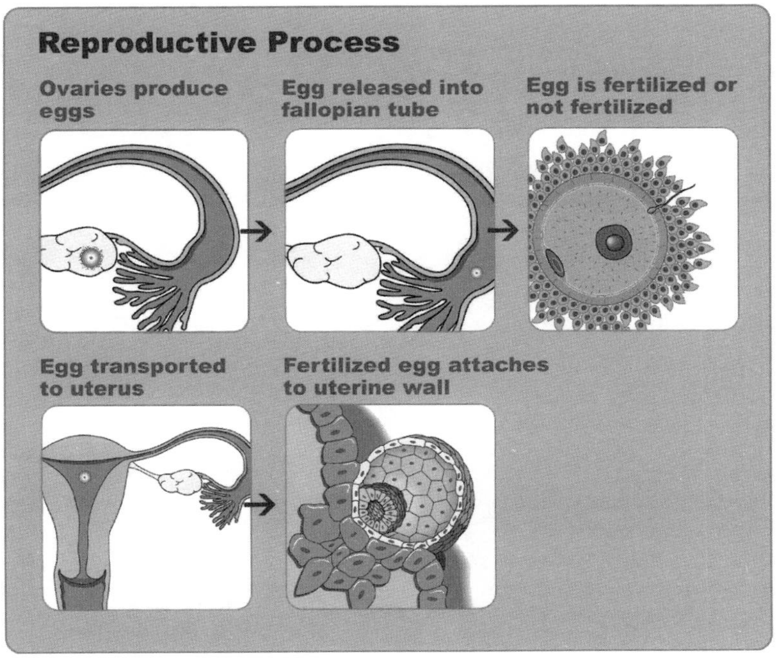

The **ovaries** are paired organs that not only produce gametes (oogenesis) but are also responsible for the production of the two female hormones: estrogen and progesterone. They are similar to the gonads in the male. **Ovaries** are oval in shape and measure approximately 3.5 cm long, 2 cm wide, and 1 cm thick. They are positioned on either side of the uterus. Each ovary has an outer cortex and an inner medulla. The connective tissue of the cortex is called its **stroma**, and throughout the stroma are many ovarian follicles in various stages of development.

Normally only one ovarian follicle develops or matures each month. During maturation, the follicle enlarges and develops a second layer. This mature follicle measures approximately 1 cm in diameter and is called a **graafian follicle**. During ovulation the surface of the follicles gives way and allows the ovum to escape. The ruptured follicle then develops into a **corpus luteum**, which produces progesterone, inhibin, relaxin, and limited amounts of estrogen. **Progesterone** and **inhibin** prevent further follicles from developing when the corpus luteum is under development. **Relaxin** helps to prevent uterine contractions so the chances of fertilization are increased. Once fertilization takes place, the placenta takes over hormone secretion.

Once the ovum is released it enters the nearest open end of 1 of 2 fallopian tubes. The **fallopian tubes** (also called uterine tubes, oviducts, or salpinges) transport the ovum to the uterus. Each fallopian tube is narrow, smooth, and muscular, measuring approximately 10 cm in length. The lumen of each tube is lined with cilia and epithelial cells. The narrow isthmus of each tube opens directly into the uterus. The longest, dialated portion of the tube is called the **ampulla**, while the funnel-shaped distal end is the infundibulum.

I. MATCHING.
Put the following steps in order from 1 to 4.

1. ____
2. ____
3. ____
4. ____

A. corpus luteum is formed
B. ovarian follicle is produced
C. progesterone and inhibin suppress additional follicle maturation
D. graafian follicle is formed

FALLOPIAN TUBES, UTERUS, AND VAGINA

I. **MATCHING.**
In the blanks provided below, refer to the image and enter the letter for the term corresponding term to the following numbers.

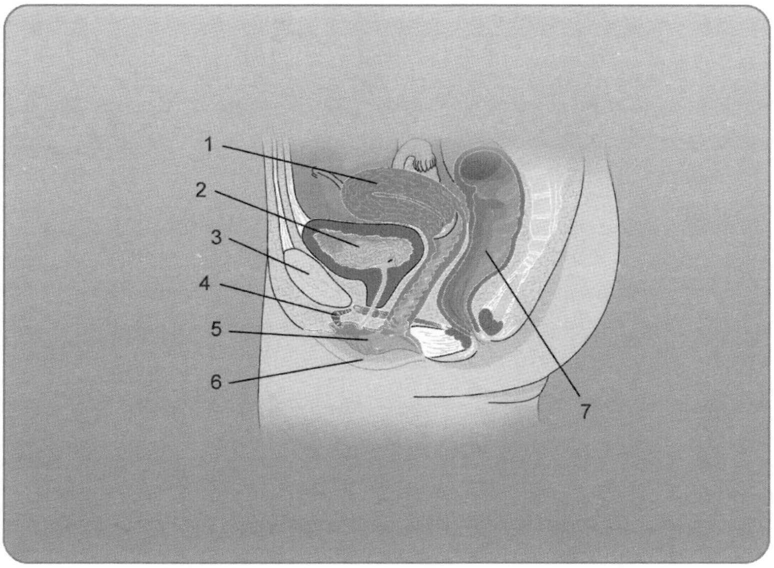

1. ___
2. ___
3. ___
4. ___
5. ___
6. ___
7. ___

A. clitoris
B. urinary bladder
C. rectum
D. uterus
E. labium majus
F. symphysis pubis
G. labium minus

FEMALE SUPPORTING STRUCTURES

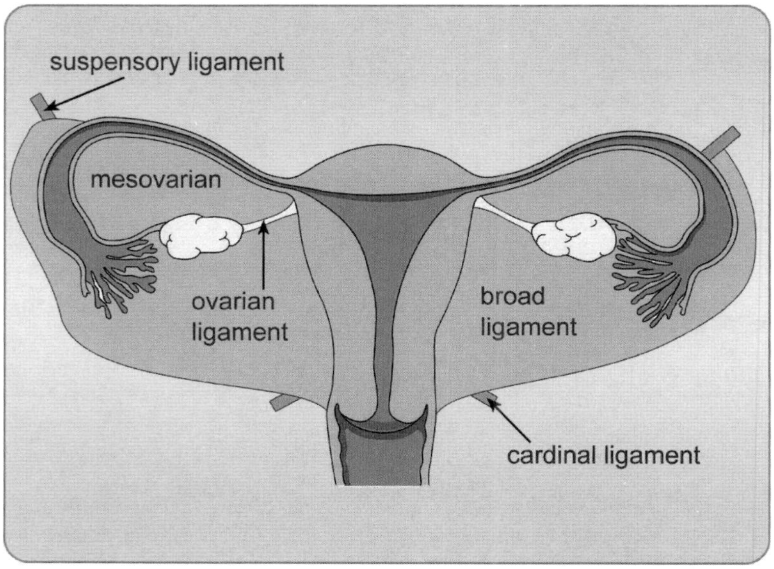

The **uterus** is located in the pelvic cavity between the rectum and the bladder. It is able to expand during pregnancy, so it has mobility, although maintaining its normal position is vital to fertilization. Several ligaments (8) help maintain the normal uterine position in the abdomen even when its position alters due to changes in the bladder, rectum and during pregnancy. The eight uterine ligaments are the broad ligaments (2), uterosacral ligaments (2), posterior ligament, anterior ligament, and round ligaments (2).

The **broad ligaments** create a partition of the pelvic cavity and suspend the uterus. The uterosacral ligaments connect to the sacrum, providing support from the back. The anterior ligament is located on the front of the uterus, extending to the bladder. The posterior ligament is located on the back of the uterus, extending to the front of the rectum. The round ligaments consist of flattened bands situated between the broad ligament and the uterine tubes. They exit the pelvic cavity through the inguinal canals and end at the **labia majora**.

EXTERNAL FEMALE ORGANS

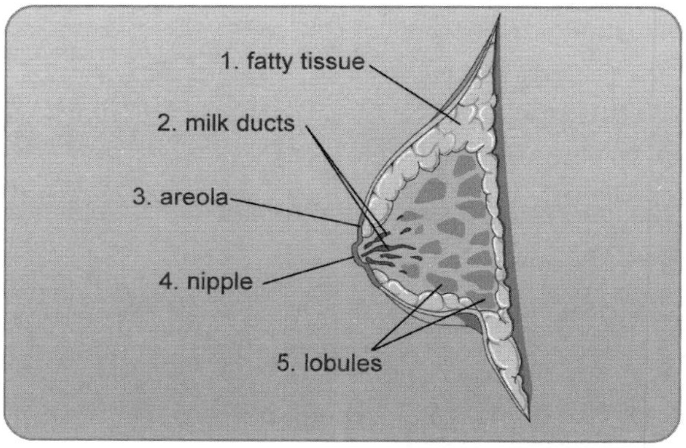

The other organs of the female reproductive system are the external genitalia, also called the **vulva**. The vulva consists of the **mons pubis**, a pad of connective tissue that covers the symphysis pubis and (after puberty) supports the coarse pubic hair. The **labia majora** (plural) are two longitudinal folds of skin comprised of adipose and muscular tissue. They are continuous with the mons pubis and eventually form the perineum (the area between the thighs to the anus). The labia majora are covered with hair and contain multiple sebaceous glands, which secrete a greasy, lubricating substance.

The **labia minora** (plural) are two smaller longitudinal folds located between the labia majora. They are hairless, contain sebaceous glands, and split to form the **prepuce** (fold of skin) that covers the clitoris. The **clitoris**, a small rounded structure made up of erectile tissue and sensitive epithelium, is found at the upper portion of the vestibule (the cleft between the labia into which both the vagina and urethra open).

You may remember from your study of the skeletal system that the pelvis includes the hip bones, the pubic bones, and the symphysis pubis, the fibrocartilaginous joint formed by the junction of the pubic bones.

There are several openings on the vulva: the external urinary meatus for excretion of urine; the vaginal orifice; and the ducts from the vestibular glands. The **hymen** is a membrane surrounding or partially covering the vaginal orifice. The **greater vestibular glands (Bartholin glands)** are located on each side to the vaginal orifice, while the ducts of the **lesser vestibular glands (Skene glands)** are located near the urinary meatus. These glands produce fluids important for intercourse, similar to the bulbourethral glands in the male.

And finally, also included in the female reproductive system are the **mammary glands**. Structurally, these glands within the **breasts** are modified sweat glands and are actually a part of the integumentary (skin) system. Functionally, however, they are associated with the reproductive system because they secrete milk for nourishment of infants (a process called lactation). Each gland is composed of 15 to 20 lobes with a duct that opens at the tip of the **nipple**. The nipple itself is partially composed of erectile tissue and is surrounded by a circular area, the **areola**, that is usually darker in pigment than the surrounding skin.

I. TRUE/FALSE.
Mark the following true or false.

1. The labia minora support coarse pubic hair after puberty.
   - ○ true
   - ○ false

2. The clitoris is a small, rounded structure made up of erectile tissue and epithelium.
   - ○ true
   - ○ false

3. The mons pubis is a pad of connective tissue that covers the symphysis pubis.
   - ○ true
   - ○ false

4. The labia majora contain sebaceous glands which secrete a greasy, lubricating substance.
   - ○ true
   - ○ false

5. The vulva is the area between the thighs to the anus.
   - ○ true
   - ○ false

II. **FILL IN THE BLANK.**

In the blanks provided below, refer to the above image and enter the term corresponding to the following numbers. Use the word(s) in the box to fill in the blanks.

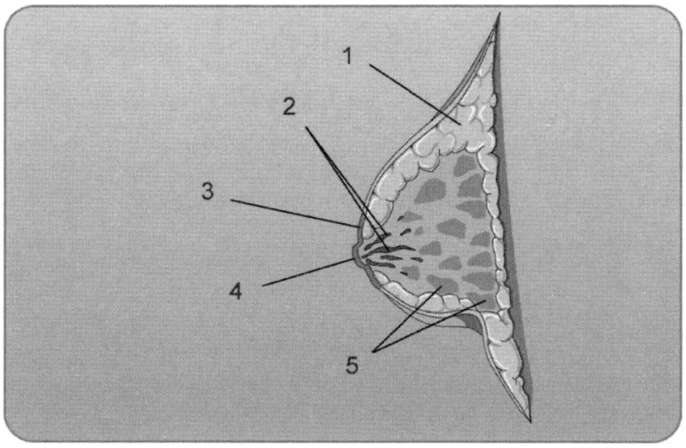

1. ________________
2. ________________
3. ________________
4. ________________
5. ________________

nipple
lobules
fatty tissue
areola
milk ducts

FEMALE REPRODUCTIVE ANATOMY - LESSON 1

eggs: Gametes or ova.

estrogen: A female hormone secreted by the ovary, it is responsible for typical female sexual characteristics.

progesterone: A female hormone that prepares and maintains the uterus for pregnancy.

mesentery: A double layer of peritoneum that acts as a structural support for the ovaries.

mesovarium: The fold of peritoneum connecting the ovary with the wall of the abdominal cavity.

suspensory ligament: A fold of peritoneum that extends out from the ovary to the wall of the pelvis. (Also called infundibulopelvic ligament.)

ovarian ligament: A fibrous ligament that connects the ovary to the lateral surface of the uterus. (Also called utero-ovarian ligament.)

cortex: Outer portion of an organ.

medulla: Inner part of an organ.

stroma: The connective tissue of the cortex that contains many ovarian follicles in various stages of development.

graafian follicle: Matured ovarian follicle that produces the female hormone estrogen.

corpus luteum: The ruptured ovarian follicle that produces the female hormone progesterone.

oviducts: Another name for the fallopian tubes.

ampulla: The longest portion of the fallopian tube.

infundibulum: The funnel-shaped distal end of the fallopian tube.

FEMALE REPRODUCTIVE ANATOMY - LESSON 2

fundus: The uppermost portion of the uterus.

proliferative: A stage in the menstrual cycle where the endometrium rapidly regenerates and the blood supply increases.

fornix: A recessed area around the cervix.

medulla: Inner part of an organ.

vestibular: Lubricating glands for the fornix.

Bartholin's gland: Lubricating glands for the fornix.

vulva: Part of the female reproductive system called the external genitalia.

mons pubis: A pad of connective tissue that covers the symphysis pubis and (after puberty) supports the coarse pubic hair.

perineum: The area between the thighs to the anus.

sebaceous glands: Glands which secrete a greasy, lubricating substance.

prepuce: A covering fold of skin of the clitoris.

mammary: Glands located within the breasts that are modified sweat glands.

integumentary: The skin.

lactation: The secretion of milk from the breasts for nourishment of infants.

areola: A circular pigmented area that surrounds the nipple.

REVIEW: FEMALE REPRODUCTIVE ANATOMY

I. MULTIPLE CHOICE.
Choose the best answer.

1. A mature follicle.
   - ◯ mons pubis
   - ◯ estrogen
   - ◯ graafian follicle
   - ◯ progesterone

2. A pad of connective tissue covering the symphysis pubis.
   - ◯ perineum
   - ◯ mons pubis
   - ◯ oviducts
   - ◯ gametes

3. The reproductive system can be divided into the internal organs and the _______.
   - ◯ mons pubis
   - ◯ internal genitalia
   - ◯ external genitalia
   - ◯ perineum

4. A covering fold of skin.
   - ◯ prepuce
   - ◯ follicle
   - ◯ mesentery
   - ◯ cortex

5. The distal end of the uterine tube.
   - ◯ areola
   - ◯ perineum
   - ◯ ova
   - ◯ infundibulum

6. A circular pigmented area.
   - ◯ areola
   - ◯ pubis
   - ◯ ampulla
   - ◯ vestibular

7. The longest portion of the fallopian tube.
   - ◯ Bartholin's gland
   - ◯ vulva
   - ◯ ampulla
   - ◯ areola

8. The connective tissue of the cortex.
   - ◯ stroma
   - ◯ sebaceous
   - ◯ mesentery
   - ◯ vulva

9. The uppermost portion of the uterus.
   - ◯ stroma
   - ◯ corpus luteum
   - ◯ oviducts
   - ◯ fundus

10. Another term for the external genitalia.
   - ◯ ova
   - ◯ vulva
   - ◯ gametes
   - ◯ lactation

11. The ovaries are located on either side of the uterus and are supported by this.
   - ◯ menses
   - ◯ perineum
   - ◯ mesentery
   - ◯ medulla

12. A gland that lubricates the vagina during sexual excitement.
   - ◯ Bartholin gland
   - ◯ secretory phase
   - ◯ fornix
   - ◯ cortex

13. The first of the female hormones.
   - ◯ progesterone
   - ◯ estrogen
   - ◯ stroma
   - ◯ ova

14. Glands that secrete a greasy substance.
- ◯ lactation
- ◯ menses
- ◯ sebaceous
- ◯ mesovarium

15. A ligament that comprises the mesentery.
- ◯ mesovarium
- ◯ gametes or ova
- ◯ oviducts
- ◯ fornix

16. The inner portion of an ovary.
- ◯ prepuce
- ◯ areola
- ◯ mons pubis
- ◯ medulla

17. The ruptured follicle that generates progesterone.
- ◯ mesovarium
- ◯ fornix
- ◯ corpus luteum
- ◯ menses

18. The area between the thighs.
- ◯ vulva
- ◯ symphysis pubis
- ◯ perineum
- ◯ cortex

19. The cyclic discharge of blood and tissues from the uterus.
- ◯ menstruation
- ◯ mons pubis
- ◯ secretory phase
- ◯ ampulla

20. Another name for #19.
- ◯ menses
- ◯ lactation
- ◯ secretory phase
- ◯ mesovarium

21. The secretion of milk.
- ◯ menses
- ◯ lactation
- ◯ milk ducts
- ◯ secretory phase

22. Modified sweat glands.
- ◯ mammary glands
- ◯ Bartholin's glands
- ◯ sebaceous glands
- ◯ sweat glands

23. The outer surface of an ovary.
- ◯ cortex
- ◯ fornix
- ◯ medulla
- ◯ follicle

24. The recessed area around the cervix.
- ◯ prepuce
- ◯ vortex
- ◯ fornix
- ◯ mons pubis

25. Another term for fallopian tubes.
- ◯ mammary glands
- ◯ oviducts
- ◯ tubal ligation
- ◯ mesovarium

26. The joint formed by a union of the pubic bones by thick fibrocartilage.
- ◯ mons pubis
- ◯ mesentery
- ◯ secretory phase
- ◯ symphysis pubis

27. The middle stage through which the uterine lining progresses.
   - ◯ secretory phase
   - ◯ lactation
   - ◯ menses
   - ◯ oviducts

28. The main product of the ovaries.
   - ◯ areola
   - ◯ gametes or ova
   - ◯ estrogen
   - ◯ progesterone

MALE REPRODUCTIVE ANATOMY - LESSON 1

The primary function of the male reproductive system, as stated earlier, is to perpetuate the species. This is done through the creation and transportation of **sperm**. Most of the structures and organs shown have an important role in this process. The main structures of the male reproductive system are: testes, reproductive ducts, accessory reproductive glands, and supporting structures.

The **testes**(singular: testis) are the male gonads (gamete-producing glands). These are contained in a sac-like structure called the **scrotum**. The **cremaster** and **dartos muscles** flex to pull the scrotum close to the body or relaxe to regulate the temperature of the testes. Normally there are two testes, each in its own compartment and separated by the longitudinal median septum. Each testis is surrounded by connective tissue called the **tunica albuginea**. The testes are further divided into compartments called **lobules**, which contain the **seminiferous tubules** where the spermatozoa are produced. The sperm pass from these tubules into the rete testis and then into the efferent ductules to complete the maturation process before leaving the testes via the epididymis.

MALE REPRODUCTIVE ANATOMY - LESSON 2

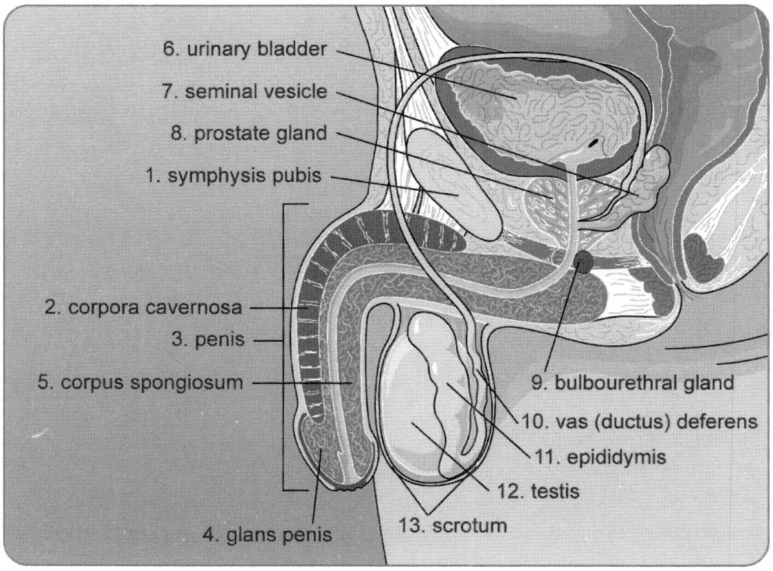

The **epididymis** is part of the reproductive ducts within the male reproductive system. It consists of a very coiled tube that fits snugly over the upper end of each testis. Sperm from the efferent ductules are stored in the epididymis before ejaculation. The total length of each epididymis is 20 feet. The sperm spend about 3 weeks maturing in the epididymis.

The **vas deferens** (also called the ductus deferens) is a continuation of the epididymis that ascends to the urethra. It passes out of the scrotum and into the abdominal cavity through an inguinal canal. It is part of the spermatic cord that also includes blood vessels, nerves, and a lining that all function closely with the testis. Once it reaches the abdominal cavity, the vas deferens separates from the rest of the spermatic cord and crosses the ureter to reach the posterior side of the urinary bladder. Here it becomes part of the ejaculatory duct, where it passes through the prostate gland and terminates in the urethra.

MALE REPRODUCTIVE ANATOMY - LESSON 3

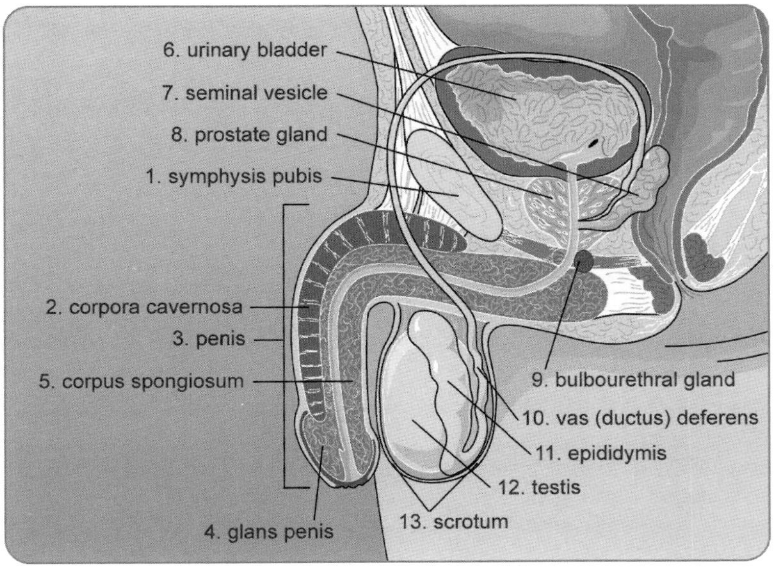

The **accessory glands**—namely the seminal vesicles, prostate gland, and bulbourethral glands—secrete additives to the sperm that strengthen and protect them. These secretions, together with the sperm, are called **semen**. The **seminal vesicles** are glands found immediately beneath the bladder. They secrete a sticky, alkaline, yellow substance that assists in sperm movement and longevity. It is the union of the seminal vesicles and the vas deferens that make up the ejaculatory ducts. The **prostate gland** surrounds the urethra at the base of the bladder. It is a singular gland made up of many small glands and muscle fibers enclosed in a dense connective tissue. The prostate secretes a thin, milky, alkaline substance that assists in sperm motility. The alkaline nature of the seminal fluid protects the sperm from the acidic environment of the female vagina.

Finally, there are two **bulbourethral glands** (also called Cowper glands), each approximately the size of a pea, located inferior to the prostate. Their ducts open into the urethra where they secrete a mucoid substance before ejaculation, coating the lining of the urethra in order to further protect the sperm.

The supporting structures of the male reproductive system are the scrotum, penis, and spermatic cords. The ideal temperature for sperm formation is about 3 degrees Celsius below normal body temperature. Therefore, the testes are held outside of the body in the scrotum. The **scrotum** is a pouch of skin containing two sacs that are separated by a septum. Each sac contains a testis, epididymis, and the lower part of a spermatic cord. The spermatic cords enclose the vas deferens, blood vessels, lymphatic's, and nerves. They are located in the inguinal canal, between the scrotum and abdominal cavity.

The **penis** is made up of three cylindrical masses of erectile tissue. Two lateral cylinders are called the **corpora cavernosa** and, a third, medial one called the corpus spongiosum, the distal part of which forms the glans penis. The glans penis is covered by a loose-fitting casing known as the **prepuce** or foreskin. The urethral opening, or external meatus, is used to excrete both urine and seminal fluid.

MALE ACCESSORY GLANDS AND SUPPORTING STRUCTURES

I. MATCHING.
Match the correct term to the definition.

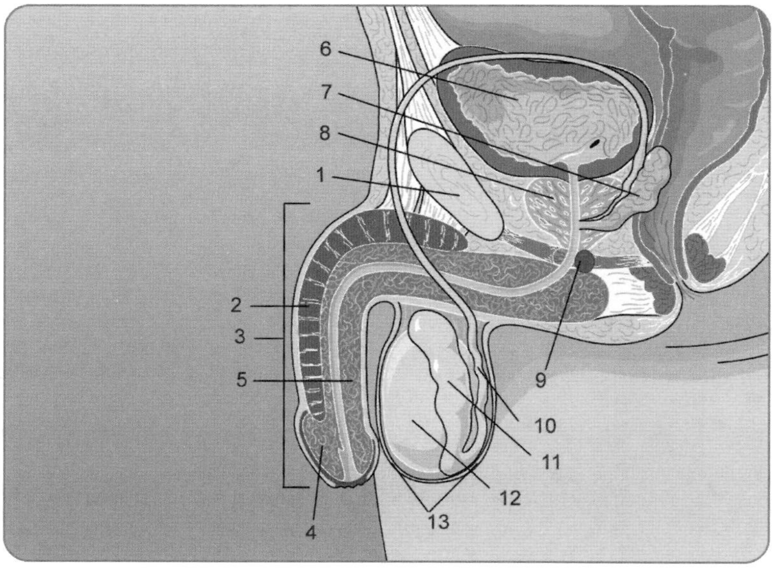

1. ___
2. ___
3. ___
4. ___
5. ___
6. ___
7. ___
8. ___
9. ___
10. ___
11. ___
12. ___
13. ___

A. prostate gland
B. corpora cavernosa
C. epididymis
D. corpus spongiosum
E. vas (ductus) deferens
F. glans penis
G. seminal vesicle
H. symphysis pubis
I. scotrum
J. bulbourethral gland
K. penis
L. testis
M. urinary bladder

MALE REPRODUCTIVE ANATOMY TERMINOLOGY

gonads: Gamete-producing glands.

median septum: The separation between the two testes.

tunica albuginea: Connective tissue that surrounds each testis.

seminiferous tubules: The area where the spermatozoa are produced.

rete testis: The network of canals that the sperm run through.

efferent ductules: The area that the rete testis empties into.

dartos: A muscle in the scrotal wall that responds to temperature changes and moves the position of the testes within the scrotum.

cremaster: One of the muscles, attached to the spermatic cord, that responds to temperature changes and moves the position of the testes within the scrotum.

spermatic cord: A group of structures that go through the inguinal canal to the testis. The structures include the vas deferens, arteries, veins, lymphatic vessels, and nerves.

semen: The combination of secretions from the seminal vesicles, prostate gland, and bulbourethral glands with sperm.

Cowper gland: Two bulbourethral glands, each approximately the size of a pea, which are located inferior to the prostate.

urethra: A 20-cm long S-shaped tube that connects the urinary bladder and ejaculatory ducts to the outside of the body.

meatus: The end of the urethra.

prepuce: A retractable fold of skin at the tip of the penis, also called foreskin.

circumcision: The removal of the prepuce.

REVIEW: MALE REPRODUCTIVE ANATOMY

I. MULTIPLE CHOICE.
Choose the best answer.

1. One of the scrotal wall muscles.
   - ◯ dartos
   - ◯ urethra
   - ◯ rete testis
   - ◯ vas deferens

2. Also called bulbourethral glands.
   - ◯ tunica albuginea
   - ◯ rete testis
   - ◯ circumcision
   - ◯ Cowper glands

3. The removal of the prepuce.
   - ◯ resection
   - ◯ epididymis
   - ◯ rete testis
   - ◯ circumcision

4. Secretions from the glands, in combination with the spermatozoa.
   - ◯ sperman
   - ◯ seeman
   - ◯ semen
   - ◯ seman

5. A very coiled tube located at the upper end of each testis that is approximately 6.5 meters in length.
   - ◯ epididmis
   - ◯ epididymis
   - ◯ epididimys
   - ◯ epidydimis

6. A continuation of the epididymis that goes up and into the urethra.
   - ◯ vas deferens
   - ◯ prepuce
   - ◯ vasideferens
   - ◯ rete testis

7. The foreskin of the penis.
   - ◯ glans penis
   - ◯ prepuce
   - ◯ epididymis
   - ◯ dartos

8. The connective tissue that surrounds the testis.
   - ◯ tunica albuginea
   - ◯ tunica testiculosa
   - ◯ tunica spongosa
   - ◯ tunica testosterosa

9. The place in the body where the sperm are produced.
   - ◯ sperm tubules
   - ◯ semen tubules
   - ◯ seminiferous tubules
   - ◯ epididymis

10. After production, the sperm pass directly into this structure.
   - ◯ right testis
   - ◯ left testes
   - ◯ Cowper glands
   - ◯ rete testis

UNIT 13

The Integumentary System and Special Sensory Organs

THE INTEGUMENTARY SYSTEM AND SPECIAL SENSORY ORGANS – INTRODUCTION

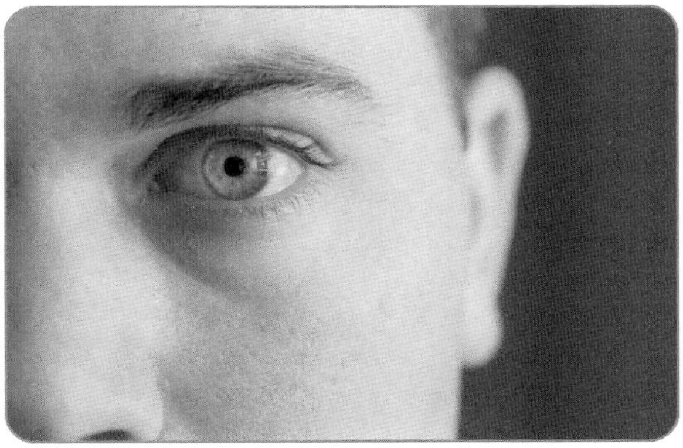

The senses of sight, smell, taste, hearing, and touch are important tools in relating the body and its internal systems to the external world. The anatomical parts that perform these functions are not individually or collectively part of any single system, but their role is unique and important to carry out the functions that allow for interaction between the body and the environment. Three primary sensory organs will be covered in this unit: the skin, eyes, and ears (including the related mouth and nose). The mouth is responsible for taste, but its anatomy is relatively simple and was covered in earlier units.

The senses facilitate interaction with the external world by alerting us to danger, drawing us to nutritional sources, allowing us to communicate, transmitting information important to our cognitive functions, and so forth. Without sight, one would never see a magnificent sunset; without hearing, one would not experience the exhilaration of beautiful music; without touch, one would miss the luxurious softness of a puppy's fur; without smell, one would never enjoy the scent of roses, and food would only taste half as good; and without taste, well, what would life be without sweets?

Maintaining proper function of these sensory receptors may not be vital to the sustenance of life itself, but it does add substantially to human convenience, contentment, and quality of life.

SKIN

The **skin** is the largest human organ, covering approximately 3,000 square inches on an average adult. It is considered an organ because it is made up of several kinds of tissues that are structurally arranged to work together.

> **Highlights**
>
> The skin has six functions:
>
> 1. Protection of body from disease and injury
> 2. Prevention of dehydration
> 3. Regulation of body temperature
> 4. Reception of stimuli
> 5. Regulation of body fluids
> 6. Selective absorption

The skin covers the entire external surface of the body and, along with its associated structures (**hair**, **glands**, and **nails**), it constitutes the **integumentary system**. This system accounts for approximately 7% of the body's weight and performs six important functions:

1. **Protection of the body from disease and external injury.** The tough outer layer of skin is adapted to withstand abrasion and penetration of pathogens. The pigmented layer protects the body from the damaging effects of ultraviolet light.
2. **Prevention of dehydration.** The outer layer of the skin is essentially waterproof, protecting the body from desiccation (the act of drying up) on land and from absorption when immersed in water.
3. **Regulation of body temperature.** Evaporative cooling is made possible by the secretion and evaporation of perspiration (sweat glands). Vasoconstriction of the capillaries assists in warming of the body, while vasodilation assists in cooling it.
4. **Reception of stimuli.** The skin is rich with sensory receptors specialized for touch, pressure, temperature, and pain.

5. **Regulation of body fluids.** The skin performs an excretory function to eliminate excess water, salts, and other metabolic wastes.
6. **Selective absorption.** Some substances that are beneficial to the body can penetrate through the skin, such as gases, vitamins, and hormones. This explains the effectiveness of medicinal patches.

I. TRUE/FALSE.
Mark the following true or false.

1. The integumentary system accounts for approximately 7% of the body's weight.
   - ◯ true
   - ◯ false

2. The skin is considered an organ.
   - ◯ true
   - ◯ false

3. The outer layer of the skin is very susceptible to disease and external injury.
   - ◯ true
   - ◯ false

4. The skin helps get rid of excess water, salts, and other metabolic wastes.
   - ◯ true
   - ◯ false

5. The skin is impenetrable and cannot absorb substances.
   - ◯ true
   - ◯ false

CROSS SECTION OF THE SKIN

The skin, while it may appear to be a single layer, is made up of two layers called the epidermis and dermis. The **epidermis** is the outermost layer (-epi meaning “over” or “upon”) and is made of epithelial tissue. It contains no blood vessels. There are many cell types that make up the epidermis. The more important ones are the **keratinocytes**, which form the outer layer of the skin; the **melanocytes**, or pigmentation cells; the **Langerhans** cells, which play a role in immunity; and the **Merkel** cells, which aid in light touch reception. The ability of the epidermal cells to quickly repair and reproduce is vital for providing protection to the underlying structures.

The **dermis** is made up of fibrous tissue, and contains some nerves, blood vessels and muscles. The dermis determines the depth of the “total skin” covering the body-the thickest being on the back and the thinnest on the eyelids. The two layers which make up the dermis are the papillary and reticular layers. The **papillary layer** gives a ridged appearance to the epidermis, most visible on the fingers and toes. The **reticular layer** is made up of collagenous and elastic fibers, providing strength and elasticity. There are neural receptors in the dermis, such as **Pacinian corpuscles**, which provide the sensation of deep touch. Hair follicles and sebaceous and sweat (**sudoriferous**) glands are also found in the dermis. The basement membrane that binds the epidermis to the dermis is called the **dermoepidermal junction**, or DEJ.

Skin cross section is pictured below with the major structures identified. Study the figure and enter the terms in the blanks provided.

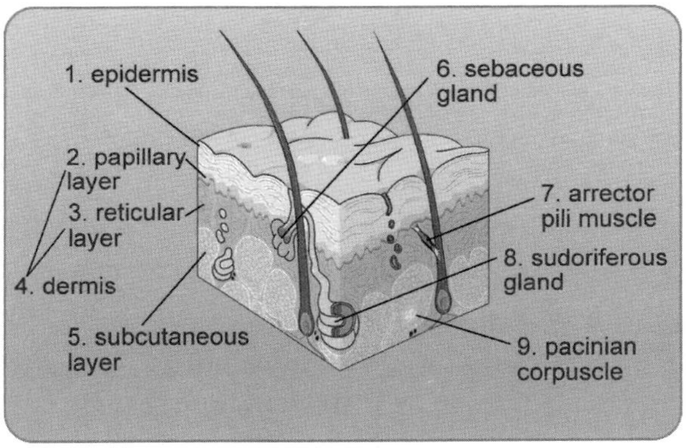

I. **FILL IN THE BLANK.**

In the blanks provided below, refer to the above image and enter the term corresponding to the following numbers. Use the word(s) in the box to fill in the blanks.

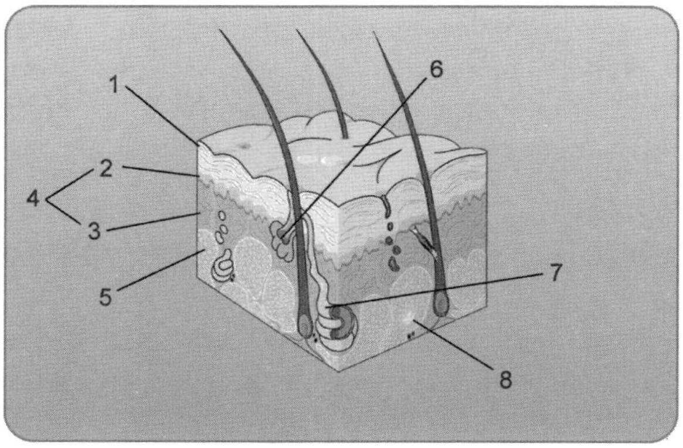

1. ______________
2. ______________
3. ______________
4. ______________
5. ______________
6. ______________
7. ______________
8. ______________
9. ______________

subcutaneous layer
sudoriferous gland
reticular layer
pacinian corpuscle
sebaceous gland
epidermis
arrector pili muscle
papillary layer
dermis

HAIR AND NAILS - LESSON 1

The integumentary system also includes hair and nails which are components that originate in the skin. As mentioned earlier, the hair follicles originate in the dermis. The hair protrudes from the epidermis. The primary function of hair is protection. Hair on the scalp and eyebrows protects against sunlight. The hair inside the nostrils, as well as the eyelashes, protects against airborne particles. Much like the epidermis, the growth of hair takes place within the deeper layer, and the cells die as they are pushed away. It is at this point that the hair becomes visible.

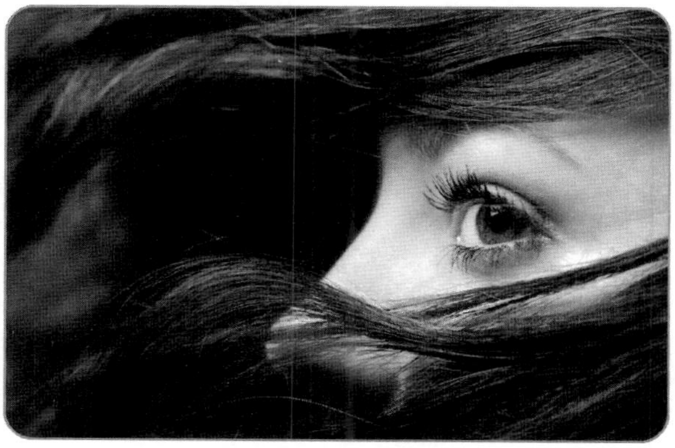

Sebaceous glands, or oil glands, and the smooth muscles called **arrector pili** are associated with hair. The arrector pili muscles are involuntary and respond to thermal or psychological stimuli. When these muscles contract, the hair is pulled into a vertical position, causing the phenomenon called "goose bumps" or chills. This is depicted as number 7 in the graphic on the previous page.

We are born with approximately 5 million hair follicles—100,000 of which are on the scalp. No additional hair follicles are formed after birth.

HAIR AND NAILS - LESSON 2

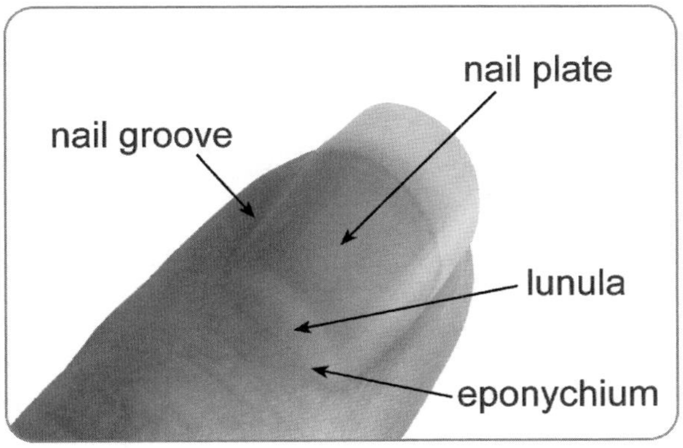

Nails are found on the distal ends of the fingers and the toes. They protect the digits. In the case of the fingers, nails help to grasp and pick up small objects. Nails are formed from a hardened layer of the epidermis called **keratin**.

The **nail body** (also called the nail plate) is the visible part of the nail, and the remainder of the nail lies behind the cuticle. The nail bed is the layer of epithelium under the nail plate, and it contains blood vessels, nerves, and melanocytes.

In addition to the functions mentioned above, the overall appearance of the skin and nails can aid in diagnosing problems or injuries to other body systems. The color of the skin can indicate a variety of illnesses, such as pale skin during shock or anemia, flushed red skin with a fever, or the greenish hue accompanying digestive complaints.

Yellowish or split nails can indicate nutritional deficiencies, and a bluish tint to the nails is a sign of inadequate oxygenation of the blood.

I. **MULTIPLE CHOICE.**
Choose the best answer.

1. The hair and nails are part of the (◯ skin, ◯ integumentary, ◯ cells and tissues, ◯ epithelial) system.

2. The (◯ nail, ◯ nail bed, ◯ nail plate , ◯ nail cuticle) contains blood vessels and nerves.

3. Hair, the primary function of which is to protect from airborne particles, is located (◯ on the scalp, ◯ on the extremities , ◯ inside the nostrils, ◯ inside the intestines).

REVIEW: SKIN

I. MATCHING.
Match each labeled structure to the correct term.

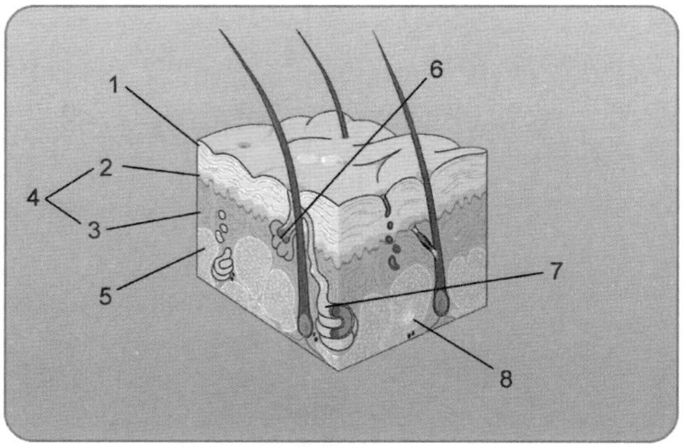

1. ___
2. ___
3. ___
4. ___
5. ___
6. ___
7. ___
8. ___
9. ___

A. sudoriferous gland
B. reticular layer
C. pacinian corpuscle
D. sebaceous gland
E. epidermis
F. arrector pili muscle
G. papillary layer
H. dermis
I. subcutaneous layer

II. MATCHING.
Match the correct term to the definition.

1. ___ the membrane that binds the epidermis to the dermis
2. ___ substance that makes toe and finger nails
3. ___ connective tissue that surrounds organs
4. ___ provides protection from sunlight
5. ___ secretion
6. ___ lines intestines and blood vessels

A. fascia
B. smooth muscle tissue
C. glandular epithelial tissue
D. keratin
E. hair
F. dermoepidural junction

III. MULTIPLE CHOICE.
Choose the best answer.

1. Tissues are made up of _____.
   - ◯ similar organs that perform a similar function
   - ◯ similar structures that are found in the same body region
   - ◯ similar cells that perform a similar function
   - ◯ similar fibers that perform a specific function

2. The largest organ in the body is the _____.
   - ◯ heart
   - ◯ skin
   - ◯ liver
   - ◯ large intestine

SPECIAL SENSORY ORGANS - EARS AND EYES

Two important sensory receptors are the ears and eyes. They help us react to the environmental stimuli through sound and sight. In many cases, they help us avoid dangerous situations. Both senses also elicit emotions when we hear familiar voices or when we view images of pleasant objects.

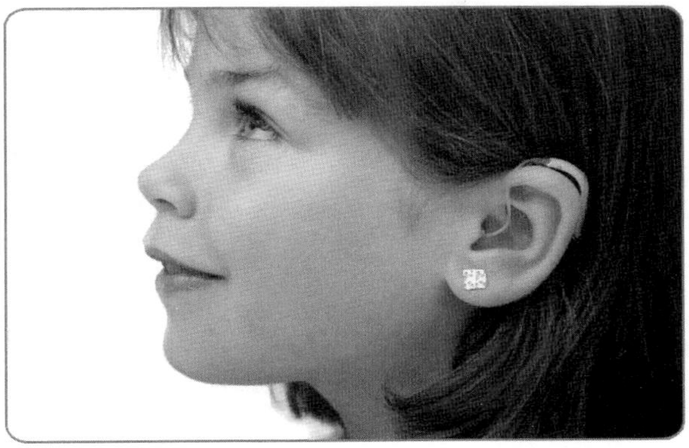

EXTERNAL STRUCTURES OF THE EYE

Humans have two eyes set in the front of the skull just far enough apart to achieve stereoscopic vision. It is this three-dimensional effect that enables us to assess depth. The eyeball of an adult is approximately 1 inch in diameter and is protected in the head by the bones of the skull. The bone cavity that holds the eyeball, called the **orbit**, is lined with a layer of protective fat. About 4/5 of the eye is positioned inside the orbit.

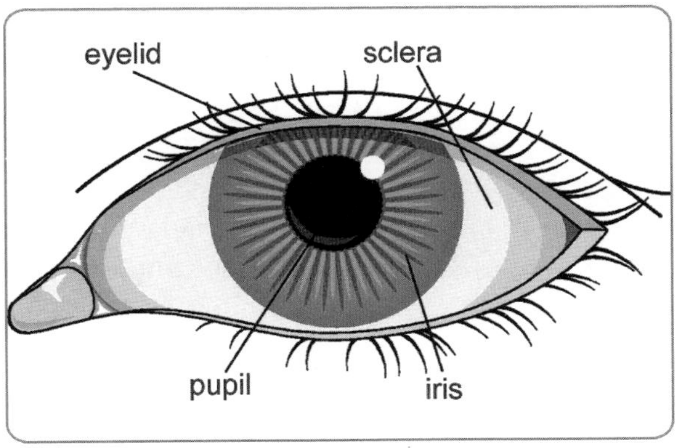

The external structures serve to protect the more delicate inner eye components. These are the eyebrows, eyelids (also called palpebrae), eyelashes, and the ducts that produce tears (lacrimal glands). Specifically, the **eyebrows** shade the eyes from the sun and prevent perspiration or other objects from getting into the eyes.

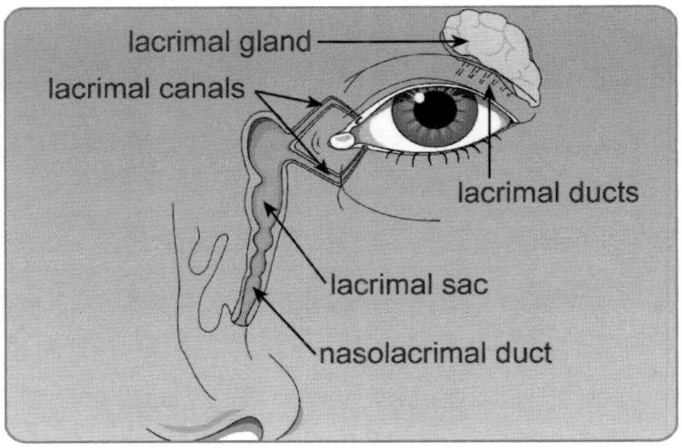

Each eyelid has many lashes to protect the eye from airborne objects. The **eyelids** also protect the eyeball from **desiccation** (drying up) by reflexively blinking approximately every seven seconds. The eyelids also close reflexively if an object is moving towards the eye. There are two muscles of note involved with the function of the **palbebrae**, or eyelids. The **levator palpebrae superioris muscle** acts to open the eye by raising the superior eyelid. The **orbicularis oculi** muscle is a facial muscle the closes the eye. The **conjunctiva** is a thin mucous membrane that lines the interior surface of the eyelid and the exposed surface of the eyeball. The superior and inferior eyelids meet at the **medial canthus**, just lateral to the nose, and the **lateral canthus** at each lateral corner of the eye.

Tears secreted from the **lacrimal gland** and transported through the **lacrimal duct** constantly moisten and clean the exposed portion of the eyeball. All of these aid in the prevention of damage to the eye and preservation of vision.

I. **MULTIPLE CHOICE.**
Choose the best answer.

1. The (◯ eyelashes, ◯ eyelids, ◯ eyebrows, ◯ lacrimal glands) help shade the eyeballs from the sun.

2. On average the eyelid blinks approximately (◯ every 60 seconds, ◯ every seven seconds, ◯ every 15 seconds, ◯ more than seven times per second).

EYE MUSCLES

The six extraocular muscles are attached to the orbit and are crucial to eye movement. Four **rectus muscles** (**superior**, **inferior**, **medial**, and **lateral**) attach to the sclera and rotate or tilt the eyeball in the direction their name indicates. The superior and inferior oblique muscles each pull the eye laterally, superiorly and inferiorly respectively.

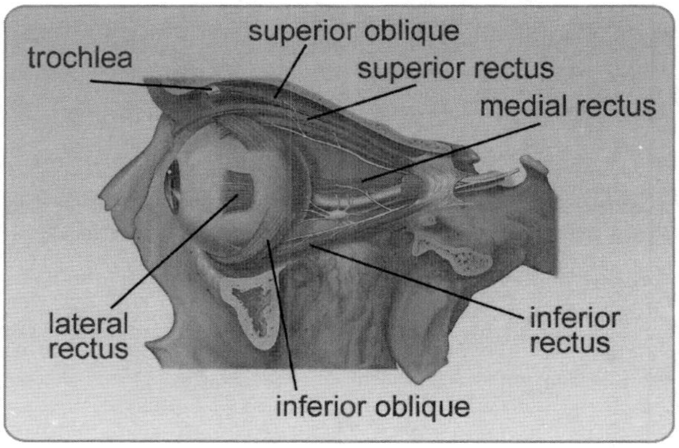

The **trochlea** is a fibrous loop in the eye socket through which the superior oblique muscle passes before attaching to the eye. It is the trochlea attachment that limits the degree to which we can rotate our eyes upward and downward.

Highlights

The anatomy of the trochlea was not fully understood until about 1982.

I. MATCHING.
Match the correct term to the definition.

1. ___ medial rectus muscle
2. ___ trochlea
3. ___ inferior oblique muscle

A. limits the amount of downward and upper eye rotation
B. rotates the top of the eye away from the nose
C. moves the eye toward the nose

II. MULTIPLE CHOICE.
Choose the best answer.

1. Depth perception is enhanced by the (◯ shape of the eyes, ◯ placement of the eyes in the skull, ◯ lateral rectus muscle, ◯ trochlea).

INTERNAL EYE STRUCTURES AND EYESIGHT

Anatomically, the eye consists of two main cavities: the anterior and posterior. The **anterior chamber** includes the structures from the lens forward and contains the aqueous humor (watery material). The **posterior cavity** occupies the space behind the lens and contains vitreous humor (gelatin-like material). Both the **aqueous** and **vitreous humors** are important to help the eyeball maintain normal pressure, avoiding collapse of the structure.

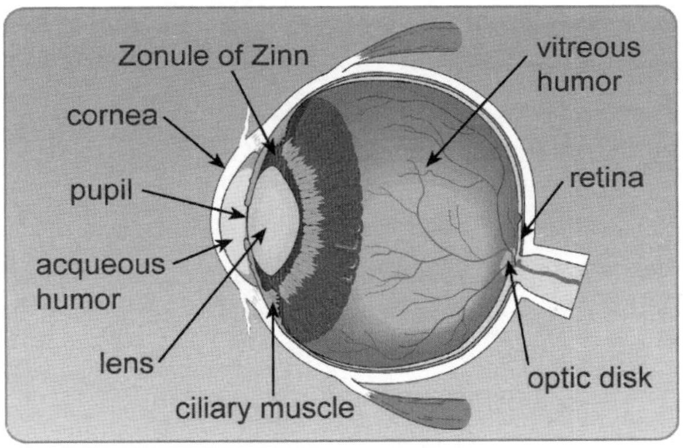

The major internal structures of the eye are shown in the image. These parts all play a critical role in how we see. There are four processes that take place to form an image on the retina:

1. light passes through the **cornea** (refraction)
2. the **lens** focuses the light (accommodation via the suspensory ligaments and **ciliary muscle**)
3. the **pupil** constricts to further focus the rays (constriction via the iris)
4. both eyes move inward simultaneously to provide binocular vision (convergence)

The suspensory ligament of the lens is also called the zonule of Zinn.

The **retina** contains specialty cells called rods and cones. The **rods** help us see in low light and the cones, more active during higher light levels, help determine color. There are more rods than cones in the retina. The **macula** of the retina acts like a “sunblock” and absorbs excess ultraviolet light. At the center of the macula is the highest concentration of cone cells in the eye called the **fovea**. The fovea is responsible for central, high-resolution vision.

From the rods and cones, bipolar cells pass impulses to the **ganglion neurons**, which direct the impulses to the optic disk, the small circular area located in the posterior of the eyeball. From there the fibers emerge through small holes in the sclera and become the optic nerve. The process is very complex, and any deviation along the route of vision can lead to abnormal vision. More details about vision are discussed in the Pathophysiology module.

REVIEW: EYE

I. MATCHING.
Match the correct term to the definition.

1. ____ the muscles of the eye
2. ____ the outermost layer of the eyeball
3. ____ the aqueous humor is located here
4. ____ a jelly-like substance behind the lens
5. ____ the transparent structure that forms the anterior portion of the eye
6. ____ muscle on the top of the eye, innervated by a cranial nerve

A. anterior cavity
B. cornea
C. superior rectus muscle
D. sclera
E. ocular muscles
F. vitreous humor

II. MULTIPLE CHOICE.
Choose the best answer.

1. The _____ limits the degree in which we can rotate our eyes upward and downward.
   - ◯ inferior rectus muscle
   - ◯ superior rectus muscle
   - ◯ trochlea
   - ◯ suspensory lens ligament

2. The lacrimal duct secretes _____.
   - ◯ aqueous humor
   - ◯ lymph fluid
   - ◯ periorbital fat
   - ◯ tears

3. What is another term for palpebrae?
   - ◯ eyebrows
   - ◯ eyelids
   - ◯ eyelashes
   - ◯ eye sockets

4. What part of the eye has the most cones?
   - ◯ optic disk
   - ◯ fovea
   - ◯ macula
   - ◯ zonule of Zinn

EAR, NOSE, AND THROAT

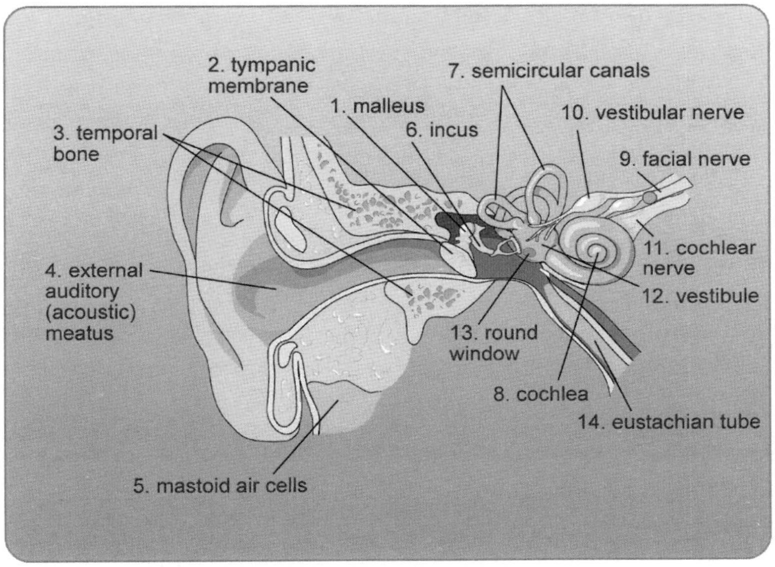

The ear is closely associated with the nose and throat, both anatomically and structurally. As a result, diseases of these structures are diagnosed and treated by a specialist called an **otorhinolaryngologist.** (This is taken from the combining forms for ear (*ot/o*), nose (*rhin/o*) and throat or larynx (*laryng/o*) respectively.) All three of these structures are associated with senses, namely hearing, smell, and taste.

Smell, or **olfaction**, is not nearly as developed in humans as it is in other animals. We do not rely on smell to communicate or locate food sources. In fact, it is probably the least important of all the senses in terms of both maintaining proper body function and enhancing the quality of life. The olfactory sense detects the presence of odors and relatively quickly accommodates to them. Think about it. Only very strong odors maintain our attention for longer than a few minutes (skunk, sewage, burning). Other less obtrusive odors quickly leave the consciousness. However, if you leave the immediate vicinity of the odor and return to it later, you are again alert to the presence of the odor. Olfaction is very closely related to the sense of taste. In fact, if your nose is "plugged" with a cold or other disorder, you often cannot taste or even recognize foods that you usually enjoy. The olfactory or first cranial nerve perceives and relays information assimilated during olfaction. Some odors can also activate the fifth cranial nerve and cause reactionary responses. For example, pepper can cause sneezing, onions can make the eyes water, and ammonia (such as in smelling salts) can revive an unconscious person.

The sense of taste, called **gustation**, is primarily accomplished in the mouth, and especially the tongue. The receptors that make taste possible are called taste buds. These receptors perceive five taste sensations: sweet, sour, salty, bitter, and savory (or "umami"). The receptors responsible for receiving the information necessary to identify these individual taste sensations are localized on specific regions of the tongue. The structures of the tongue, soft palate, and oropharynx are part of both the digestive and respiratory systems and were covered in those chapters.

The most complex of the three structures treated within the medical specialty of otorhinolaryngology, both anatomically and functionally, is the ear. Although it is primarily associated with hearing, the ear actually has two important functions in the human body: it receives sound and maintains balance. There are specialized structures within the ear that perform these different functions. Sensations received by the ear are transmitted to the brain via the eighth cranial nerve. Anatomically the ear is divided into three major areas: the external ear, the middle ear, and the inner ear.

I. TRUE/FALSE.
Mark the following true or false.

1. Gustation is another word for the sense of smell.
   - ◯ true
   - ◯ false

2. Olfaction is closely related to gustation.
   - ◯ true
   - ◯ false

3. The first cranial nerve perceives and relays information assimilated during olfaction.
   - ◯ true
   - ◯ false

4. Some odors can activate the fifth cranial nerve and cause reactionary responses.
   - ◯ true
   - ◯ false

5. The receptors that make taste possible are called olfactories.
   - ◯ true
   - ◯ false

EAR

The external ear consists of the auricle (pinna) and the external auditory meatus. The auricle (or pinna) is the visible fleshy appendage attached to the side of the head. This is a funnel of elastic cartilage both covered and lined by skin. The external auditory (or acoustic) meatus is a slightly S-shaped canal about 1 cm in length that extends from the outside into the temporal bone of the skull. The skin that lines the meatus contains oil glands and specialized wax-secreting glands that produce cerumen (known to lay people as earwax). This acts as an insect repellent. The function of the external ear is to conduct sound waves through a gas medium to the structures of the middle ear.

Highlights

External ear: Conducts sound waves to the structures of the middle ear.

Middle ear: Receives sound waves, amplifies sound, protects ears from loud sounds, equalizes pressure.

Inner ear: Contains functional organs for hearing and equilibrium.

The middle ear receives the sound waves through a solid medium. The tympanic membrane receives the impulses coming in from the meatus and vibrates to set the ossicles in motion. The three ear ossicles are the malleus, incus, and stapes. These tiny bones are also called the hammer, anvil, and stirrup. They act as levers to amplify the sound received from the meatus up to twenty times. The innermost portion of the stapes attaches to the oval window in the inner ear. There are two small muscles that are attached to the malleus and stapes, which contract automatically to protect the ear from loud sounds. The middle ear is connected to the nasopharynx by the eustachian tube. It is this connection that equalizes air pressure on either side of the tympanic membrane.

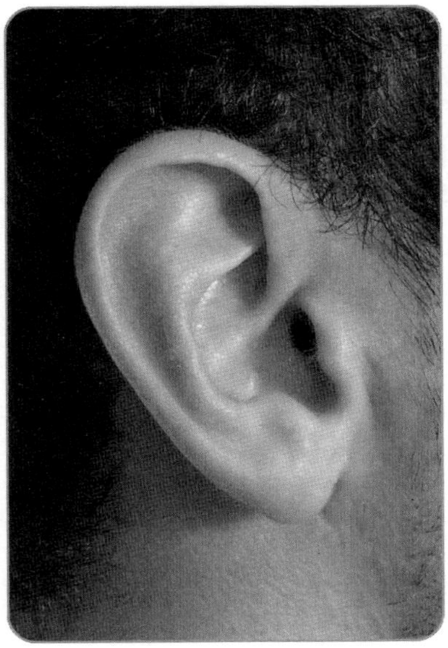

The inner ear, also called the labyrinth, contains the functional organs for hearing and equilibrium. It consists of two parts, an outer bony labyrinth that encloses a membranous labyrinth. The membranous labyrinth consists of tubular chambers that contain a fluid. A fluid also fills the space between the bony labyrinth and the membranous labyrinth. These two fluids provide a liquid medium for conduction of the vibrations involved in hearing and maintaining equilibrium. The bony portion of the inner ear is divided into three areas: the vestibule, semicircular canals, and cochlea. The vestibule is the central portion and contains the round window. The semicircular canals are primarily responsible for maintaining balance, and the cochlea is the structure involved in hearing. Receptor cells for hearing are located within the cochlear duct. A membrane extends inside the cochlear duct to form a canopy over the hair cells on the membranous floor of this duct. As the hair cells vibrate against this canopy, the mechanical forces of sound vibrations are transformed into electrical sensory impulses that are carried to the brain for interpretation.

The ear, much like the eye, has many built-in protective features to preserve its delicate structures and important function. The external auditory meatus and pinna are designed to not only collect sound waves, but to also prevent objects and particles from entering the ear. The excretion of the ceruminous glands, muscles which autonomically contract, and position of the inner ear are also protective features. Additionally, the tympanic membrane has an unusual ability to repair itself. A ruptured "eardrum" can actually be completely healed within a single day without any outside intervention.

Despite the built-in preserving components of the ear, it is still susceptible to disease, trauma, degeneration, and malfunction.

THE MIDDLE EAR

The middle ear is a hollow cavity of the temporal bone, extending from the tympanic membrane to the oval window of the **cochlea**. It is also called the **tympanic cavity**. The middle ear receives acoustic energy via the **tympanic membrane**, which vibrates to set the auditory bones (ossicles) in motion. The eardrum is attached to the **malleus** (hammer) that connects to the **incus** (anvil) that in turn connects to the **stapes** (stirrup). The innermost portion of the stapes attaches to the oval window in the inner ear. The middle ear is connected to the nasopharynx by the **eustachian tube**. It is this connection that equalizes air pressure on either side of the tympanic membrane.

There are two small muscles that are attached to the malleus and stapes, which contract automatically to protect the ear from loud sounds.

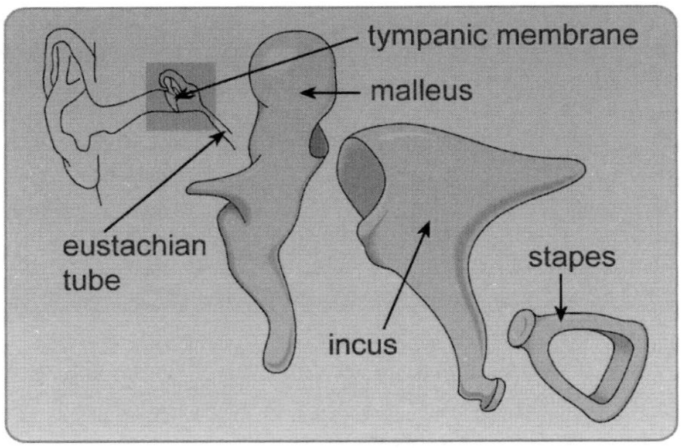

I. **MATCHING.**
Match the correct term to the definition.

1. ___ tympanic membrane
2. ___ stapes
3. ___ malleus
4. ___ eustachian tube
5. ___ incus

A. equalizes air pressure
B. also known as the anvil
C. initiates movement of the ossicles
D. ossicle attached to the oval window of the cochlea
E. ossicle attached to the eardrum

THE INNER EAR

The **inner ear**, also called the labyrinth, contains the functional organs for hearing and equilibrium. It consists of two parts: an outer bony labyrinth that encloses a membranous labyrinth. The membranous labyrinth consists of tubular chambers that contain a fluid called endolymph. Another fluid, called perilymph, fills the space between the bony labyrinth and the membranous labyrinth. These two fluids provide a liquid medium for vibration conduction involved in hearing and maintaining equilibrium. The bony portion of the inner ear is divided into three areas:

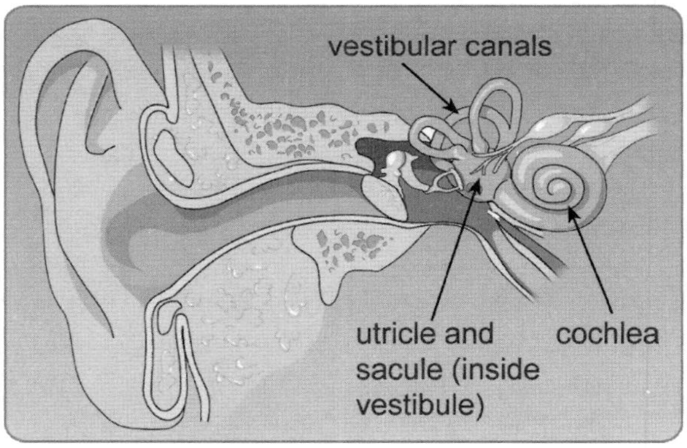

- the vestibule
- semicircular canals
- cochlea

The **vestibule** is the central portion and contains the oval and round windows to the cochlea. The oval window is attached to the stapes of the middle ear. The stapes vibrates against the oval window, producing movement of the fluid within the **cochlea** and causing the round window to bulge outward. The bulging causes a reaction in the cochlea's basilar membrane's hair cells, which are indirectly connected to the cochlear nerve. From there, impulses pass to the brain stem. The auditory area of the temporal lobe of the brain is the final receptor of the impulses, producing the sensation of sound.

The **semicircular canals** and their fluid, the **endolymph**, are structures that help us maintain static and dynamic equilibrium. **Static equilibrium** is the ability to sense the position of the head relative to gravity as well as acceleration or deceleration of the body (such as riding in a car). **Dynamic equilibrium** is the ability to maintain balance when sudden movement of the head or body occurs.

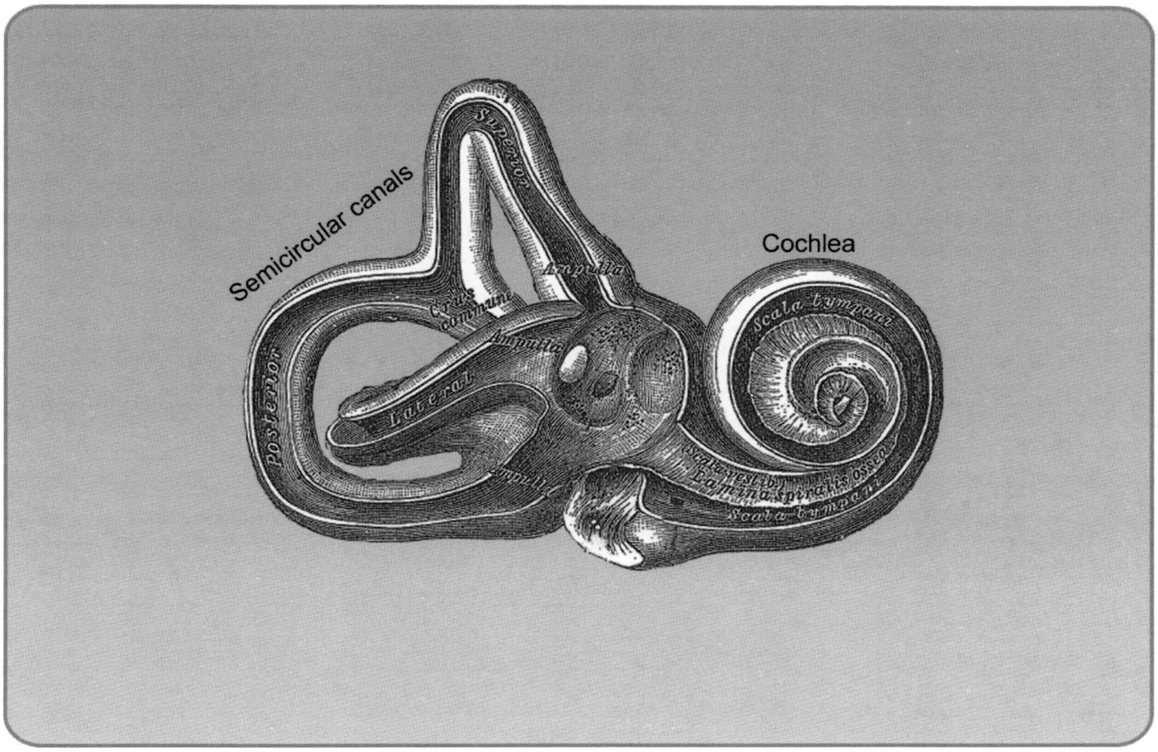

I. MULTIPLE CHOICE.
Choose the best answer.

1. The part of the inner ear concerned with maintaining balance is the (◯ cochlea, ◯ semicircular canals, ◯ perilymph, ◯ bony vestibule).

2. The oval window is (◯ connected to the stapes of the middle ear, ◯ connected to the anvil of the inner ear, ◯ connected to the incus of the inner ear, ◯ bony vestibule).

ANSWER KEY

Structural Organization of the Body

LEVELS OF STRUCTURAL ORGANIZATION

I. MATCHING.

1. D. made up of several organs which have a common function
2. B. responsible for all of the movement of the body
3. F. made up of groups of cells and the materials surrounding them
4. A. molecules combine together to form this level
5. E. supports structure and function
6. C. protects cavities and organ structures from injury and fluid loss

DIRECTIONAL TERMS

I. MULTIPLE CHOICE.

1. ventral
2. lateral
3. anterior
4. inferior
5. proximal
6. dorsal
7. medial
8. posterior

COMBINING DIRECTIONAL TERMS

I. FILL IN THE BLANK.

1. ventrolateral
2. inferoposterior
3. posteroinferior
4. superolateral
5. lateroposterior
6. mediolateral
7. inferomedial
8. superoinferior
9. anteromedial
10. dorsoflexion
11. distocervical
12. anterolateral

REGIONS, QUADRANTS, AND LANDMARKS

I. MULTIPLE CHOICE.

1. left upper quadrant
2. below the jaw
3. upper middle abdominal-pelvic region

The Skeletal System

BONE FORMATION AND DEVELOPMENT

I. MATCHING.

1. G. cells that the body has programmed to create bones
2. A. bone-forming cells that secrete a matrix which becomes calcified
3. B. former osteoblasts that are surrounded by bone matrix and have calcified
4. D. the first formation of bone
5. C. large multinucleated cells that reabsorb bone matrix
6. E. bone that has ossified and calcified
7. F. bone formation

BONE LANDMARKS AND FEATURES

I. MULTIPLE CHOICE.

1. Bone marking
2. Bone type
3. Bone marking
4. Bone marking
5. Bone type
6. Bone marking
7. Bone type
8. Bone type
9. Bone marking
10. Bone marking
11. Bone type
12. Bone marking
13. Bone type
14. Bone marking
15. Bone marking
16. Bone marking
17. Bone marking

REVIEW: BONES

I. MATCHING.

1. F. rounded projections that are often part of the articular surface of a bone
2. E. an opening or hole in a bone that allows the passage of nervous and/or vascular tissue
3. B. the terminal end of a long bone
4. G. the elongated middle portion or shaft of a long bone
5. D. connected at a joint or junction
6. C. also called compact bone, it forms the protective outer layer around every bone in the body and is composed of osteons
7. A. also called spongy bone, it contains a mesh-like network of bone tissue that is not composed of osteons

II. MULTIPLE CHOICE.

1. red blood cells
2. white blood cells
3. carry oxygen from the lungs to the rest of the body
4. help fight infections and aid the immune system
5. are capable of producing all other types of blood cells
6. white blood cells
7. white blood cells
8. mineral
9. thrombocytes
10. rigidity and strength

REVIEW: AXIAL AND APPENDICULAR SKELETON

I. MULTIPLE CHOICE.

1. appendicular
2. appendicular
3. axial
4. axial
5. appendicular
6. appendicular
7. axial
8. appendicular
9. axial
10. axial
11. appendicular
12. axial
13. appendicular
14. appendicular

MAIN CRANIAL BONES AND SUTURES

I. FILL IN THE BLANK.

1. parietal
2. temporal
3. frontal
4. occipital

II. FILL IN THE BLANK.

1. coronal suture
2. sagittal suture
3. lambdoid suture
4. parietal bone
5. frontal bone
6. temporal bone

REVIEW: THE SKULL

I. FILL IN THE BLANK.

1. coronal suture
2. sphenoid bone
3. nasal bone
4. frontal bone
5. temporal bone
6. nasal concha
7. maxilla
8. parietal bone
9. squamous suture
10. lambdoid suture
11. occipital bone
12. mastoid process
13. styloid process
14. condyloid process
15. coronoid process
16. supraorbital foramen
17. lacrimal bone
18. zygomatic bone
19. vomer
20. mandible

VERTEBRAL COLUMN

I. MATCHING.

1. G. lower back
2. F. between the bones of the spine
3. B. the neck
4. E. connects to the ribs
5. D. join
6. A. triangular shaped
7. C. tailbone

REVIEW: AXIAL SKELETON

I. FILL IN THE BLANK.

1. cervical
2. thoracic
3. intervertebral discs
4. coccyx
5. cervical
6. dagger
7. floating
8. manubrium
9. xiphoid process
10. spinal cord

II. MATCHING.

1. B. 27 bones
2. D. 6 bones
3. A. 26 bones
4. C. 7 bones

BONES OF THE SHOULDER

I. MATCHING.

1. B. collar bone
2. D. where the head of the humerus rests
3. A. upper arm bone
4. E. shoulder blade
5. C. medial end

II. MULTIPLE CHOICE.

1. long bone
2. S
3. humerus
4. epicondyle
5. scapula

BONES OF THE ANTEBRACHIUM

I. MATCHING.

1. B. pinky-side bone
2. E. prominence
3. C. point of the elbow
4. D. joint of ulna and radius
5. A. thumb-side bone

II. MULTIPLE CHOICE.

1. ulna
2. radius
3. malleolus
4. tuberosity
5. styloid process

HAND AND WRIST BONES

II. MATCHING.

1. C. wrists
2. A. hands
3. B. fingers

HIP BONES AND FEMUR

I. MATCHING.

1. B. thigh bone
2. D. lower part of the "eye mask"
3. C. the head of the femur fits into this
4. E. hip bone
5. A. kneecap

II. MULTIPLE CHOICE.

1. ischium
2. trochanter
3. acetabulum
4. medial and lateral epicondyles
5. femur

LOWER LEG AND FOOT BONES

I. MATCHING.

1. B. feet bones
2. A. ankle bone(s)
3. D. toes
4. E. protect the ankle
5. C. larger lower leg bone

II. MULTIPLE CHOICE.

1. 14
2. fibula
3. tibia
4. epicondyle
5. tibia

The Muscular System

FUNCTION AND TYPES

I. MATCHING.

1. D. Allow human skeleton movement
2. F. Maintain a sitting position
3. E. Allow for smooth movement when bending or twisting joints
4. B. When muscles contract and produce heat
5. C. Primary muscles allowing voluntary movement of the body
6. G. Muscles lining the walls of internal organs
7. A. Muscle found only in the heart

SMOOTH MUSCLE

I. MULTIPLE CHOICE.

1. resistant to fatigue
2. striations
3. the eye
4. peristalsis
5. greater length than width

NAMING MUSCLES

I. MATCHING.

1. B. Shape
2. C. Location
3. D. Attachment
4. E. Size
5. A. Orientation of fibers
6. G. Relative position
7. F. Function

MUSCLES OF THE FACE AND HEAD

I. FILL IN THE BLANK.

1. frontalis
2. temporalis
3. orbicularis oculi
4. buccinator
5. orbicularis oris
6. triangularis
7. procerus
8. nasalis
9. levator labii superioris
10. zygomaticus major
11. masseter
12. platysma

II. MULTIPLE CHOICE.

1. orbicularis oculi
2. triangularis
3. frontalis
4. platysma
5. buccinator
6. nasalis
7. levator labii superioris
8. orbicularis oris
9. masseter
10. zygomaticus major
11. temporalis
12. procerus

MUSCLES OF FACIAL EXPRESSION AND MASTICATION

I. SPELLING.

1. mentalis
2. depressor
3. pterygoid
4. labii
5. risorius
6. anguli
7. inferioris

MUSCLES OF THE NECK

I. FILL IN THE BLANK.

1. sternocleidomastoid
2. levator scapula
3. trapezius
4. digastric
5. hyoglossus
6. omohyoid
7. sternohyoid

MUSCLES OF THE ANTERIOR TORSO

I. FILL IN THE BLANK.

1. trapezius
2. deltoid
3. pectoralis major
4. serratus anterior
5. linea alba
6. sternocleidomastoid
7. external oblique
8. umbilicus (belly button) OR umbilicus
9. rectus abdominis

MUSCLES OF THE POSTERIOR TORSO

I. FILL IN THE BLANK.

1. trapezius
2. deltoid
3. infraspinatus
4. teres minor
5. teres major
6. latissimus dorsi

7. gluteus medius
8. supraspinatus
9. rhomboideus (major)
10. erector spinae group
11. lumbar aponeurosis

MUSCLES OF THE ARM

I. FILL IN THE BLANK.

1. coracobrachialis
2. brachialis
3. hypothenar muscles
4. palmar aponeurosis
5. abductor pollicis brevis
6. flexor retinaculum
7. palmaris longus
8. flexor carpi radialis
9. brachioradialis
10. biceps brachii
11. triceps
12. flexor carpi ulnaris
13. flexor digitorum superficialis

ACTIONS OF ARM MUSCLES

I. MULTIPLE CHOICE.

1. supinate
2. pollex
3. anconeus
4. extensor digiti minimi
5. thenar
6. brevis
7. coracobrachialis
8. retinaculum
9. biceps
10. pronator teres
11. extensor digitorum communis
12. palmaris longus
13. triceps
14. flexor digitorum profundus

MUSCLES OF THE LEG

I. FILL IN THE BLANK.

1. adductor magnus
2. semitendinosus
3. semimembranosus
4. gluteus maximus
5. greater trochanter
6. iliotibial tract
7. biceps femoris

II. FILL IN THE BLANK.

1. tensor fasciae latae
2. sartorius
3. rectus femoris
4. vastus lateralis
5. iliopsoas
6. pectineus
7. adductor longus
8. gracilis
9. vastus medialis

MUSCLES OF THE LOWER LEG

I. FILL IN THE BLANK.

1. peroneus longus
2. peroneus brevis
3. lateral malleolus
4. extensor digitorum longus
5. anterior tibialis
6. tibia
7. gastrocnemius
8. soleus
9. extensor hallucis longus
10. medial malleolus

REVIEW: MUSCLE ANATOMY

I. FILL IN THE BLANK.

1. face
2. arm
3. leg
4. face
5. neck
6. face
7. arm
8. back
9. face
10. face
11. arm
12. arm
13. back OR torso
14. neck OR face
15. neck
16. arm
17. arm
18. face
19. back
20. leg
21. leg
22. face
23. leg
24. arm
25. face
26. face
27. leg
28. face
29. leg
30. torso
31. neck
32. arm
33. leg
34. leg
35. face
36. leg
37. leg
38. back
39. face
40. torso
41. arm
42. back
43. leg

II. MULTIPLE CHOICE.

1. pronator teres
2. biceps
3. mentalis
4. gluteus maximus
5. extensor digiti minimi
6. extensor hallucis longus
7. lumbar aponeurosis
8. rhomboideus
9. deltoid
10. lateral and medial pterygoid
11. lateral malleolus
12. levator labii superioris
13. triceps
14. external oblique
15. orbicularis oris
16. Achilles tendon
17. greater trochanter
18. superolateral
19. semimembranosus
20. proprioception
21. flexor carpi radialis
22. gracilis
23. biceps femoris
24. gluteus medius
25. brevis
26. musculoskeletal system
27. posteroanterior

The Joints

THE JOINTS – INTRODUCTION

I. TRUE/FALSE.

1. true
2. true
3. false
4. true
5. false

II. FILL IN THE BLANK.

1. synovial
2. suture and syndesmosis
3. cartilaginous
4. biaxial
5. ligaments

JOINT MOVEMENT

I. MATCHING.

1. E. unbending
2. B. bending
3. C. moving away from midline
4. D. adding a part back to the body
5. A. circling

II. FILL IN THE BLANK.

1. flexion OR adduction
2. extension OR adduction
3. circumduction
4. extension OR abduction
5. flexion OR adduction

IV. MATCHING.

1. D. flexing the toe
2. C. pointing the toe
3. E. around an axis
4. B. lying face up
5. A. lying face down

V. FILL IN THE BLANK.

1. prone
2. rotation
3. plantar flexion
4. dorsiflexion
5. supine

VI. MULTIPLE CHOICE.

1. Movement of the foot that brings the top of the foot closer to the leg.
2. move with ease
3. flexion
4. movement in a circle
5. prone
6. joint
7. fibrous, cartilaginous, synovial
8. synovial joints
9. multiaxial
10. somewhat moveable

LIGAMENTS

I. MATCHING.

1. A. shaped like a cross
2. E. curved or bow-shaped ligament
3. B. support
4. D. like a raven's beak
5. C. indirect

II. FILL IN THE BLANK.

1. coracoid
2. accessory
3. cruciate
4. arcuate
5. collateral

III. MATCHING.

1. C. sickle-shaped
2. A. the neck
3. F. between bones
4. E. three cornered
5. D. groin area
6. B. lengthwise

IV. FILL IN THE BLANK.

1. longitudinal
2. falciform
3. interosseous
4. nuchal
5. triquetral
6. inguinal

The Circulatory System

BLOOD

I. FILL IN THE BLANK.

1. plasma
2. five
3. CBC
4. erythrocytes

ERYTHROCYTES, LEUKOCYTES, AND THROMBOCYTES

I. MULTIPLE CHOICE.

1. leukocytes
2. megakaryocytes
3. erythrocytes
4. white blood cells
5. to carry oxygen

II. FILL IN THE BLANK.

1. crit
2. segs
3. basos
4. eos
5. lymphs

HEART

I. FILL IN THE BLANK.

1. clenched fist
2. pulmonary trunk
3. aorta
4. systole
5. diastole

ANATOMY OF THE HEART

I. FILL IN THE BLANK.

1. aorta
2. left pulmonary artery
3. left atrium
4. mitral valve
5. aortic valve
6. left ventricle
7. apex
8. right ventricle
9. pulmonary valve
10. tricuspid valve
11. right atrium

LAYERS OF THE HEART

I. TRUE/FALSE.

1. false
2. true
3. false
4. true
5. true

HEART CHAMBERS AND VALVES

I. MULTIPLE CHOICE.

1. right ventricle
2. ventricles
3. semilunar valves
4. atrioventricular valve

CONTRACTION AND RHYTHM OF THE HEART

I. MATCHING.

1. B. systole phase
2. B. systole phase
3. A. diastole phase
4. B. systole phase
5. A. diastole phase

ARTERIES AND VEINS

I. MATCHING.

1. C. arteries
2. B. veins
3. D. capillaries
4. A. heart

CARDIOVASCULAR TERMINOLOGY

I. MULTIPLE CHOICE.

1. plasma
2. mediastinum
3. systole
4. plasma
5. capillaries
6. platelets
7. hematocrit
8. differential
9. diastole
10. eosinophils
11. erythrocytes
12. hemoglobin

ARTERIES

I. FILL IN THE BLANK.

1. aorta
2. function
3. subclavian
4. the same

CONDUCTION MECHANISM OF THE HEART

I. MATCHING.

1. E. sinoatrial node (pacemaker)
2. C. internodal fibers (pathway)
3. B. atrioventricular node
4. J. atrioventricular bundle (bundle of His)
5. D. right and left bundle branches
6. F. Purkinje fibers
7. G. right atrium
8. I. left atrium
9. A. interventicular septum
10. H. apex

BLOOD CIRCULATION

I. MATCHING.

1. B. vein that does not directly connect to the vena cava
2. A. largest artery in the body
3. C. largest vein in the body

REVIEW: THE HEART

I. MATCHING.

1. H. aorta
2. E. right atrium
3. G. tricuspid valve
4. I. chordae tendinae
5. A. pulmonary valve
6. K. right ventricle
7. J. ventricular septum
8. D. left ventricle
9. C. mitral valve
10. B. left atrium
11. F. left plumonary artery

II. MATCHING.

1. E. blood enters the right atrium
2. B. blood flows through tricuspid valve
3. C. blood enters right ventricle
4. G. blood flows through pulmonary valve
5. H. blood goes through the pulmonary artery to the lungs
6. I. blood enters left atrium
7. D. blood flows through mitral valve
8. F. blood enters left ventricle
9. J. blood flows through aortic valve
10. A. blood is distributed by the aorta to the body

ARTERIES OVERVIEW

I. MULTIPLE CHOICE.

1. ascending aorta
2. aortic arch
3. aorta

ARTERIES OF THE BRAIN

I. MULTIPLE CHOICE.

1. Circle of Willis
2. Circle of Willis

ARTERIES OF THE HEAD AND NECK

I. FILL IN THE BLANK.

1. posterior auricular
2. external carotid
3. internal carotid
4. vertebral
5. common carotid
6. superficial temporal

7. maxillary
8. superior labial
9. inferior labial
10. facial
11. lingual

II. MULTIPLE CHOICE.

1. ophthalmic
2. vertebral
3. facial
4. labial
5. auricular

REVIEW: ARTERIES OF THE UPPER EXTREMITY

I. FILL IN THE BLANK.

1. brachial
2. humeral circumflex
3. deep brachial
4. ulnar recurrent
5. interosseous
6. palmar arch
7. metacarpal
8. common palmar digitals
9. princeps pollicis
10. radial

AORTA AND THORACIC ARTERIES

I. MULTIPLE CHOICE.

1. ascending aorta
2. aortic arch
3. aorta

VEINS OF THE CARDIOVASCULAR SYSTEM

I. MULTIPLE CHOICE.

1. venules
2. superficial veins
3. sinuses
4. head, arms, and thoracic cavity (except the lungs)
5. inferior vena cava

REVIEW: VEINS

I. FILL IN THE BLANK.

1. internal jugular
2. saphenous
3. brachiocephalic
4. external jugular
5. diploic
6. supratrochlear
7. retromandibular
8. basilic
9. cephalic
10. median cubital
11. median antebrachial
12. hemiazygos
13. azygos

II. MULTIPLE CHOICE.

1. plexus
2. greater saphenous
3. inferior vena cava

THE LYMPHATIC SYSTEM – LESSON 2

I. MATCHING.

1. C. thymus
2. D. tonsils
3. B. spleen
4. A. bone marrow

REVIEW: THE LYMPHATIC SYSTEM

I. MULTIPLE CHOICE.

1. lymphoid tissue
2. thoracic duct
3. superior vena cava

The Nervous System

NERVOUS TISSUE AND NEURONS

I. FILL IN THE BLANK.

1. dendrites
2. nucleus
3. dendrites
4. axon terminal
5. terminal branches
6. axon
7. cell body
8. nucleolus

II. MULTIPLE CHOICE.

1. visceral sensory
2. somatic
3. somatic sensory and visceral sensory
4. within the ventral body cavity
5. afferent
6. nervous tissue
7. 100 years
8. nucleus
9. dendrite
10. axon
11. mixed nerves

REVIEW: NERVOUS SYSTEM ANATOMY

I. MULTIPLE CHOICE.

1. gyri
2. pons
3. neuron
4. meninges
5. cerebrum
6. choroid plexus
7. fissures
8. splenium of corpus callosum
9. medulla oblongata
10. mesencephalon
11. sulci
12. arachnoid
13. commissure
14. cerebellum
15. dura mater
16. corpus callosum
17. optic chiasm
18. diencephalon
19. mesencephalon
20. pia mater
21. corpora quadrigemina
22. pituitary

BRAIN ANATOMY

I. FILL IN THE BLANK.

1. frontal lobe
2. temporal lobe
3. pituitary gland
4. infundibulum
5. mammillary body
6. pons
7. facial nerve
8. vestibulocochlear nerve
9. glossopharyngeal nerve
10. vagus nerve
11. hypoglossal nerve
12. accessory nerve
13. spinal cord
14. medulla
15. cerebellum
16. abducens nerve
17. trochlear nerve
18. trigeminal nerve
19. oculomotor nerve
20. optic tract
21. optic chiasm
22. optic nerve
23. olfactory bulb
24. filaments of olfactory nerve

II. MULTIPLE CHOICE.

1. cauda equina
2. olfactory
3. vagus nerve
4. trigeminal
5. vestibulocochlear
6. optic nerve
7. conus medullaris
8. abducens
9. hypoglossal nerve
10. filum terminale
11. oculomotor nerve
12. glossopharyngeal

III. MATCHING.

1. A. The sense of smell.
2. L. Vision.
3. C. This nerve controls all movement of the eyeballs.
4. K. This is a very small nerve, both sensory and motor, which innervates the superior oblique muscle of the eye.
5. I. This is the largest of the cranial nerves. It is primarily sensory, but does send motor impulses to the muscles of mastication (chewing).
6. D. This is a small nerve that provides both motor and sensory innervation to the lateral rectus eye muscle.
7. H. This is a mixed nerve. The motor fibers innervate facial, scalp, and superficial neck muscles. The salivary glands are also innervated by this. The sensory fibers arise from the taste buds on the tongue.
8. B. Hearing and equilibrium.
9. G. This is mixed nerve that innervates the tongue and pharynx.
10. E. This arises from the medulla and has both motor and sensory fibers which serve autonomic organs of the thoracic and abdominal cavities.
11. J. This is a motor nerve only. It innervates the muscles of the pharyngeal region as well as the sternocleidomastoid and trapezius muscles.
12. F. This supplies motor fibers to the muscles of the tongue.

SENSORY AND MOTOR COMMUNICATION

I. MATCHING.

1. A. Somatic Sensory
2. C. Somatic Motor
3. B. Visceral Sensory
4. D. Visceral Motor

REVIEW: THE PERIPHERAL NERVOUS SYSTEM

I. FILL IN THE BLANK.

1. brain
2. conus medullaris
3. filum terminale
4. cauda equina
5. second lumbar

II. MULTIPLE CHOICE.

1. 31
2. cranial
3. autonomic nervous
4. both Central Nervous and Peripheral Nervous Systems

III. MATCHING.

1. B. tibial nerve
2. C. median nerve
3. D. sciatic nerve
4. B. tibial nerve
5. A. femoral

The Digestive System

MOUTH AND ASSOCIATED ORGANS

I. FILL IN THE BLANK.

1. labia
2. vestibule
3. oral cavity proper
4. stratified squamous epithelium
5. red margin
6. vermilion border
7. labial frenulum

PALATE

II. FILL IN THE BLANK.

1. gingivae (gums)
2. hard palate
3. uvula
4. gingivae (gums)
5. inferior labial frenulum
6. superior labial frenulum
7. superior labia (upper lip)
8. soft palate
9. posterior wall oropharynx
10. tongue
11. vestibule
12. inferior labia (lower lip)

III. MULTIPLE CHOICE.

1. viscera
2. lumen
3. oral cavity
4. buccal
5. gut
6. abdomen

ANATOMY OF THE TONGUE

II. FILL IN THE BLANK.

1. lingual tonsils
2. circumvallate papillae
3. fungiform papillae
4. epiglottis
5. lingual tonsils
6. sulcus terminalis
7. filiform papillae

III. MULTIPLE CHOICE.

1. papillae
2. lingual
3. lingual frenulum

TEETH

I. FILL IN THE BLANK.

1. crown
2. neck
3. root canal
4. root
5. enamel
6. dentin
7. dentin tubules
8. pulp cavity
9. gingiva
10. cementum
11. bone

PHARYNX

I. MULTIPLE CHOICE.

1. oropharynx
2. epiglottis

ALIMENTARY CANAL

I. FILL IN THE BLANK.

1. tunica mucosa
2. tunica submucosa
3. tunica muscularis
4. tunica serosa

STRUCTURES OF THE ALIMENTARY CANAL

I. MULTIPLE CHOICE.

1. parietal peritoneum
2. gastroenterology
3. serosa
4. absorption
5. omentum
6. secretion
7. serosa
8. alimentary canal
9. muscularis
10. retroperitoneal
11. dorsal mesentery
12. 30 feet
13. submucosa
14. distention
15. collagen
16. peristalsis
17. secretory
18. greater omentum
19. support

REVIEW: UPPER DIGESTIVE STRUCTURES

I. SPELLING.

1. papillae
2. gastroenterology
3. distention OR distension
4. lingual
5. peritoneum
6. mucosa
7. mesentery
8. omentum
9. lumen
10. peristalsis

II. MATCHING.

1. G. tunica serosa
2. B. omentum
3. D. lumen
4. J. retroperitoneal
5. A. oral cavity
6. F. abdomen
7. E. greater omentum
8. C. gut
9. I. lingual
10. H. buccal

III. MULTIPLE CHOICE.

1. gastroenterology
2. parietal peritoneum
3. papillae
4. viscera
5. absorption
6. lingual frenulum
7. collagen
8. peristalsis
9. 30 feet
10. support

MAJOR STRUCTURES OF THE DIGESTIVE SYSTEM

I. FILL IN THE BLANK.

1. pharynx
2. liver
3. gallbladder
4. duodenum
5. ascending colon
6. cecum
7. appendix
8. rectum
9. parotid (salivary) gland
10. esophagus
11. stomach
12. pancreas
13. transverse colon
14. descending colon
15. sigmoid colon
16. small intestine

MOUTH AND ESOPHAGUS

I. MATCHING.

1. E. passageway for the respiratory and digestive system
2. A. small, fleshy mass hanging from the soft palate
3. C. extends from the soft palate in the mouth to the level of the hyoid bone
4. B. lid-like structure that hangs over the entrance to the larynx
5. D. part of the alimentary canal that connects the pharynx to the stomach

STOMACH

I. MATCHING.

1. A. dome-shaped portion of stomach
2. C. controls opening into the small intestine
3. B. controls opening into the stomach

LARGE GLANDULAR ORGANS OF THE DIGESTIVE SYSTEM

I. FILL IN THE BLANK.

1. pancreas
2. liver
3. gallbladder

REVIEW: DIGESTIVE STRUCTURES

I. MULTIPLE CHOICE.

1. splenic flexure
2. duodenum
3. ileocecal valve
4. splenic flexure
5. rectum
6. appendix
7. epiglottis
8. stomach
9. esophagus

II. FILL IN THE BLANK.

1. pharynx
2. liver
3. gallbladder
4. duodenum
5. ascending colon
6. cecum
7. appendix
8. rectum
9. parotid (salivary) gland
10. esophagus
11. stomach
12. pancreas
13. transverse colon
14. descending colon
15. sigmoid colon
16. small intestine

The Respiratory System

RESPIRATION

I. FILL IN THE BLANK.

1. sinuses
2. oral cavity
3. epiglottis
4. thyroid cartilage
5. vocal folds
6. esophagus
7. trachea
8. lungs
9. heart
10. diaphragm

GROSS RESPIRATORY

I. FILL IN THE BLANK.

1. nasal cavity
2. external naris
3. larynx
4. trachea
5. right pulmonary bronchus
6. hard palate
7. soft palate
8. pharynx
9. lungs
10. left pulmonary bronchus

II. FILL IN THE BLANK.

1. lower
2. upper
3. upper
4. lower
5. upper
6. upper
7. lower
8. lower
9. upper
10. upper

NASAL CAVITY

I. TRUE/FALSE.

1. true
2. false
3. true

SINUS CAVITIES

I. FILL IN THE BLANK.

1. frontal sinuses
2. ethmoid sinus cells
3. maxillary sinuses
4. turbinates

PHARYNX

I. FILL IN THE BLANK.

1. laryngopharynx
2. nasopharynx
3. pharynx
4. oropharynx

LARYNX AND TRACHEA

I. FILL IN THE BLANK.

1. hyoid bone
2. thyrohyoid membrane
3. thyroid cartilage
4. trachea

II. FILL IN THE BLANK.

1. hyoid bone
2. epiglottis
3. thyroid cartilage
4. esophagus
5. trachea

BRONCHI

I. FILL IN THE BLANK.

1. trachea
2. bronchial tubes
3. secondary bronchus
4. tertiary bronchus

REVIEW: THE LUNGS AND THORACIC CAVITY

I. MATCHING.

1. C. lower trachea
2. D. lobes
3. B. carina
4. A. lung lingula
5. E. bronchus

The Endocrine System

THYROID AND PARATHYROID GLANDS

I. FILL IN THE BLANK.

1. hyoid bone
2. thyroid cartilage
3. right lobe of thyroid gland
4. left lobe of thyroid gland
5. isthmus of thyroid gland

II. FILL IN THE BLANK.

1. thyroid hormone
2. iodine
3. larynx
4. thyrocalcitonin
5. parathyroid

ADRENAL GLANDS

I. MATCHING.

1. C. left adrenal gland
2. A. pancreas
3. E. left kidney
4. D. right kidney
5. B. right adrenal gland

PANCREAS

I. MATCHING.

1. B. endocrine
2. A. exocrine
3. B. endocrine
4. B. endocrine

GONADS (MALE AND FEMALE)

I. FILL IN THE BLANK.

1. ductus deferens
2. epididymis
3. testes

PINEAL GLAND, DUODENUM, AND PLACENTA

I. FILL IN THE BLANK.

1. epiphysis
2. thymus
3. melatonin
4. placenta

The Urinary System

KIDNEYS

I. MULTIPLE CHOICE.

1. renal hilum
2. renal
3. outer cortex and inner medulla
4. nephrons
5. behind the peritoneal cavity

URETERS, BLADDER, AND URETHRA

I. FILL IN THE BLANK.

1. bladder
2. trigone
3. micturition
4. calices
5. voiding

URINARY ANATOMY

I. FILL IN THE BLANK.

1. adrenal gland
2. kidney
3. ureter
4. urinary bladder
5. urethra

REVIEW: URINARY ANATOMY

I. MULTIPLE CHOICE.

1. urinary bladder
2. micturition
3. cortex
4. retroperitoneal
5. hilum
6. urethral orifice
7. nephr/o
8. column of Bertin
9. ureter
10. medulla
11. adrenal glands

The Reproductive System

OVARIES AND FALLOPIAN TUBES

I. MATCHING.

1. B. ovarian follicle is produced
2. D. graafian follicle is formed
3. A. corpus luteum is formed
4. C. progesterone and inhibin suppress additional follicle maturation

FALLOPIAN TUBES, UTERUS, AND VAGINA

I. MATCHING.

1. D. uterus
2. B. urinary bladder
3. F. symphysis pubis
4. A. clitoris
5. G. labium minus
6. E. labium majus
7. C. rectum

EXTERNAL FEMALE ORGANS

I. TRUE/FALSE.

1. false
2. true
3. true
4. true
5. false

II. FILL IN THE BLANK.

1. fatty tissue
2. milk ducts
3. areola
4. nipple
5. lobules

REVIEW: FEMALE REPRODUCTIVE ANATOMY

I. MULTIPLE CHOICE.

1. graafian follicle
2. mons pubis
3. external genitalia
4. prepuce
5. infundibulum
6. areola
7. ampulla
8. stroma
9. fundus
10. vulva
11. mesentery
12. Bartholin gland
13. estrogen
14. sebaceous
15. mesovarium
16. medulla
17. corpus luteum
18. perineum
19. menstruation
20. menses
21. lactation
22. mammary glands
23. cortex
24. fornix
25. oviducts
26. symphysis pubis
27. secretory phase
28. gametes or ova

MALE ACCESSORY GLANDS AND SUPPORTING STRUCTURES

I. MATCHING.

1. H. symphysis pubis
2. B. corpora cavernosa
3. K. penis
4. F. glans penis
5. D. corpus spongiosum
6. M. urinary bladder
7. G. seminal vesicle
8. A. prostate gland
9. J. bulbourethral gland
10. E. vas (ductus) deferens
11. C. epididymis
12. L. testis
13. I. scotrum

REVIEW: MALE REPRODUCTIVE ANATOMY

I. MULTIPLE CHOICE.

1. dartos
2. Cowper glands
3. circumcision
4. semen
5. epididymis
6. vas deferens
7. prepuce
8. tunica albuginea
9. seminiferous tubules
10. rete testis

The Integumentary System and Special Sensory Organs

SKIN

I. TRUE/FALSE.

1. true
2. true
3. false
4. true
5. false

CROSS SECTION OF THE SKIN

I. FILL IN THE BLANK.

1. epidermis
2. papillary layer
3. reticular layer
4. dermis
5. subcutaneous layer
6. sebaceous gland
7. arrector pili muscle
8. sudoriferous gland
9. pacinian corpuscle

HAIR AND NAILS – LESSON 2

I. MULTIPLE CHOICE.

1. integumentary
2. nail bed
3. inside the nostrils

REVIEW: SKIN

I. MATCHING.

1. E. epidermis
2. G. papillary layer
3. B. reticular layer
4. H. dermis
5. D. sebaceous gland
6. F. arrector pili muscle
7. A. sudoriferous gland
8. C. pacinian corpuscle
9. I. subcutaneous layer

II. MATCHING.

1. F. dermoepidural junction
2. D. keratin
3. A. fascia
4. E. hair
5. C. glandular epithelial tissue
6. B. smooth muscle tissue

III. MULTIPLE CHOICE.

1. similar cells that perform a similar function
2. skin

EXTERNAL STRUCTURES OF THE EYE

I. MULTIPLE CHOICE.

1. eyebrows
2. every seven seconds

EYE MUSCLES

I. MATCHING.

1. C. moves the eye toward the nose
2. A. limits the amount of downward and upper eye rotation
3. B. rotates the top of the eye away from the nose

II. MULTIPLE CHOICE.

1. placement of the eyes in the skull

REVIEW: EYE

I. MATCHING.

1. E. ocular muscles
2. D. sclera
3. A. anterior cavity
4. F. vitreous humor
5. B. cornea
6. C. superior rectus muscle

II. MULTIPLE CHOICE.

1. trochlea
2. tears
3. eyelids
4. fovea

EAR, NOSE, AND THROAT

I. TRUE/FALSE.

1. false
2. true
3. true
4. true
5. false

THE MIDDLE EAR

I. MATCHING.

1. C. initiates movement of the ossicles
2. D. ossicle attached to the oval window of the cochlea
3. E. ossicle attached to the eardrum
4. A. equalizes air pressure
5. B. also known as the anvil

THE INNER EAR

I. MULTIPLE CHOICE.

1. semicircular canals
2. connected to the stapes of the middle ear

APPENDIX

Laboratory RESULT INQUIRY

Pat: [redacted] Age/Sex: [redacted] HID: AFH
Account: [redacted] Loc: LAB (OPD)
Phys: [redacted]
Tests: (all)
Patient Phone #: [redacted]

F47563 COLL: [redacted] 20:59 REC: [redacted] 21:06 PHYS: [redacted]

Test	Flag	Result	Reference	Units
CBC				
WBC	H	20.8	[5.0-19.5]	10^3/uL
RBC		4.80	[3.00-5.40]	10^6/uL
HGB		14.0	[10.0-18.0]	g/dL
Hematocrit		41.4	[31.0-55.0]	%
MCV		86.3	[85.0-123.0]	fL
MCH		29.2	[28.0-40.0]	pg
MCHC		33.9	[32.0-36.0]	g/dL
RDW	H	17.0	[11.3-15.6]	%
Platelets	H	602	[150-400]	10^3/uL
MPV		8.5	[6.6-10.1]	fL
MANUAL DIFF				
Diff Type		Manual		
% Segmented Neutrophils		43	[14-44]	%
% Band Neutrophils		7	[6-13]	%
% Lymphocytes		45	[41-71]	%
% Monocytes		5	[0-10]	%
Absolute Neutrophils	H	10.4	[1.5-10.0]	10^3/uL
Absolute Lymphs		9.4	[2.0-17.0]	10^3/uL
Absolute Monos		1.0	[0.3-2.7]	10^3/uL
RBC Morphology		Normocytic, Normochromic	[NCNC]	
Atypical Lymphocytes*		1+	[NEG]	
Platelet Estimation		Agrees with count	[PLTOK]	